Medication Safety Officer's Handbook

Connie M. Larson, PharmD

Associate Director of Pharmacy, Safety and Quality
Medication Safety Officer
University of Illinois Hospital & Health Sciences System
Clinical Assistant Professor of Pharmacy Practice
University of Illinois at Chicago College of Pharmacy
Chicago, IL

Deb Saine, MS, RPh, FASHP, FSMSO

Program Manager, Medication Safety
Winchester Medical Center
Winchester, VA

American Society of Health-System Pharmacists®
Bethesda, MD

Any correspondence regarding this publication should be sent to the publisher, American Society of Health-System Pharmacists, 7272 Wisconsin Avenue, Bethesda, MD 20814, attention: Special Publishing.

Director, Special Publishing: Jack Bruggeman

Acquisitions Editor: Robin Coleman

Editorial Project Manager: Ruth Bloom

Editorial Resources Manager: Bill Fogle

Cover Design and Layout: Carol A. Barrer

Page Design: DeVall Advertising

Library of Congress Cataloging-in-Publication Data

Medication safety officer's handbook / editors, Connie M. Larson, Deb Saine.

p. ; cm.

Includes bibliographical references and index.

ISBN 978-1-58528-210-4 (alk. paper) -- ISBN 978-1-58528-357-6 (PDF format)

I. Larson, Connie M. II. Saine, Deb R. III. American Society of Health-System Pharmacists.

[DNLM: 1. Medication Errors--prevention & control. 2. Medication Systems, Hospital--standards. 3. Medication Systems, Hospital--organization & administration. 4. Quality Assurance, Health Care--methods. 5. Safety Management--methods. WX 179]

610.28'9--dc23

2012045835

ISBN 978-1-58528-210-4

Dedication

This book is dedicated to medication safety officers and other medication and patient safety leaders. May you find inspiration and motivation to carry on this important work.

To the patients and families who have experienced a medication error, we are committed to working for a safer health care system for all.

—Connie Larson and Deb Saine

I would like to dedicate this book to Toby Clark for encouraging and fostering my interest in medication safety work by creating a medication safety officer position for me many(!) years ago. Also, I would like to thank my children, Julia, Emma, and Jack for their love and ongoing support.

—Connie

To my mom, the first pharmacist I ever knew, and my dad, who guided me with wisdom and love.

—Deb

Table of Contents

Preface

Welcome to our world! The medication safety officer's arena is a fascinating, challenging, dynamic space. As medication safety officers, we need to combine our specialized knowledge of medications with expertise in quality improvement principles as well as leadership skills to bring people together toward a common goal: keeping our patients free from harm. We both received questions such as "Where do I start," "What do I need to know?" We realized that there was no resource with the right balance of information. The idea of a how-to guide seemed like the ideal way to help practitioners dedicated to medication safety work. The *Medication Safety Officer's Handbook* is a resource that not only helps get you started but takes you down the path to safety.

The *Handbook* is structured to provide a guide for both new and current medication safety officers. But even if you don't have the title, certainly all health care professionals have a responsibility to improve medication safety wherever we practice. We wrote this book as a go-to resource in approaching and handling problems and challenges in your workplace. There are practical tools and tips for everyone interested in medication safety work and quality improvement in general. We have provided examples from a variety of places that you will be able to apply or adapt for your own workplace.

We found authors as excited as we are about medication safety to share their expertise and ideas. Our goal was to include key topics vital to the medication safety officer and provide a blend of knowledge, responsibilities, tools, and tips from people in the field. We feel this book distinguishes itself by providing direction for the unique role and responsibilities of a medication safety officer while providing practical strategies for applying the concepts of medication safety work into your daily practice.

Questioning minds wanted to know, and the answers may be found in the following pages:

- What are MSO responsibilities?
- There are so many things to do—how do I prioritize?
- With no formal authority, how do I make change happen?
- What should I include in a medication safety assessment for a formulary review?
- Help! How do I design a template for a modified root cause analysis?
- What should I include in a medication safety orientation for staff?

- Where can I find more information on a medication safety topic?
- Alphabet soup! What do all these acronyms mean?

Looking at the completed work, it does beg the question: Can anyone be and do all these things? Do not be intimidated! Even in the best-case scenario, with plenty of help, no one can be an expert on all things. The good news is you don't have to know it all—we've given you the resources and information from a variety of dedicated people to help you do your job better and improve medication safety in your workplace.

Medication safety is a journey! To quote Margaret Mead:

> *Never doubt that a small group of thoughtful, committed citizens can change the world; indeed, it's the only thing that ever has.*

Connie M. Larson

Deb Saine

May 2013

Contributors

L. Hayley Burgess, PharmD
Director of Medication Safety and System Innovations
Clinical Services Group
HCA Management Service
Nashville, TN

Kathryn A. Crea, PharmD, BCPS
Director of Accreditation and Patient Safety Officer
Riverside Methodist Hospital—OhioHealth
Columbus, OH
Assistant Professor
University of Findlay College of Pharmacy
Findlay, OH

Lynn E. Eschenbacher, PharmD, MBA
Assistant Director, Clinical Services
Director, PGY-1 Pharmacy Residency Program
Chair, ASHP Section of Inpatient Care Practitioners
WakeMed Health & Hospitals
Raleigh, NC

Sarah Hein, PharmD
Medication Safety Specialist
Tampa General Hospital
Tampa, FL

Joanne G. Kowiatek, RPh, MPM, FASHP
Oncology Consultant Pharmacist
UPMC CancerCenter
Pittsburgh, PA

Connie M. Larson, PharmD
Associate Director of Pharmacy, Safety and Quality
Medication Safety Officer
University of Illinois Hospital & Health Sciences System
Clinical Assistant Professor of Pharmacy Practice
University of Illinois at Chicago College of Pharmacy
Chicago, IL

Karla M. Miller, PharmD, BCPP
Assistant Vice President
Pharmacy Services & Clinical Therapeutics
Clinical Services Group
HCA Management Service
Nashville, TN

Marjorie Shaw Phillips, MS, RPh, FASHP
Pharmacy Coordinator, Clinical Research & Education
Georgia Regents Medical Center Pharmacy
Clinical Professor of Pharmacy Practice
University of Georgia College of Pharmacy
Augusta, GA

Deb Saine, MS, RPh, FASHP, FSMSO
Program Manager, Medication Safety
Winchester Medical Center
Winchester, VA

Susan J. Skledar, RPh, MPH, FASHP
Associate Professor
School of Pharmacy
University of Pittsburgh
Clinical Pharmacist
UPMC Pharmacy Health System Formulary
Management/Drug Use Policy Team
University of Pittsburgh Medical Center
Department of Pharmacy
Pittsburgh, PA

Ann E. Wehmeyer, PharmD, BCPS
Senior Patient Safety Specialist
Department of Performance Improvement and Clinical Effectiveness
Rush University Medical Center
Chicago, IL

Lisa M. Hanlon Wilhelm, BS Pharm, RPh
Medication Safety and Compliance Specialist
Penn State Hershey Medical Center
Department of Pharmacy
Hershey, PA

Acknowledgments

We thank our contributors for sharing their collective experience, insight, and wisdom as medication safety leaders. It's been a long journey—thank you for your perseverance! We especially appreciate the assistance of Ruth Bloom, project editor extraordinaire—we couldn't have done it without you. Special kudos to Jack Bruggeman and Bill Fogle at ASHP. Their dedication and encouragement was instrumental in bringing this project to completion.

Connie would like to acknowledge the many practitioners she has worked with through the years. My first months working as a pharmacist were an invaluable experience, working with great people that helped me envision and realize the kind of pharmacist I wanted to be: caring and mindful. Thank you to Trish Balow for supporting my ideas as well as contributing valuable information to enhance our medication safety program. To Gloria Sporleder and Agnes Dominic, the two best technicians in the world: thanks for all your help and ideas over the years. Also, thank you to my director, Andrew Donnelly, for his ongoing support and encouragement for the MSO position.

Deb would like to acknowledge the pharmacy directors with whom she has worked. To Bill Herbert from Madison: thank you for your vision—you created a pharmacist position dedicated to medication safety in 1990, before MSOs were widely known. Thanks for the opportunity to embark on what has become a career-defining path. To Bob Theriault from Lebanon: thanks for the autonomy—you allowed me free reign to explore and develop our medication safety officer position, helping me grow it into a force for positive change. I especially appreciate your "permission" to "stay late and work hard." To Tonya Smith and Bonnie Pitt from Winchester: thank you for supporting my professional service and leadership activities. You've encouraged me to explore and experience a variety of medication safety practices both across the country and abroad. I would like to acknowledge the inaugural members of the Medication Safety Section Advisory Group (SAG). Our insightful discussions greatly expanded my knowledge base and helped bring medication safety to the forefront of pharmacy practice. Thank you, with much love, to my children, Beth, Julie, and Kevin, for accepting "the book" as a regular presence in our lives. Lastly, thank you to my husband, Pat, for his inspiration, advice, and always—for the adventure.

Getting Started

Deb Saine and Connie M. Larson

CHAPTER 1

"Medicine used to be simple, ineffective, and relatively safe. Now it is complex, effective, and potentially dangerous."

—Professor Sir Cyril Chantler[1]

Introduction

The above statement by Professor Chantler can certainly apply to medication use today. The Institute of Medicine (IOM) Committee on Identifying and Preventing Medication Errors estimates a hospitalized patient experiences at least one medication error per day. Furthermore, the IOM reports at least 25 percent of all medication-related injuries are preventable. In the United States alone, at least 1.5 million preventable adverse drug events (ADEs) occur each year, at a cost of over 3.5 billion (2006) dollars.[2] Mortality rates attributed to ADEs range between 1 and 2.45 percent.[3,4] The imperative for action to prevent harm related to medication use is undeniable.

"The foundation of a successful medication safety program is a dedicated, willing pharmacist leader."[5] This premise is supported by the IOM, the National Quality Forum (NQF), and the American Society of Health-System Pharmacists (ASHP).[2,6,7] A leader committed to advancing medication safety will deliver the focus and expertise necessary to enhance an organization's patient safety outcomes. The medication safety officer (MSO), a position dedicated to patient safety efforts to reduce the risks of medication use, will fulfill this essential role.

Scope of Practice

What are the expectations and the boundaries for the MSO's work? In the chapter "Action Agenda for Health Care Organizations," the IOM Committee on Identifying and Preventing Medication Errors recommends "advocate for a medication safety officer with responsibility for improving medication safety throughout the hospital."[2] The NQF-endorsed Practice 18 Objective states, "Pharmacy leadership structures and systems ensure a multidisciplinary focus and a streamlined operational approach to achieve organization-wide safe medication use."[6] The ASHP Statement on the Role of the Medication Safety Leader provides an excellent concise overview of the MSO role (see Appendix 1-A). The statement asserts, "The scope of a medication safety leader's responsibilities reaches into every corner of the health-care system and encompasses many roles, such as educator, preceptor, mentor, detective, compliance officer, risk manager, engineer, accountant, statistician, computer analyst, and counselor."[7] The MSO's scope is comprehensive, intended to span the entire medication-use process as practiced by every participant discipline, across the entire organization.

Stated simply, the MSO's mission is to prevent patient harm. Consider the National Patient Safety Foundation's (NPSF) statement "Patient safety has to do primarily with the avoidance, prevention, and amelioration of adverse outcomes or injuries stemming from the processes of health care itself."[9] Note that the emphasis of safety is on *outcomes*, rather than concentrating on *preventing errors*. This is a key concept for the MSO to understand. The MSO's mission, then, may be focused to state: avoid, prevent, and ameliorate adverse outcomes or injuries (e.g., patient harm) stemming from the medication-use process. The *medication-use process* includes procedures and systems used to provide medication therapy to patients such as medication procurement, storage, prescribing, transcribing, preparing, dispensing, administration, documentation, and monitoring. This mission frames the overarching goal and guides the MSO's decisions and actions.

The NPSF further recognizes that safety ". . . is more than the absence of adverse outcomes and it is more than avoidance of preventable errors or occurrences. Safety does not reside in a person, device, or department."[9] This correlates well with the MSO's broad scope of practice in medication safety, as described above. The MSO must also address issues and occurrences encompassing errors and deviations, risky situations, and near misses, as well as events resulting in adverse outcomes. To improve safety, the MSO will explore relationships between systems and their elements.

The MSO's approach to medication safety may be portrayed as a pyramid (see Figure 1-1). In a broad sense, it describes the MSO's activities in pursuit of his or her mission. The levels of the pyramid are not mutually exclusive, as the MSO will be addressing multiple issues concurrently. This short discussion provides an overview of the tactics used by the MSO; concepts and specific MSO actions are presented in more detail in subsequent chapters.

A successful medication safety program depends on the presence of a *safe culture*.[2,5,6,10-12] Culture is so vital to improving safety that it tops the lists of the "Model

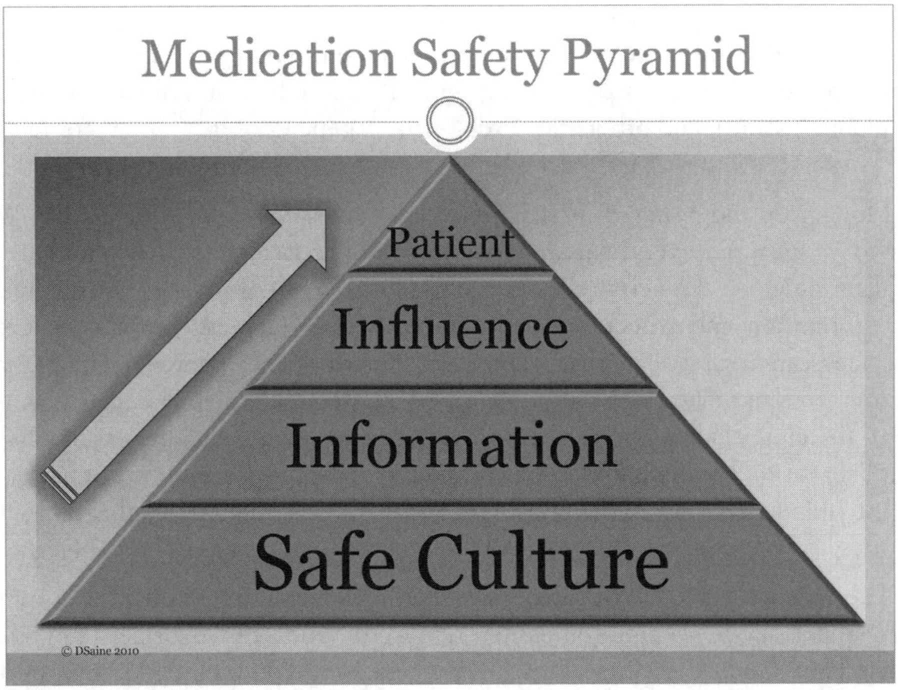

Figure 1-1. Medication safety pyramid.
Source: Courtesy of Deb Saine.

Strategic Plan for Medication Safety"[13] and the Agency for Healthcare Research and Quality's (AHRQ) "30 Safe Practices for Better Health Care."[14] Developing and enhancing a culture in which medication safety thrives are fundamental to the MSO's functions—thus, they comprise the base of the pyramid. When possible, the MSO should try to integrate strategies to enhance the culture of safety with other tasks or responsibilities. Perspectives on culture and the MSO's role are described in Chapter 5.

The next section of the pyramid, *Information,* reflects the MSO's use of internal and external information, and information on standards of care to direct his or her activities. "Strategic goals related to medication safety should be based on an assessment of internal medication-use processes and capabilities, external influences on medication safety, patient needs, and the health care marketplace as it relates to medication use."[15] MSOs must strive to understand the nature of events and the safety environment in their own organizations to prioritize and strategize actions to improve safety.[7,10-13, 16,17] At the same time, it is essential for the MSO to develop and maintain medication safety expertise through continuous professional development, and awareness of external events and developments in the patient safety field.[7] Michael Cohen, President of the Institute for Safe Medication Practices, points out the importance of this by observing "Unfortunately, there are too many in health care who feel that if it hasn't happened to them, the adverse experiences of others do not apply." The MSO should also be familiar with standards of care as a basis for medication safety enhancement. Examples include the best practice recommendations of professional organizations (e.g., ASHP), accreditation standards (e.g., The Joint Commission), and other standards-setting agencies (e.g., Centers for Disease Control and Prevention). Chapter 2 begins to discuss these concepts in more detail.

Moving up the pyramid, it is time for action: *Influencing Practice Change.* With little to no authority over the many disciplines and departments participating in the medication-use process across the organization, the MSO cannot simply "command" a transformation, and expect it to occur. As the MSO, you must combine leadership skills, medication safety expertise, experience in performance improvement methods, and teamwork to influence practice changes to improve safety.[7] Influencing change is one of the most challenging aspects of the MSO's role and is addressed in Chapter 3. Collaboration is essential to improving safety.[5,6,11,12,18,19] Through culture change and use of information and data, the MSO must shape and guide medication safety ventures, *must influence them*, to reach the pinnacle of the pyramid: *Patient Safety*.

The patient is placed at the top of the pyramid, as the subject of the MSO's primary goal: patient safety, keeping the patient safe from harm. It emphasizes the patient-centered mission of the MSO. The commitment we make to patient safety must be explicit and visible in the organization—the highpoint, or the top, of the pyramid.

Job Description

The MSO is "a clinical practitioner designated by an organization to serve as the authoritative expert in safe medication use."[7] Other titles used to describe this role include medication safety leader, medication safety manager, medication safety coordinator, medication safety clinical specialist, medication safety pharmacist, and director of medication safety. A job description will help communicate the vision for this role, expectations for performance, and the relationships to others within the organization. It also serves as a written document to describe responsibilities, qualifications, and reporting relationships and is typically required during development of a new MSO position. Reviewing existing job descriptions can also be helpful when updating or enhancing the MSO's role. The intent of this chapter is to give a general sense of the scope and intent for this position, with the understanding that the culture and organizational structure will directly impact the responsibilities and opportunities for the MSO. When considering this position's scope of responsibilities as you develop a proposal to administration, you will wonder how you managed to get along without this dedicated person!

Reporting Structure

The MSO may serve an individual hospital, a group of organizations at a health system level, or a more diverse collection of organizations at a corporate level. Reporting structures vary for the MSO, as the position continues to evolve within health care organizations. At hospital or health system settings, the MSO most commonly reports to one of four areas: Pharmacy, Patient Safety/Risk Management, Quality Improvement, or a senior administrator (e.g., vice president, chief medical officer). Because the MSO's reporting process depends a great deal on the organization's culture, structure, and hierarchy, there could be more than one reporting line. While the optimal placement has not been studied, there are some factors for consideration.

Patient safety, the freedom from accidental injury due to medical care or medical errors[8]—is an essential organizational priority. Medication safety, which may be defined as the freedom from accidental injury due to medical care or medical errors *during the medication-use process*, deserves the same prioritization, given the scope of medication use in patient care and the frequency and severity of potential harm. It follows that the MSO should be placed high in the organizational chart to work collaboratively with the patient safety officer (PSO). Reporting to senior leadership offers the MSO the attendant authority and empowerment to facilitate change. This also allows the MSO to align concerted safety efforts with other key leaders, such as the chief nursing officer (CNO), chief pharmacy officer (CPO), and chief executive officer (CEO). A suggested structure for this paradigm is shown in Figure 1-2.

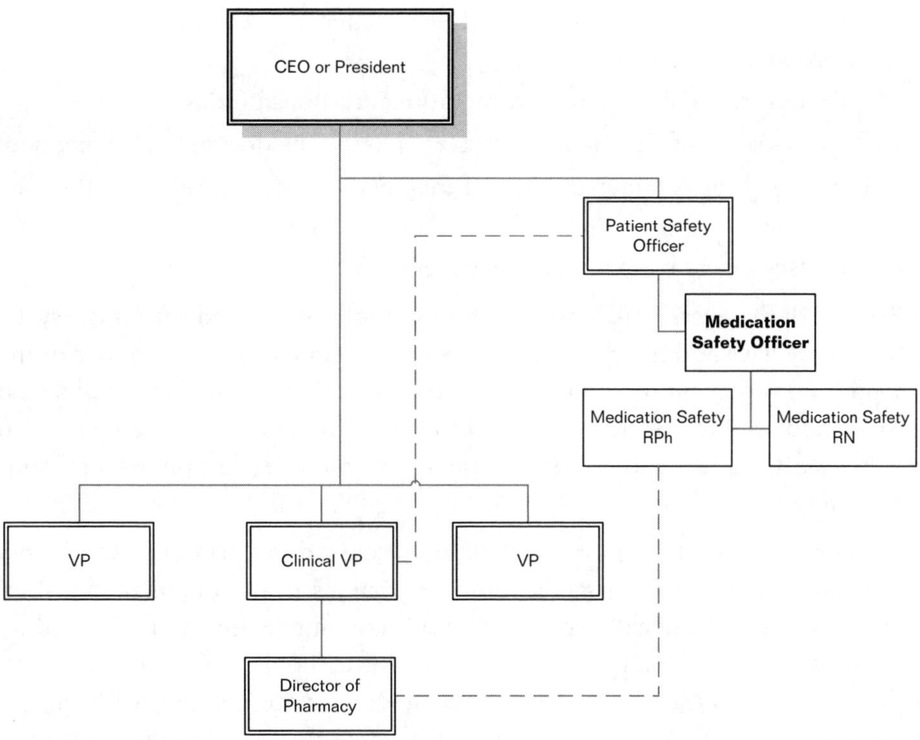

Figure 1-2. Safety organization chart.
Source: Used with permission of Bill Wightkin, A.T. Still University, School of Osteopathic Medicine in Arizona.

Within a department, a position generally has a direct report based on the specific department's hierarchy. An MSO based in a department most often reports to the director or leader of that area. In the pharmacy department, it is common for the MSO to report to the director of pharmacy. Other department leaders for MSO reporting include the director of quality and safety or the director of performance improvement. Some MSOs report to leadership at the vice president level, gaining strategic advantages discussed above.

There are potential benefits (and conversely, challenges) for the MSO reporting structure within or external to the pharmacy department.

Potential benefits of reporting within the pharmacy department include:

- Elevated attention to medication safety through MSO involvement in department leadership, operations, clinical services, and business decisions
- Enhanced understanding of pharmacy operations by MSO and ability to design safety systems and resolve identified risks
- Close working relationships with pharmacy staff
- Increased access by pharmacy department to MSO expertise

Potential benefits of reporting outside the pharmacy department include:

- Fosters an interdisciplinary approach to medication safety
- Eliminates conflicts of interest with departmental agendas, such as financial or production decisions
- Freedom from daily pharmacy operational responsibilities
- Removes potential for medication safety focus to be diverted to staffing duties
- Enhances MSO's understanding of the perspectives and roles of other disciplines
- Increases access by external departments to MSO expertise

Because of the overall responsibility for oversight of the medication-use system, the MSO may have additional reporting lines. For example, you may have a primary (or solid line) reporting relationship with the director of pharmacy, with secondary (or dotted line) reporting to the director of performance improvement. Matrix reporting is often a reflection of the organization's management philosophy and its patient safety structure.

A committee structure, more thoroughly discussed in Chapter 2, should be in place to directly oversee the medication-use systems in the organization. As the MSO, you should take a leadership role on this committee, generally referred to as the Medication Safety Committee (MSC). The MSC should report to the Pharmacy and Therapeutics (P&T) Committee, as a subcommittee charged with ensuring medication safety throughout the organization. The P&T also has responsibility to medical staff leadership to keep physician leadership informed of P&T activities, and they may solicit feedback from that group prior to making decisions that could impact physician practices (e.g., therapeutic interchanges). Another reporting line could be the organization's Patient Safety Committee or other similarly named committee (e.g., Safety Council).

Authority

Overall, the most important aspect of any type of structure is to make sure identified problems/issues are brought to the attention of the appropriate level of authority. For you to be effective in this role, it is critical to establish a sufficient level of authority. The MSO must have the support of the organization's administration to conduct investigations, interview staff, and coordinate process improvement activities. A close relationship with the Safety/Risk Management department would help to facilitate these types of activities. Safety/Risk Management is generally the department that has responsibility for coordinating patient safety investigations, and the MSO should be the primary authority on incidents involving medications. A committee structure is best for authorizing and approving process improvements and final action plans, and the MSC would be the appropriate multidisciplinary committee. Committee involvement is discussed in Chapter 2.

Responsibilities

Regardless of organizational structure, this position involves a wide variety of activities. There will be general day-to-day activities related to review and investigation of reported medication errors and then time-specific activities related to oversight of the medication system utilizing an MSC. In general, any activities related to medication use should be considered under the MSO's jurisdiction. Even though this concept seems obvious, medication-use discussions can take place in a myriad of settings within an organization without the MSO's knowledge. It becomes important then for the MSO to have knowledge of critical medication-use activities. Some are obvious, some not. The entire medication-use process, comprised of formulary system, storage, ordering, verification, preparation, dispensing, and administration and monitoring, has potential safety issues.

Medication-use discussions within the organization include traditional committee structures sanctioned by the medical staff and other ad hoc or work-groups for specific projects. Some organizations are good at identifying committee charges/activities and communicating this information to key stakeholders so it is important to know your organization's culture and communication style. The depth of the MSO's activities in any given situation or medication-related committee may depend on the workload or the group's representation. You may find your participation in various meetings may be frequently requested. Prioritization is important in determining what activities to participate in as it is difficult, if not impossible, to be involved in every meeting. In a process where roles and responsibilities are clearly defined, the MSO may be able to provide a consultation instead of direct participation.

The MSO's responsibilities may be categorized in five broad areas: leadership, medication safety expertise, influencing practice change, research, and education.[7]

The details for each section may be found in Appendix 1-A. A summary of responsibilities within each area follows.

Leadership

- Establish the vision for a safe medication use system
- Develop the medication safety plan
- Lead activities to achieve the vision and plan
- Support and enhance a culture of safety

Medication Safety Expertise

- Serve as expert resource for medication safety
- Recommend safe systems design, including technology and practice changes
- Facilitate management of medication-related risks and adverse events
- Lead medication safety committee

Influencing Practice Change

- Foster a comprehensive and interdisciplinary approach to medication safety actions
- Collaborate with departments and groups to apply risk reduction strategies
- Align and integrate medication safety into the organization's strategic plan
- Employ quality improvement methodologies to improve processes

Research and Education

- Participate in external event reporting programs
- Integrate medication safety into orientation and training for all providers
- Conduct research and contribute to literature on medication safety
- Educate colleagues, students, residents, and other health care professionals

Job descriptions often call for a more granular description of responsibilities, activities, or tasks. Key activities for the MSO include the following:

- Reviews and analyzes medication errors and ADEs
- Ensures compliance with medication safety regulations and standards
- Serves as chair for the MSC
- Serves as a resource to the organization and community on medication safety matters
- Assists in the development and review of medication-use pharmacy and hospital- and system-level policies, and their implementation
- Guides the design, implementation, and maintenance of safe medication systems in the organization

- Monitors the external environment for best practices and evaluates them for implementation in the organization
- Provides direction for prioritization of the organization's medication system improvement projects
- Facilitates or develops a structured approach for employee orientation and training for pharmacy staff and others involved in the medication-use process related to medication safety as it applies to the specific job category
- Provides ongoing medication safety education for pharmacy staff and other health care professionals to promote safe medication practices
- Facilitates availability of educational programs and materials to improve medication safety and regulatory compliance
- Participates in departmental and interdisciplinary hospital, health system, and regional committees related to emergency medications, drug shortages, adverse events, medication errors, policy review, technology, safe medication use, and patient safety
- Analyzes current medication-use practices that may contribute to medication errors using quality improvement methodologies, facilitates process and system changes to reduce the likelihood of occurrence/recurrence of error

A review of 30 job descriptions dated between 2002 and 2012 for hospital or health-systems MSOs revealed that expectations continue to evolve. Activities related to enhancing or building a *Just Culture* (see Chapter 5 for more discussion of Just Culture) and participation in technology planning and safety assessments were more likely to be found in more recent job descriptions than earlier examples. Recent job summaries reflected a more comprehensive approach to the position. The range of hospital or health-system experience listed in job qualifications ranged from 0 to 10 years, with a median of 5 years. Sample job descriptions are provided in Appendix 1-B. Appendix 1-C demonstrates alignment of MSO responsibilities with an organizational strategic plan.

Attributes of the MSO

Possession of certain attributes will improve the MSO's effectiveness. Your strengths should include the abilities to anticipate error and hazards and mitigate potential harm. A wide variety of skills is necessary to hone these abilities, including cognitive skills, such as situational awareness, and social/interpersonal skills, such as teamwork.[20] Attributes for success[7,20-22] may be categorized as knowledge, skills, and abilities (KSAs), and are presented below. In this format, *knowledge* refers to the understanding of an organized body of information; *skills* denote proficiency or expertise in the subject matter; and *abilities* signify the capacity to perform an activity or task. As a current or prospective MSO, you will benefit from evaluating your KSAs for professional development opportunities.

Knowledge

The MSO should have a broad understanding of:

- All aspects of the medication-use system
- Health care technologies used in the medication-use process
- Pharmaceutical care
- Clinical expertise
- Culture of safety, Just Culture concepts
- Change management concepts
- Holistic nature of health care systems
- Concepts of risk and prioritization, statistics, population data
- Performance improvement methodologies and tools
- Framework for human error
- Basic principles of human factors
- Medication safety resources
- Standards of practice related to medication use
- Accreditation process, standards, and regulations

Skills

The MSO should demonstrate excellence in the following skills:

- Leadership
- Verbal communication and presentation (small and large group)
- Written communication, editing
- Active listening
- Time management
- Project management
- Analytical
- Safe system/process design

Abilities

The MSO should possess the ability to perform the following:

- Facilitate practice change
- Collaborate with staff at all levels
- Effectively provide education
- Synthesize solutions
- Apply standards of practice to improve safety
- Apply defined strategies and protocols
- Function proactively vs. reactively
- Write clear and concise policy and procedures

- Recognize risks, anticipate errors
- Analyze systems and evaluate data

Education and Professional Development

During the evolution of the MSO position (early 1990s to early 2000s), those serving as MSOs relied largely on health care system experience, continuing education offerings, and mentorship to build their expertise. Medication safety is now part of didactic and experiential education, with diverse professional development offerings for practitioners in a variety of disciplines. As the field remains quite dynamic, this section gives a general overview of possibilities, and the reader is encouraged to seek current information at the time of reading.

Topics related to medication safety are integrated into accredited Doctor of Pharmacy degree programs through the core curriculum and pharmacy practice experiences. The Accreditation Council for Pharmacy Education (ACPE) lists "medication safety" as a distinct clinical science section in its 2011 curriculum guidance document.[23] Safety topics include causes of medication errors, systems approaches to medication errors, human factors, error reduction strategies, pharmacy leadership in medication safety, and quality improvement methods. ACPE also suggests that students should participate in identifying and reporting medication errors and adverse drug reactions and participate in activities regarding accreditation and regulatory safety requirements during their advanced pharmacy practice experiences (APPEs).

The ACPE notes that separate medication safety courses are not mandated, but the expectation is that the subject matter be addressed adequately in the curriculum. Some schools provide dedicated medication safety courses and may include opportunities for advanced practice experiences to strengthen the foundation in medication safety. Although the Doctor of Pharmacy graduate should be familiar with medication safety concepts, the content, intensity, and depth of this medication safety education is not adequate to prepare the graduate for the MSO position.

All ASHP postgraduate year one (PGY1) residency programs include an educational outcome related to medication safety.[24] This gives the resident opportunities for deeper understanding of medication safety principles and to actively participate in an organization's improvement activities. Preceptors may include discussions of concepts such as system error, process-mapping, error categorization, human factors, and Just Culture. The goals, objectives, and in particular, the instructional objectives, articulated in the ASHP accreditation standard requirements provide guidance to develop an effective introduction to medication safety for the resident.

Completion of a postgraduate year two (PGY2) pharmacy residency in medication-use safety is recommended for those interested in becoming an organization leader in this area. Based on the outcomes of this program, graduates will be qualified to:[24]

- Function as an effective leader for medication-use safety

- Serve as an authoritative resource on medication-use safety for the organization
- Develop a vision of an ideal safe medication-use system for the organization
- Represent the medication-use safety perspective to the organization's design of its technology and automation systems
- Conduct planning for the pursuit of the organization's vision of a safe medication-use system
- Collect medication-use data and use appropriate data analysis techniques to identify needed improvements in the medication-use system
- Manage changes in the medication-use system
- Conduct medication-use safety research

Formal programs, such as fellowships, offer intensive learning experiences related to medication safety. While some concentrate on medication safety, others may provide a more broad perspective in patient safety. A summary of programs currently available is provided in Table 1-1.

Demonstration of competency may be identified through credentialing programs. The American Society of Medication Safety Officers (ASMSO) has announced the Board Certified Medication Safety Specialist (BCMSS) credential, with the first examination to be available in 2013.[25] The BCMSS establishes core competency domains for medication safety, and sets an expected proficiency level. It also strives to validate a candidate's medication safety knowledge and skill set for employers. The National Association for Healthcare Quality (NAHQ)'s Certified Professional in Healthcare Quality (CPHQ) is another certification program of interest for the MSO.[26] Although not specific to medication safety, the content outline for CPHQ certification addresses many MSO tasks and responsibilities such as leadership, information management, quality improvement, and patient safety. The Certified Professional in Patient Safety (CPPS) credential identifies professionals competent in patient safety science and human factors engineering who can effectively plan and implement patient safety initiatives. The Certification Board for Professionals in Patient Safety (CBPPS) , established by the NPSF, oversees this credentialing process.[27]

Continuing education (CE) programs on various aspects of medication safety have proliferated within the last decade. This may be related to increased interest in safety and related research and publications, primed by the 2000 IOM report "To Err Is Human: Building a Safer Health System" and those published subsequently. The field of patient safety, including medication safety, has snowballed, with increased attention by accrediting organizations. Some states now require a defined number of hours of CE in medication safety for relicensure. The Accreditation Council for Pharmacy Education (ACPE) CE Universal Activity Number topic designator "05" indicates the program is related to patient safety. CE programs are provided in a number of formats, encompassing home study and live presentations via teleconference, webinar, and meetings.

Table 1-1. MSO Professional Development Programs

Program	Duration	Focus	For More Information
Medication Safety Pharmacy Fellowship at Saint Vincent Hospital/MCPHS	24 months	Medication safety, education, and clinical research	http://www.stvincenthospital.com/professionals/pharmacy-fellowship.aspx
Purdue University Community Practice Research Fellowship Program/MS in Pharmacy Practice with an Emphasis in Medication Safety	24 months	Medication safety; community pharmacy services	http://www.phpr.purdue.edu/residencies/snyder.pdf
ISMP Safe Medication Management Fellowships	12 months	Medication safety	http://ismp.org/profdevelopment/managementfellowship.asp
FDA/ISMP Safe Medication Management Fellowship	12 months	Medication safety; regulatory experience	http://ismp.org/profdevelopment/fdaismpfellowship.asp
AHA-NPSF Comprehensive Patient Safety Leadership Fellowship	12 months	Patient safety; transformational change	http://www.hpoe.org/PSLF/PSLF_main.shtml
ISMP International Mentorship Program	4 weeks	Group and individual learning projects (international participants travel to U.S.)	http://ismp.org/Consult/internationalExperience.asp
IHI Patient Safety Executive Development Program	7 days	Patient safety leadership	http://www.ihi.org/offerings/Training/PatientSafetyExecutive/2013patientsafetyexecutivedevelopment/Pages/default.aspx
ISMP Practitioner in Residence Program	5 days	Individualized program—medication safety	http://ismp.org/Consult/practitioner.asp
UW Systems Engineering Initiative for Patient Safety Short Course	4–5 days	Applies engineering approaches to patient safety	http://cqpi.engr.wisc.edu/shortcourse_home
ISMP Medication Safety Intensive	2 days	Medication safety; medication safety oversight	http://ismp.org/educational/MSI/default.asp

ISMP, Institute for Safe Medication Practices; FDA, Food and Drug Administration; AHA, American Hospital Association; NPSF, National Patient Safety Foundation; IHI, Institute for Healthcare Improvement; MCPHS, Massachusetts College of Pharmacy and Health Sciences; UW, University of Wisconsin.

Education and professional development opportunities include college of pharmacy curricula, postgraduate programs, intensive options, and CE offerings. MSOs are encouraged to use information in the responsibilities and attributes sections to assess areas for professional development and to seek opportunities to meet those needs. In turn, the MSO should endeavor to inspire every practicing pharmacist to engage in medication safety professional development.

Summary

The MSO position is critical for enhancing medication safety in an organization. Their leadership encompasses the entire medication-use process across the organization. A pyramid approach incorporating safe culture, use of information, and influencing change may be used to reduce patient harm related to medication use. The position must be structured to ensure comprehensive scope and adequate authority to carry out responsibilities in areas of leadership, medication safety expertise, influencing practice change, research, and education. Self-assessment of key attributes and ability to perform MSO job responsibilities should be used to drive professional development. By effectively identifying and addressing medication safety concerns and proactively providing direction to safeguard the medication-use system, the MSO will be an organization's highly valued asset. This position's challenges will be considerable, but the rewards of making important changes that improve the safety and well-being of patients and staff are immeasurable.

References

1. Chantler C. The role and education of doctors in the delivery of healthcare. *Lancet.* 1999;353:1178-1181.
2. Committee on Identifying and Preventing Medication Errors, Board on Health Care Services, Institute of Medicine. Aspden P, Wolcott JA, Bootman JL et al., eds. *Preventing Medication Errors.* Washington, DC: The National Academies Press; 2007.
3. Bates DW, Cullen DJ, Laird N, et al. Incidence of adverse drug events and potential adverse drug events. Implications for prevention, ADE Prevention Study Group. *JAMA.* 1995; 274:29-34.
4. Classen DC, Pestotnik SL, Evans RS, et al. Adverse drug events in hospitalized patients. Excess length of stay, extra costs, and attributable mortality. *JAMA.* 1997;277:301-306.
5. Burgess LH, Cohen MR, Denham CR. A new leadership role for pharmacists: A prescription for change. *J Patient Saf.* 2010;6:31-37.
6. National Quality Forum (NQF). Safe practices for better healthcare—2010 update: A consensus report. Available at: http://www.qualityforum.org/Publications/2010/04/Safe_Practices_for_Better_Healthcare_%e2%80%93_2010_Update.aspx. Accessed November 8, 2012.
7. ASHP statement on the role of the medication safety leader. In: Hawkins B, ed. *Best practices for hospital and health-system pharmacy: positions and guidance documents of ASHP, 2012–2013 ed.* Bethesda, MD: American Society of Health-System Pharmacists; 2012:201-4.
8. Committee on Quality of Health Care in America, Institute of Medicine. Kohn L, Corrigan J, Donaldson M, eds. *To err is human: building a safer health system.* Washington, DC: The National Academies Press; 2000.

9. The National Patient Safety Foundation. Agenda for research and development in patient safety. Available at: http://www.npsf.org/wp-content/uploads/2011/10/Agenda_for_RD_in_Patient_Safety.pdf. Accessed November 19, 2012.
10. Mark SM, Weber RJ. Developing a medication patient safety program—infrastructure and strategy. *Hosp Pharm*. 2007;42(2):149-156.
11. Cohen MM, Kimmel NL, Benage MK, et al. Medication safety program reduces adverse drug events in a community hospital. *Qual Saf Health Care*. 2005;14:169-174.
12. Brennan C, Donnelly K, Somani S. Needs and opportunities for achieving optimal outcomes from the use of medicines in hospitals and health systems. *Am J Health-Syst Pharm*. 2011; 68:e50-60.
13. American Hospital Association, Health Research & Educational Trust and the Institute for Safe Medication Practices. Pathways for medication safety: Leading a strategic planning effort. Available at: http://www.ismp.org/tools/pathwaysection1.pdf. Accessed November 19, 2012.
14. Agency for Healthcare Research and Quality (AHRQ). 30 safe practices for better health care. Available at http://www.ahrq.gov/qual/30safe.pdf. Accessed November 19, 2012.
15. Smetzer JL. Managing medication risks through a culture of safety. In: Cohen MR, ed. *Medication Errors*. 2nd ed. Washington, DC: American Pharmacists Association; 2007;605-654.
16. Kowiatek JG, Weber RJ, Skledar SJ, et al. Medication safety manager in an academic medical center. *Am J. Health-Syst Pharm*. 2004:61:58-64.
17. Mark SM, Weber RJ. Developing a medication patient safety program, part 2: Process and implementation. *Hosp Pharm*. 2007;42:207-215.
18. Chisholm-Burns MA, Lee JK, Spivey CA, et al. US pharmacists' effects team members on patient care: Systematic review and meta-analyses. *Med Care*. 2010;48:923-933.
19. Sutker WL. The physician's role in patient safety: What's in it for me? *Proc (Bayl Univ Med Cent)*. 2008;21(10):9-14.
20. Taylor-Adams S, Brodie A, Vincent C. Safety skills for clinicians: An essential component of patient safety. *J Patient Saf*. 2008;4:141-147.
21. Kowiatek J. Establish a successful medication safety program. *Pharm Purch Prod*. 2011;8:6-9.
22. Saine D. Navigating the seven c's of a medication safety pharmacist. *Pharm Purch Prod*. 2007;4: 6-7.
23. Accreditation Council for Pharmacy Education. Accreditation standards and guidelines for the professional program in pharmacy leading to the doctor of pharmacy degree, effective February 14, 2011. Available at: https://www.acpe-accredit.org/pdf/S2007Guidelines2.0_ChangesIdentifiedInRed.pdf. Accessed November 24, 2012.
24. American Society of Health-System Pharmacists. Residency Accreditation. Available at http://www.ashp.org/menu/Accreditation/ResidencyAccreditation.aspx. Accessed November 26, 2012.
25. American Society of Medication Safety Officers. Certification. Available at: http://asmso.org/node/5. Accessed November 26, 2012.
26. National Association for Healthcare Quality. CPHQ Certification. Available at: http://www.nahq.org/certify/content/index.html. Accessed November 26, 2012.
27. Certification Board for Professionals in Patient Safety. The CPPS Examination. Available at: http://cbpps.org/cpps-exam/. Accessed November 26, 2012.

Appendix 1-A

ASHP Statement on the Role of the Medication Safety Leader

Position

The American Society of Health-System Pharmacists (ASHP) believes that medication safety is a fundamental responsibility of all members of the profession of pharmacy. For a medication safety program to succeed, however, it is essential that there be an innovative leader to set a vision and direction, identify opportunities to improve the medication-use system, and lead implementation of error-prevention strategies. The medication safety leader's role includes responsibility for leadership, medication safety expertise, influencing practice change, research, and education. ASHP believes that because of their training, knowledge of the medication-use process, skills, and abilities, pharmacists are uniquely qualified to fill the roles and meet the responsibilities of the medication safety leader in hospitals and health systems.

Background

Hospital and health-system pharmacists have improved pharmacy systems over the past 60 years to reduce the risk that medications could harm patients. Medication safety was at the heart of such historic innovations in pharmacy services as unit-dose systems, decentralized clinical pharmacy services, and intravenous admixture services. The crucial leadership role of pharmacists in medication safety has been summarized as follows:

> Pharmacy leadership is the core of a successful medication safety program. Pharmacy leaders can play an enormously important role in performance improvement. They can be part of the senior leadership team's DNA because their impact and view go far beyond the walls of the pharmacy.... Pharmacists can play an important role as leaders to reduce patient safety risks, optimize the safe function of medication management systems, and align pharmacy services with national initiatives that measure and reward quality performance.[1]

The landmark Institute of Medicine (IOM) report *To Err Is Human: Building a Safer Health System*[2] generated major patient safety initiatives by government agencies, regulatory and accrediting bodies, professional and organizational associations, and health care organizations. The Joint Commission (TJC) National Patient Safety Goals (NPSGs)[3] are an example of a response to the original IOM report. The Pharmacy Practice Model Initiative (PPMI)[4] and the National Quality Forum (NQF) Safe Practice 18[5] incorporate medication safety principles to ensure optimal patient safety and outcomes.

The medication safety leader (also referred to as a medication safety officer, medication safety manager, or medication safety coordinator, among other titles) is a clinical practitioner designated by an organization to serve as the authoritative expert in safe medication use. Traditionally, the medication safety leader has been a clinical pharmacist or manager within the department of pharmacy, although the position is sometimes filled by a nurse or physician. The medication safety leader may report to the organization's risk management department, its office of quality, or to a senior administrator (e.g., hospital vice president, chief medical officer, or chief executive officer). Reporting outside the pharmacy department may foster interdisciplinary approaches to medication safety. Medication safety leadership may encompass a single hospital or a group of organizations (e.g., spanning a health system or at a corporate level of a larger organization). Regardless of organization size, it is critical that the fundamentals of medication safety are the central component of the medication safety leader's job function. Although medication safety leaders may have other responsibilities in smaller institutions, medication safety should remain their core responsibility, and they must be strategically positioned and empowered to lead efforts to reduce the risks of medication use.

The characteristics of a medication safety leader include:

1. A strong understanding of the facility's internal systems and processes developed through firsthand experience, observations, medication-use evaluations, interviews, and data analysis for a spectrum of patient populations (e.g., pediatric, geriatric, cardiac, oncology).
2. Clinical expertise and a broad understanding of health care systems and processes to facilitate accurate interpretation of clinical events.
3. Knowledge of and experience with all aspects of the medication-use system, including procurement, prescribing, transcribing, preparation, distribution, administration, documentation, and monitoring.
4. Strong analytical skills and an understanding of statistics, population data, and the concepts of risk and prioritization.
5. Knowledge of performance improvement methodology and tools, including root cause analysis (RCA), failure mode and effects analysis (FMEA), cause-and-effect diagramming, process-flow mapping, and methods for monitoring projects and measuring the progress of performance improvement initiatives.
6. Three or more years of post-training health-system practice experience.
7. Demonstrated leadership skills.
8. Excellent small and large group presentation skills.
9. Excellent verbal communication skills, especially the ability to communicate to all types of health care providers, as individuals as well as in small and large groups.
10. Excellent writing and editing skills.

11. Strong personal belief that resolving the problem of medication errors is a systems issue and not an individual health care provider issue.
12. Ability to function proactively rather than reactively.
13. Strong personal belief in the concept of a "just culture"[6] that enhances transparency, opens participation to all health care professionals, and fosters a "lessons learned" environment in an organization's medication-error reporting system.
14. Understanding of concepts and application of safety principles, continuous quality improvement, and human factors engineering.
15. Appropriate assertiveness.
16. A passion for medication safety and improving patient outcomes.
17. Proven success in working with interdisciplinary teams and engaging diverse groups.
18. Strong personal belief in engaging patients as part of the health care team.
19. Eagerness to learn from events outside one's own facility (e.g., through external sources of information) to apply learning about what went wrong in order to identify and remedy possible system weaknesses to prevent patient harm.[7]

The scope of a medication safety leader's responsibilities reaches into every corner of the health care system and encompasses many roles, such as educator, preceptor, mentor, detective, compliance officer, risk manager, engineer, accountant, statistician, computer analyst, and counselor. A typical day may include attending safety rounds, precepting pharmacy students and residents, writing policies, reviewing adverse drug reactions and medication error reports, developing error-prevention strategies, leading process improvement teams, implementing action items, reviewing smart pump libraries, ensuring safe use of automated medication dispensing systems, assessing the safety of replacement drug products during drug shortages, orienting new professional staff, assisting with medication reconciliation, conducting tracers to ensure compliance with accreditation standards (e.g., TJC medication management standards and NPSGs), working with practitioners to resolve acute events, attending medical staff meetings, or educating the corporate board on the culture of safety. Most medication safety leaders quickly find themselves involved in many projects and committees as well as serving as the contact person when nursing, pharmacy, or medical staff have questions or problems. The medication safety leader needs a solid understanding of patient safety principles and must have the ability to prioritize work activities to have a positive impact on the safety of patient care. The medication safety leader should strive to acquire additional skills crucial to success, such as presentation and communications skills, as well as expertise in process improvement methodologies such as Six Sigma and Lean. Formalized training in medication safety can be achieved through residency, fellowship, certificate programs, and other methods of continuing education. ASHP supports the expansion of pharmacy education and postgraduate residency training to include an emphasis on medication safety.[8]

Responsibilities of Medication Safety Leaders

Medication safety leaders must collaborate with all types of health care professionals, support staff, and management, and consider all components of the medication-use process in both inpatient and clinic settings in order to improve medication safety. The medication safety leader's role includes responsibility for leadership, medication safety expertise, influencing practice change, research, and education.

Leadership. To provide leadership, the medication safety leader will:

1. Develop a vision of an ideal safe medication-use system for the organization.
2. Oversee the planning, creation, review, and refinement of a medication safety plan.
3. Proactively develop and lead implementation of error-prevention strategies based on practice standards, literature review, medication safety tools, and analysis of the organization's medication safety data.
4. Participate in the planning, design, and implementation of the organization's medication-use technology and automation systems.
5. Build a culture of safety through "lesson learned" education and communication across the entire organization.
6. Oversee processes to collect information on the organization's medication errors and system failures to ensure that they are captured and barriers to reporting are addressed.
7. Ensure compliance with state and federal regulatory and legal requirements relating to medication safety, and assist in the accreditation process by ensuring that the organization's medication-use processes meet applicable medication management standards and NPSGs.

Medication Safety Expertise. In the role of medication safety expert, the medication safety leader will:

1. Serve as an authoritative resource on medication safety for the organization.
2. Contribute the medication safety perspective for technology initiatives.
3. Contribute the medication safety perspective to internal and external emergency preparedness planning.
4. Serve as an internal consultant to investigate medication safety events or issues and develop recommendations for action.
5. Serve as the chair of the Medication Safety Committee, whose duties may include setting the agenda, reviewing general and specific error reports, and examining the progress of projects and initiatives assigned to the medication safety team.

6. Be knowledgeable in the application and use of a variety of quality improvement methodologies and tools (e.g., FOCUS-PDCA or Lean methodologies, root cause analysis, failure mode and effects analysis).
7. Collect, review, and analyze, as the leader of review teams, the organization's medication-use, medication error, adverse drug reaction, and continuous quality improvement data (e.g., markers of adverse drug events, smart pump event data, triggers and surveillance information, and automated dispensing system and bedside barcode scanning reports) and use appropriate data analysis techniques to identify needed improvements and develop high-leverage error-reduction strategies.
8. Predict and prepare to manage medication safety issues caused by potential or actual drug product shortages and the use of replacement drug products.
9. Maintain knowledge of trends and developments in the patient safety field through continuous professional development; reading articles, journals, and related material; attending appropriate seminars, conferences, or educational programs; and utilization of information from the Institute of Safe Medication Practices (ISMP) National Medication Error Reporting Program, the Food and Drug Administration (FDA) MedWatch program, and similar programs.
10. Participate at a local and national level in patient safety and medication safety organizations and initiatives.

Influencing Practice Change. To influence practice change, the medication safety leader will:

1. Collaborate with other departments (e.g., pharmacy, risk management, and patient safety), hospital or health-system senior leadership, frontline staff, and nursing and medical staff leadership to identify and prioritize safety issues and develop risk-reduction strategies using the methods listed above to identify opportunities to improve medication safety.
2. Manage changes in the medication-use system to enhance medication safety, ensure that appropriate measures are taken to address and resolve medication safety issues, and see that hospital staff and faculty are supported in providing safe care for patients.
3. Work closely with others (e.g., the patient safety officer) to integrate medication safety into the overall strategic plan for patient safety and coordinate medication safety initiatives with organizational patient safety initiatives.
4. Participate in or lead multidisciplinary hospital and health-system committees concerned with medication errors, adverse drug events and reactions, near misses, policy review, safe medication use, new product review, and patient safety to identify risk points and prioritize system improvements to reduce the potential for medication error and patient harm.

5. Consult with and advise specific clinical teams and the hospital and health system generally on opportunities and strategies to improve patient care.
6. Encourage organization-wide medication error reporting through an established and accepted error reporting system that utilizes appropriate error detection methods (e.g., trigger tools) and through other appropriate avenues such as the Pharmacy & Therapeutics Committee, Medication Safety Committee, or Patient Safety Committee.
7. Develop effective methods for spreading best medication-use practices throughout the organization.
8. Use continuous quality improvement principles to assess and report on the status of efforts to improve medication safety.
9. Periodically review and update clinical decision support tools to alert staff to high-risk situations and educate staff as needed.

Research and Education. To further research and education regarding medication safety, the medication safety leader will:

1. Design and assist in the implementation of education and orientation programs in safe medication use, including:
   - development of competency assessment for staff tasks related to medication safety (e.g., use of smart pumps and automated medication dispensing systems);
   - education of health care providers, other pertinent staff, and (as possible) patients to ensure they are competent in safe medication-use practices; and
   - provision of effective ongoing programs and presentations related to safe medication use to diverse audiences (e.g., nursing, pharmacy, respiratory care, and medical staff).
2. Share information about actual or potential medication errors or harm with safety organizations such as the Institute for Safe Medication Practices (ISMP), the FDA, drug or product manufacturers, and state error reporting programs.
3. Conduct medication-use safety research through well-designed, externally validated studies, and implement evidence-based practices for medication safety.
4. Contribute to the literature on medication safety.
5. Provide medication safety education to pharmacy colleagues, students, and residents, as well as other health care professionals.
6. Integrate medication safety into orientation and training for all health care providers who participate in the medication-use process.

Conclusion

ASHP believes that pharmacists, as experts on medication use, are uniquely qualified to serve as medication safety leaders. Medication safety leaders articulate the vision and direction for improving the safety of the medication-use system to prevent patient harm. The medication safety leader's role includes responsibility for leadership through direction and prioritization, medication safety expertise, influencing practice change, research, and education. Through analysis of the organization's medication safety data and literature review, the medication safety leader will lead development and implementation of proactive error-prevention strategies and build a culture of safety across the organization.

References

1. Burgess LH, Cohen MR, Denham CR. A new leadership role for pharmacists: a prescription for change. *J Patient Saf.* 2010; 6:31–7.
2. Kohn KT, Corrigan JM, Donaldson MS. *To Err Is Human: Building a Safer Health System.* Washington, DC: National Academy Press; 1999.
3. The Joint Commission. Facts about the National Patient Safety Goals. www.jointcommission.org/facts_about_the_national_patient_safety_goals/ (accessed 03 Nov 2012).
4. The consensus of the Pharmacy Practice Model Summit. *Am J Health-Syst Pharm.* 2011; 68:1148–52.
5. National Quality Forum. Safe Practices for Better Healthcare 2009 Update: A Consensus Report. Washington, DC: The National Quality Forum; 2009. Available at: www.qualityforum.org/publications/reports/safe_practices_2009.aspx (accessed 31 Jan 2012).
6. Marx D. *Patient Safety and the "Just Culture": A Primer for Health Care Executives.* New York: Columbia University Press; 2001.
7. Adapted from American Society of Health-System Pharmacists. Desired entry characteristics for those to be trained for medication-use safety coordinator positions. www.ashp.org/DocLibrary/Accreditation/Regulations-Standards/RTPEntryCharactMedUseSafety.aspx (accessed 28 Nov 2011).
8. American Society of Health-System Pharmacists. Required Educational Outcomes, Goals, and Objectives for Postgraduate Year Two (PGY2) Pharmacy Residencies in Medication-Use Safety. www.ashp.org/DocLibrary/Accreditation/Regulations-Standards/RTPObjMedicationSafety032608.aspx (accessed 03 Feb 2012).

Suggested Readings

1. Cohen MR (ed.). *Medication Errors.* Washington, DC: American Pharmacists Association; 2007.
2. Manasse HR, Thompson KK (eds.). *Medication Safety: A Guide for Health Care Facilities.* Bethesda, MD: American Society of Health-System Pharmacists; 2005.
3. Hepler CD, Segal R. *Preventing Medication Errors and Improving Drug Therapy Outcomes: A Management Systems Approach.* Boca Raton, FL: CRC Press; 2003.
4. Joint Commission Resources. *Medication Use: A Systems Approach to Reducing Errors*, 2nd ed. Oakbrook Terrace, IL: Joint Commission Resources; 2008.
5. Kohn LT, Corrigan JM, Donaldson MS (eds.). *To Err Is Human: Building a Safer Health System.* Washington, DC: National Academy Press; 1999.
6. Committee on Quality of Health Care in America, Institute of Medicine. *Crossing the Quality Chasm: A New Health System for the 21St Century.* Washington, DC: National Academy Press; 2001.
7. Committee on Data Standards for Patient Safety, Institute of Medicine. *Patient Safety: Achieving a New Standard for Care.* Washington, DC: National Academy Press; 2004.
8. Committee on the Work Environment for Nurses and Patient Safety, Board on Health Care Services, Institute of Medicine. Page A (ed.). *Keeping Patients Safe: Transforming the Work Environment of Nurses.* Washington, DC: National Academy Press; 2004.

9. Committee on Identifying and Preventing Medication Errors, Board on Health Care Services, Institute of Medicine. Aspden P, Wolcott JA, Bootman JL, et al. (eds.). *Preventing Medication Errors.* Washington, DC: National Academy Press; 2007.

Web Resources

www.ashp.org

www.ismp.org

www.safemedication.com

www.asmso.org

www.ahrq.gov

http://www.fda.gov/cder/drugSafety.htm

www.ihi.org

http://www.jointcommission.org/standards_information/npsgs.aspx

http://www.leapfroggroup.org/

www.qualityforum.org

www.nccmerp.org

www.usp.org

http://www.patientsafety.gov/

Approved by the ASHP Board of Directors on April 13, 2012, and by the ASHP House of Delegates on June 10, 2012. Developed through the ASHP Section of Inpatient Care Practitioners Section Advisory Group on Medication Safety and approved by the ASHP Council on Education and Workforce Development on February 21, 2012.

Lynn Eschenbacher, Pharm.D., M.B.A., is gratefully acknowledged for drafting this statement.

Source: Originally published in: Hawkins B, ed. *Best Practices for Hospital and Health-System Pharmacy: Positions and Guidance Documents of ASHP.* 2012–2013 ed. Bethesda, MD: American Society of Health-System Pharmacists; 2012:201-4. © 2012, American Society of Health-System Pharmacists, Inc. All rights reserved.

Appendix 1-B

Sample Job Descriptions

JOB DESCRIPTION #1

Medication Safety Officer

Position Summary

Provides a leadership role in formulating policy and instituting models that promote medication safety in all aspects of the medication management process. In conjunction with designated facility leadership, the role is responsible for coordinating all activities related to medication safety provided by the facility. These activities involve reporting, system and process evaluation, formulation of recommendations and initiatives, coordination of intervention strategies, and monitoring of activities related to medication safety. This individual is responsible for identifying key projects related to medication safety and is accountable for coordinating the implementation of these projects system-wide. This individual serves as a liaison to facility pharmacy, nursing and the medical staff leadership personnel.

Minimum Qualifications

- BS in Pharmacy and/or PharmD.
- Pharmacist with hospital pharmacy experience required.
- Individual who is detail-oriented.
- Ability to use independent judgment and communicate effectively.
- Strong leadership ability with superior communication (both verbal and-written) and presentation skills utilizing various types of media.
- Minimum of 3–5 years of hospital experience required.

Required Licensure/Certification Skills

NYS Pharmacy license or licensure eligibility. License or permit required within 6 months of hire.

Vision and Mission

Communicates a clear compelling and inspired vision and sense of organizational purpose. The successful leader takes steps to ensure that the group has the resources, authority, measurable goals, and monitoring systems necessary for high performance and sustained commitment. The effective leader sets realistic but stretch goals, monitors progress, and initiates action to effectively enlist others in the movement toward broad organizational and cultural change. Exhibits a clear understanding of health system long-term plan and how all areas contribute to health system vision. This is evidenced by the ability to clearly communicate this vision to staff and co-workers.

Accountability for Results

Achieves challenging objectives, finds better or more efficient ways of accomplishing strategic business results. Takes decisive action, manages financial and human resources to achieve objectives. Accepts ownership and accountability for decisions and performance outcomes. Anticipates roadblocks and takes decisive and timely action to remain on course to meet objectives. Pushes self and others for success. Achievement oriented, evidenced by examples of personal responsibility in significant achievements

Analytical and Systems Thinking

Utilizes analytical, conceptual and intuitive approaches when planning initiatives, addressing problems, opportunities, and situations. Makes decisions that are data driven whenever appropriate. Sets measurable outcomes for performance. Capitalizes proactively on opportunities by projecting future outcomes and risks.

Change Agent

Embraces and promotes a change-oriented culture, exhibits flexibility to adapt to and work effectively in new situations and with various individuals or groups. Strives for continuous quality improvements, evaluates current practices against best practices and changes as indicated. Promotes innovation and creativity. Appreciates different and opposing perspectives on an issue, adapts one's approach as the requirements of a situation change, and changes or easily accepts changes in one's own organization or job requirements. Enlists others, and sets personal examples of change, demonstrates expected behavior changes, celebrates successes.

Technical Skills and Job Knowledge

Demonstrates a command of the technical skills and job knowledge necessary to consistently achieve performance objectives. Applies the initiative to remain current with changing technology and operational, clinical, and technical advancements.

Judgment and Integrity and Ethics

Acts honestly and fairly in all interactions with staff and coworkers. Keeps promises and maintains confidences. Complies with organizational policies, both personally and as a manager. Is viewed as a role model by subordinates, peers, and executive management. Takes personal responsibility for actions. Implements departmental audit procedures to ensure ethical utilization of resources. Maintains professional business conduct appropriate to the position with a strong commitment to the high standards of business ethics.

Strategic Influence and Communications

The ability to communicate ideas and managerial direction to an audience in a persuasive manner in order to engender support or agreement. It involves targeting information to meet the needs of the audience, anticipating reactions, and generating support. Communicates the health system's agenda, spending the necessary time to ensure others fully understand intent, values, objectives, and outcomes. Communicates in a compelling and inspired manner, is optimistic, communicates effectively with all levels to include patients, physicians, peers, subordinates, and if applicable, community and external contacts. This is evidenced by subordinates' and coworkers' awareness of and understanding of the work unit's objectives and performance against objective.

People Skills

Works effectively with others for the common good of the organization; listens effectively, tolerates differences and promotes diversity. Recruits and retains qualified staff to meet unit objectives. Maintains a positive work environment needed to meet annual objectives. Develops staff through one-on-one coaching and performance appraisal meetings with each employee at least annually and prior to the due date. Accomplishes annual development objectives outlined in the performance appraisal within the assigned deadlines. Also promotes a cooperative work environment by effectively addressing dealing with individuals as well as issues of team morale and productivity. Actively utilizes the health system employee recognition program.

Duties and Responsibilities

- Analyzes facility reporting systems to determine their effectiveness in terms of adverse drug event capture, timeliness of reporting, and usefulness of information captured. Creates a system-wide reporting policy for adverse drug events including standardized definitions.
- Identifies best practices for medication safety. Analyzes current practices that contribute to medication errors and takes proactive steps for prevention. Collaborates with other leaders and facilitates process and system changes and reduce the likelihood of occurrence and recurrence of error.
- Provides project management and overall facilitation for prioritizing and advocating patient safety initiatives related to the design and implementation of systems and processes that support medication safety. Develops project plans and implement in a timely fashion. Responsible for the facilitation of sustainable performance post implementation.
- Reviews medication safety bulletins, alerts, or publications and conduct an assessment of the medication management systems and process to determine where opportunities for improvement exist. Formulates recommendations, obtains stakeholder support, and works with affected departments to develop an implementation and education plan. Provides education, guidance, and assistance to sites, departments, service lines, and individuals as it relates to medication safety.
- Participates in facility-based root cause analyses. Evaluates systems and process change recommendations on a system-wide level to determine where medication safety risks exist and opportunities for improvement are needed. Develops a system-wide plan for implementation of recommendations as well as increased awareness of the risks identified with this type of event.
- Performs a system-wide analysis of adverse drug events based on data reported from each facility. Identifies trends from a system-wide and facility basis to determine if corrective actions are needed. Uses expert panels to

review adverse drug events. Develops performance measures and reports on a frequent basis.

- Formulates educational sessions for nurses, pharmacists, physicians, and allied health professionals based on reports in the literature, responses to corrective action plans, and recommendations from committee activities.
- Participates on the Safety Institute meetings and updates the Committee on the status of initiatives identified in the medication safety plan.
- Establishes a system-wide working forum on medication safety. Develops and facilitates the implementation of meetings, selection of membership, agenda planning, minutes, follow-up, tracking, and timeliness across all facilities.
- Performance requires the ability to interact consistently and effectively with a large and diverse constituency consisting of members of the pharmacy profession, the nursing profession, medical and dental professionals, and administrative staff from all levels of the health system.
- Mentors pharmacy students in the areas of medication safety promotion and regulatory compliance issues.
- Direct involvement in ensuring the ongoing safety of the medical center's technology related to medications (for example, computerized physician order entry system for electronic ordering of patient medications, pharmacy computer system, automated dispensing cabinets, electronic MARs).
- Performs other duties as assigned.

Job Requirements

- Schedule: Full Time

Source: Courtesy of Rochester General Hospital, Rochester General Health System.

JOB DESCRIPTION #2

Medication Safety Officer

Reports To: Director, Medication Management, Use and Policy

Effective Date: May 17, 2011

Expectation For All Employees

To provide excellence and innovation in the care of patients, the training of health professionals and the creation and sharing of health knowledge. This institution exists to serve others and does so through the expression of our core values:

Respect To recognize the dignity of every person

Integrity To be honest, fair, and trustworthy

Stewardship To manage resources responsibly

Excellence To work at the highest level of performance, with a commitment to continuous improvement

Position Summary

Oversees the Medical Center's Medication Safety Program. Utilizes clinical expertise to facilitate accurate interpretation of clinical events. Work requires knowledge about hands-on medication prescribing, preparation, distribution, administration, and monitoring. Serves as expert, professional resource to Risk Management, Performance Improvement, and Pharmacy Department. In addition, work requires excellent presentation, writing, and verbal communication skills.

Essential Duties and Responsibilities

1. Investigates and analyzes reports of adverse drug events (adverse drug reactions, medication errors and near misses).
   a. Codes all events in Medical Center's Quality Tool, based on The Joint Commission error types and severity levels and ASHP Drug Classification system.
   b. Works with Quality Tool's Data Analyst to create specific reports based on review of reported events (e.g., error type, error source, high risk, pump setting errors).
   c. Extracts prescribing errors from Pharmacists Interventions report; analyzes by service, med type, MD, adjustment required per renal function.
   d. Provides information to appropriate Medical Center Committees or persons as requested or as deemed necessary.
   e. Uses clinical knowledge and clinical expertise to accurately interpret clinical events and determine contributing factors to errors.
   f. Works with Risk Management and Patient Safety in review of errors and near misses; recommends groups to work on specific recommendations.

g. Collects medication-use data and uses appropriate data analysis techniques to identify needed improvements in the medication-use system.

2. Identifies and implements process changes in response to preparation/dispensing errors, regulatory requirements, and emerging medication safety literature.
   a. Provides pharmacy supervisors with copies of relevant individual error reports as well as trended data.
   b. Develops tool to document investigation and counseling for each preparation/dispensing error in conjunction with supervisor.
   c. Works with pharmacy supervisors to develop and implement changes and safeguards for medication preparation/dispensing.
   d. Provides aggregated information to pharmacy staff about preparation/dispensing errors and intercepted prescribing errors.
   e. Analyzes the organization's current medication-use system compared to best practices.
   f. Facilitates safety-improvement changes in the medication-use physical environment.
   g. Reviews emerging medication safety literature such as ISMP and MedWatch Alerts and The Joint Commission Sentinel Events.
   h. Implements actions necessary to respond to emerging medication safety literature, regulatory requirements, and medication/dispensing errors.
   i. Facilitates changes in the organization's medication-use policies and procedures.
3. Represents the medication-use safety perspective to the organization's design of its technology and automation systems.
   a. Assures that all patient-specific and medication-specific information required to support effective medication-related patient-care decisions is readily available in a useful form to physicians, nurses, pharmacists, and other pertinent health care providers.
   b. In collaboration with information technology professionals, physicians, nurses, pharmacists, and other pertinent health-care providers, defines patient and medication information system requirements to support effective medication-related patient-care decisions by physicians, nurses, pharmacists, and other pertinent health care providers.
   c. Formulates a plan that assures the organization's patient and medication information system remains current.
   d. Assures that all processes and devices used for medication administration include critical consideration of medication-use safety, including the appropriate level of human factors evaluation.
   e. Implements effective safety features in devices and technology to prevent or reduce harm resulting from errors in administration of medica-

tions (e.g., soft alerts, hard alerts, point-of-care bar-coding, electronic medication administration records).

4. Leads multidisciplinary medication safety groups.
   a. Takes leadership role in institutional medication safety/patient safety committees.
   b. Develops an effective interdisciplinary committee structure to address medication-use safety issues.
   c. Leads strategic planning for medication-use safety.
   d. Leads planning activities for the achievement of short-term medication-use safety goals.
5. Educates Medical Center staff on medication safety.
   a. Provides effective medication-use safety-related education and/or training to health care professionals, and health care professionals in training.
   b. Works with patient safety groups to develop computer-based learning modules and other medication safety related education for the Medical Center.
   c. Provides medication safety-related information at various orientations.
   d. Instructs staff on the mechanics, as well as the importance, of reporting medication safety events (adverse drug reactions, medication errors, and near misses).
   e. Formulates a plan for any needed education, training, and/or assessment associated with implementation of a new or changed policy or procedure.
   f. Collaborates with others to develop and deliver education/training involved in the implementation of a changed policy or procedure.
6. Participates in scholarly/professional activities.
   a. Conducts medication-use safety and health outcomes research.
   b. Contributes to the literature on medication-use safety.
   c. Serves as a peer-reviewer to pharmacy journals.
   d. Demonstrates involvement in local, state or national pharmacy organization.
   e. Provides service/leadership on committees of professional organizations.
   f. Attends professional meetings in the capacity as presenter; committee/council/commission member; and/or elected/appointed officer.
   g. Provides presentations to health care professionals outside of the Medical Center.

Organizational Duties

1. Communicates appropriately using good interpersonal skills.
   a. Positive, professional demeanor is projected through verbal and non-verbal communications.

b. Information for patients and staff is delivered in a manner that is supportive, timely, and understandable.
c. Interpersonal conflicts are resolved using appropriate methods and organizational resources, including but not limited to Employee Relations Services and Faculty Employee Assistance Program.
d. Diverse perspectives are acknowledged; language and behaviors are modeled that build inclusiveness in the work environment.
e. Ideas and suggestions are clearly communicated.
f. Clarification of communication is requested when appropriate.

2. Serves, manages, and supports internal and external customers.
   a. Privacy is maintained at all times for patient and employee information.
   b. Actions are initiated to meet or exceed customer/co-workers expectations in delivering service by implementing the "I Make the Difference" philosophy (ownership begins with me; greet customers by making eye contact and smiling; provide positive, professional and prompt responses, e.g., helping visitors find their way; close every interaction with "Is there anything else I can do for you?").
   c. Appropriate resources throughout the organization are used consistently to meet customer needs.
   d. Relationships with staff in other work areas are fostered to meet internal and external customer needs.
   e. Positive working relationships with peers, management, and customers are maintained at all times.
   f. Organizational mission and values of respect, integrity, stewardship, and excellence are evident in behaviors.
3. Participates in performance improvement activities.
   a. Participation in performance improvement activities and initiatives is on-going.
   b. Initiative is demonstrated to proactively diagnose and resolve problems.
   c. Change is met with positive, supportive behavior.
4. Participates as a team member and is accountable for own work responsibilities.
   a. Time off is scheduled to avoid disrupting workflow.
   b. Help is offered to others to solve problems and complete tasks to facilitate communication and positive team dynamics.
   c. Productive work habits are consistently displayed.
   d. Accountability for actions and decisions is demonstrated in daily work.
   e. Feedback is solicited and accepted in a positive manner.
   f. Constructive input is offered to support the work unit.

Minimum Requirements

Advanced pharmacy degree (Doctor of Pharmacy or Master's degree). Experience: PGY1-required, PGY2 or Fellowship-preferred or equivalent hospital experience (5 years in specific practice area). License/Certification: Virginia State Board of Pharmacy License or within 60 days of hire. Job requires standing for prolonged periods. Proficient communicative, auditory and visual skills; attention to detail and ability to write legibly; ability to lift/push/pull <20 lb. May be exposed to chemicals.

General Information

The above statements are intended to describe the general nature and level of work being performed by individuals assigned to this position. They are not intended to be an exhaustive list of all duties, responsibilities, and skills required of personnel so classified.

Source: Courtesy of University of Virginia Health System.

JOB DESCRIPTION #3

Associate Director, Safety and Quality

Responsibilities

The major areas of responsibility for the Associate Director for Safety and Quality include Hospital Pharmacy's and Ambulatory Care Pharmacy's quality improvement programs, regulatory compliance, and staff development. The person in this position also serves as the Medication Safety Officer for the hospital and health sciences system and as such is responsible for coordinating the adverse drug reaction reporting program and assuming a leadership role in the medication error reporting program. This position requires collaboration with health care providers with medication-related responsibilities (e.g., physicians, nurses, pharmacists, quality management, safety and risk management) to measure and improve the safety of the organization's medication system. The person in this position also plays a major role in educating and/or advising pharmacy students and pharmacy residents/fellows as well as other health care students and residents.

Organizational Relationship

The Associate Director for Safety and Quality reports to the Director of Pharmacy Services. Recommendations made as the Medication Safety Officer are also reported to key medical center administrators, the Pharmacy and Therapeutics Committee and the Safety Committee.

Duties Specific to Quality Improvement

Maintains an active and progressive quality improvement program consistent with the goals of the department and the medical center. Responsibilities include:

- Oversee the development/assessment of a pharmacy quality program that monitors and ensures the integrity and safety of the services provided by the department.
- Assimilate the mission statement, goals, and objectives of the department into the departmental quality program.
- Assess departmental compliance with quality indicators through review of audits performed on these indicators.
- Alert management to significant problems identified during audits.
- Forward reports to appropriate individuals.
- Recommend improvement strategies to management regarding issues identified in audits and provide assistance for action plan implementation.
- Review, revise, add, and delete audits or indicators based on the needs of the department.

Duties Specific to Medication Safety Officer

The Medication Safety Officer ensures the safety of the organization's medication system and supports an environment dedicated to the safety of our patients, staff, and guests. Responsibilities include:

- Provide direction for the safety of the organization's medication system as chair of the Medication System Review Committee (MSRC).
- Coordinate medication system monitoring program for the ordering, distribution, administration, and monitoring of medications used in the hospital. Includes indicator development, auditing, evaluation, and feedback; process improvement recommendations; and staff education initiatives.
- Direct involvement in ensuring the ongoing safety of the medical center's computerized physician order entry system for electronic ordering of patient medications.
- Review medication error/adverse drug event literature, including the Institute for Safe Medication Practices' *Medication Safety Alert!* newsletter, to proactively address potential issues in the medical center.
- Review Medication Occurrence Reports and Adverse Drug Reaction Reports to identify potential system improvements and educational needs.
- Identify potential issues that may warrant root cause analysis (RCA) or failure mode and effects analysis (FMEA) and bring to the attention of the Safety and Risk Management office for authorization.
- Perform a RCA at the direction of the Safety and Risk Management office or the Medical Staff Review Board or a FMEA as recommended by MSRC.
- Oversee the development of new or revision of existing medication-related policy and procedures.
- Provide medication safety information for inclusion in newsletters and other educational efforts for staff education.
- Evaluate and procure commercially available medication- and patient safety-related educational materials including video and audio tapes, computer-assisted instructional programs, printed materials, etc.
- Provide medication safety inservices to medical center staff.
- Develop a structured approach for the post graduate on-the-job training of pharmacist practitioners, pharmacotherapists, pharmacy residents, technicians, and managers related to medication safety, incorporating the mission statement, goals, and objectives of the department where appropriate.

Duties Specific to Regulatory Compliance

- Serve as the content expert for The Joint Commission (TJC)/CMS medication management standards and regulations for the medical center.
- Provide medical center staff relevant education on the medication management standards.
- Report deficiencies in departmental compliance to Director of Pharmacy.
- Report deficiencies in medical center compliance to TJC/CMS Compliance Committee.
- Recommend improvements to achieve compliance.

- Ensure departmental and hospital compliance with all TJC and CMS requirements.

Duties Specific to Staff Development

- Oversee departmental training programs for new pharmacotherapists, pharmacists, and technicians.
- Ensure maintenance of training files for all employees, documenting participation and adherence to Illinois laws, accreditation organizations, and departmental policy.

Educational Expectations

- Participate in the education of nursing staff, medical staff, and all members of the health care team.
- Participate in hospital and departmental staff development by designing, evaluating, and providing inservices, continuing education programs, and by serving as a preceptor and role model.
- Participate in the education of Pharm.D. students, PGY1 and PGY2 residents, fellows, and other pharmacy staff by serving as a preceptor and role model as defined by the guidelines and requirements of the Department of Pharmacy Practice.

Research and Scholarship Expectations

- Facilitate the advancement of knowledge in health care by participating in research and scholarly activities.
- Attend and actively participate in departmental, college, and team meetings.
- Represent the department on university and medical center committees as assigned.
- Participate in public service events as available (e.g., brown bags, community education, etc.).

Education and Training

Graduate of approved 5- or 6-year pharmacy program. Licensed as a pharmacist by the State of Illinois or eligible for licensure. Post-graduate education (Pharm.D. or M.S.) required. At least 2 years experience as a clinical staff pharmacist, clinical pharmacist, or staff development pharmacist required. Must have a philosophy of practice in accordance with the department. This individual must be able and willing to participate in the educational missions of the college of pharmacy, pharmacy department, and the medical center.

Source: Courtesy of the University of Illinois at Chicago Medical Center, Department of Hospital Pharmacy Services.

Appendix 1-C. Alignment of MSO Responsibilities with Organizational Strategic Plan

Percent Time	Activity Detail	Departments Supported	Support of Strategic Plan
Responsibility #1. Identify best practices for medication safety across the organization. Facilitate medication process quality improvement and assurance related to medication safety indicators.			
10%	System support: EMR design/validation ■ Participated in 90% of validation sessions that touched the medication-use process ■ Participated in all FMEAs for the new medication processes ■ Facilitated two critical issues sessions during go-live ■ Provide evidence-based support, best safety practice guidance, and organizational lessons learned to design/build (go-live and ongoing) ■ Data analysis during go-live and post-go-live	■ Pharmacy ■ Nursing ■ OR ■ L&D ■ System-wide IT ■ Medical staff ■ 6 Sigma	■ *Goal:* care safety, community of caregivers, service culture ■ *Critical success factors:* public accountability ■ *Strategic areas of improvement:* reduce complications; improve on TJC, NPSG, and QI
30%	6 Sigma projects: Anticoagulation, Pump Programming, Palliative Care ■ Participated in process mapping (Anticoagulation) ■ Literature evaluation for best practice (Anticoagulation, Pump Programming, Palliative Care) ■ Participated in solution development (Anticoagulation) ■ Physician outreach (Anticoagulation) ■ Managed the measurement plan (Anticoagulation, Pump Programming) ■ Performed data analysis (Anticoagulation, Pump Programming) ■ Designed and performed the financial analysis (Anticoagulation) ■ Co-authored business plan (Anticoagulation) ■ Educated and communicated the plan through medical staff, pharmacy, and hospital committees (Anticoagulation, Pump Programming) ■ Served as temporary co-process owner (Anticoagulation)	■ Pharmacy ■ Nursing ■ OR ■ System-wide IT ■ Medical staff ■ 6 Sigma	■ *Goal:* care safety, service culture ■ *Critical success factors:* public accountability, financial stewardship ■ *Strategic areas of improvement:* reduce complications; improve on TJC, NPSG, and QI

continued

30%	Adverse Drug Event (ADE) subcommittee ■ Develop content for agenda ■ Organize ad hoc work groups to address issues identified through voluntary reporting, TJC standards, and Institute of Safe Medication Practices recommendations. ■ Literature evaluation for best practice ■ Continual maintenance of IV Drug Administration policy content and web application ■ Participate in medication management policy content development for the medical center ■ Coordinate communication between disciplines about policy/process changes.	■ Medical staff ■ Nursing ■ Pharmacy	■ *Goal:* quality care, care safety, community of care givers ■ *Critical success factors:* public accountability, physician/provider alignment ■ *Strategic areas of improvement:* reduce complications, improve on TJC, NPSG, and QI
Analyze current practices that contribute to medication errors and take pro-active steps for prevention.			
5%	Lead root cause analysis (RCA) surrounding medication events ■ Participate in fact gathering/staff interviews ■ Literature evaluation to identify best practices, if any ■ Facilitate meetings ■ Collate idea generation from RCA ■ Develop implementation plan ■ Coordinate measurements	■ Hospital administration ■ Inpatient nursing units ■ Procedural areas ■ Pharmacy	■ *Goal:* care safety ■ *Critical success factors:* public accountability ■ *Strategic areas of improvement:* reduce complications
5%	Lead/and or facilitate FMEAs and process resign for high-risk medication processes ■ Idea generation ■ Facilitate meetings ■ Coordinate development of mitigation strategies ■ Participate on behalf of patient safety in other projects' FMEAs	■ Medical staff ■ Pharmacy ■ Nursing ■ New patient care building committee ■ Outpatient medical group ■ System-wide IT	■ *Goal:* care safety ■ *Critical success factors:* public accountability ■ *Strategic areas of improvement:* reduce complications; improve on TJC, NPSG, and QI

continued

5%	Identify trends and opportunities for improvement from medication data entered into the event reporting system ▪ Generate reports ▪ Perform data analysis	▪ Nursing ▪ Pharmacy ▪ Medical staff	▪ *Goal:* care safety ▪ *Critical success factors:* public accountability ▪ *Strategic areas of improvement:* reduce complications; improve on TJC, NPSG, and QI
Advance and support the patient safety plan and the culture of safety throughout the medical center.			
5%	Provide summaries of medication error reporting, outcomes of ADE reduction projects, and communicate ongoing initiatives to promote medication safety in the microsystem ▪ Quarterly bring data to Professional Nursing Congress Pharmacy and Therapeutics, Professional Staff Quality Improvement, Quality Safety Board ▪ Attend the clinical educator's meeting monthly ▪ Medical Executive committee once per year ▪ Round with unit councils ▪ "Lifesaver" recognition letters to staff who make "great catches"	▪ Medical staff ▪ Nursing ▪ Pharmacy ▪ Hospital administration	▪ *Goal:* care safety, community of care givers ▪ *Critical success factors:* public accountability, physician/provider alignment, community of care givers ▪ *Strategic areas of improvement:* reduce complications; improve on TJC, NPSG, and QI
10%	Participate in safety rounds, tracers to identify medication safety opportunities. ▪ Interact with both management and front-line staff ▪ Listen to safety concerns raised ▪ Inquire about key medication safety issues ▪ Validate processes recently implemented ▪ Identify gaps in achieving TJC medication management standards/ safety goals	▪ Medical center ▪ Skilled nursing facility	▪ *Goal:* care safety ▪ *Critical success factors:* public accountability, community of care givers ▪ *Strategic areas of improvement:* reduce complications; improve on TJC, NPSG, and QI

EMR, electronic medical record; FMEA, failure mode and effects analysis; IT, information technology; IV, intravenous; L&D, labor and delivery; OR, operating room; NPSG, National Patient Safety Goals; QI, quality improvement; SBAR, situation background, assessment, recommendation; TJC, The Joint Commission.

Source: Courtesy of OSF Saint Francis Medical Center, Quality/Safety Department, Peoria, IL.

Getting Involved in the Organization

Lynn E. Eschenbacher

CHAPTER 2

Key Terms

Balanced Scorecard—A tool to display and link the organization's mission and vision to the strategic goals and objectives.

Dashboard—An "at-a-glance" visual display of selected metrics or key performance indicators often used to track the individual initiatives, goals, and objectives at a more local level.

Mistake/Error-Proofing—Implementation of fail-safe mechanisms to prevent errors from occurring with a process; for example, an ATM that gives the debit card back before the cash so that the card is not forgotten.

Team Charter—A written document defining a team's mission, scope, structure, and objectives; serves to communicate the team's focus and direction for team members, organizational leaders, and other work groups.

Introduction

Patient safety is the responsibility of everyone in health care. The role of the medication safety officer (MSO) is to guide and coordinate the organization's medication safety activities. To be successful, it is critical for the MSO to be involved in the organization to ensure the safe use of medications. The MSO must analyze the medication safety data to identify trends and recommend the priorities for the organization. The MSO must also be proactive to ensure that the entire medication-use process has been examined and strategies for safety are developed to prevent harm. The MSO should use tools such as safety self-assessments, literature, and events from other organizations to reflect on his or her own processes to prevent errors. Engaging key stakeholders will increase the acceptance of the priorities and result in successful implementation of improvement efforts. The core responsibilities of the

MSO in an organization include participating as a knowledge expert and a consultant on committees focused on safety, quality, technology, policies and procedures (PPs), clinical care guidelines, Joint Commission National Patient Safety Goals, and new product selection. Gaining visibility in the organization by presenting educational sessions helps to support the MSO's efforts to encourage every health care provider to participate in the improvement of safety related to medications. The MSO is a unique role that combines medication-use process and clinical expertise, process improvement methodologies, project management, leadership abilities, and interpersonal relationship skills to achieve improved outcomes for patients.

Getting Started

When starting at a new organization or new to the medication safety role, there are several key activities that should be included in the initial planning for getting involved:

- **Flowcharting the entire medication-use process.** One of the first steps should be to flowchart the entire medication-use process. "Walking" the process and developing a flowchart will allow the MSO to have a strong foundation and understanding of the medication-use process at that organization. This knowledge is essential because one of the MSO's role is to guide process improvements. If there is not a strong understanding of the process, then it is extremely difficult to participate in activities to review the system failures to ensure reduction of harm to patients.
- **Meeting with key personnel.** Arrange meetings with key individuals from different departments involved in the medication-use process including, but not limited to, risk managers, performance/quality improvement director, nurse mangers and educators, respiratory therapy director, catheterization laboratory director, lead anesthesiologist, or certified registered nurse anesthetist, and medical director. A simple face-to-face introduction starts a relationship, so that when an event occurs or proactive work is to be conducted it is not a cold call. Trust is an important component of the safety process; therefore, starting with introductions early on can help build credibility and network contacts. The MSO should also identify the different committees or teams that review and address the organization's safety. Attending meeting(s) as a guest enables the MSO to determine which committees will be valuable to join.
- **Developing a strategic plan.** An additional key activity is to develop a strategic plan and goals so the MSO performs the best job possible on projects and process planning. When getting started in the organization, it can be difficult at times to keep focused on medication safety and developing and implementing actions to prevent patient harm. Because safety is a vital part of every aspect of patient care and the medication-use process, it is very easy to be assigned more projects than it is possible to complete.

There will always be acute events that occur and the strategic plan should account for these; however, to keep focused on the goal of patient safety, it is critical that the MSO maintains a strong strategic direction.

Communication with the Organization

To improve patient safety, the MSO needs to determine the organization's priorities. Voluntarily reported medication safety events, adverse drug event/reaction surveillance (e.g., triggers), executive safety WalkRounds™,[1] automated dispensing cabinets, smart infusion pumps, electronic prescribing, pharmacy systems, and medical record coding are examples of key systems and programs that contain important medication data that can be analyzed. Each data set provides a different view of the organization's safety status, but most organizations have limited resources, and it may be necessary to select only a few of the data sources for evaluation. The following are possible approaches:

- Use the data listed above to identify several medication safety issues, then rank the frequency and severity of the issues to prioritize which to focus on first.
- Engage key stakeholders or committees for a multidisciplinary decision on which data to include for priority setting and ongoing analysis.
- Use the literature on what has been shown to cause more harm to patients.
- Use self-assessments such as the Institute for Safe Medication Practices (ISMP) Medication Safety Self-Assessment for Hospitals or the Self-Assessment for Antithrombotic Therapy.[2]

These self-assessments can help identify deficiencies as compared to best practices.

Consider focusing on high-alert medications, high-risk populations, and high-risk pharmacy processes. High-alert medications include chemotherapy, anticoagulation, insulin, and opiates. These medications may have the same frequency of events as other medications, but if an event were to occur the chance of significant patient harm is much greater. A more complete list of high-alert medications is located on the ISMP website.[3] High-risk populations include pediatrics and the elderly; high-risk areas include the neonatal intensive care unit, emergency department, and the peri-operative setting. Consider performing focused observations in these areas and attending existing quality improvement committees or developing a process to provide ongoing feedback to these areas. In addition, the sterile processing/compounding area (i.e., intravenous [IV] room or cleanroom) is a high-risk pharmacy process area. Nurses, prescribers, and patients all trust that the fluid in the IV bag is really what the label states it is after completion of the technician and pharmacist preparation processes. A visual confirmation is not possible. Safety technology focused on the sterile compounding area is relatively new and may not be used in many organizations. Therefore, it is important to review the processes in the IV preparation room and determine areas of vulnerability and opportunities for improvement. Once identified, the MSO is responsible for communicating these selected priorities to the organization and coordinating the work to focus on these priorities.

Determining the priorities is just the first step. Acting on the data and implementing changes is challenging but essential to improving the safety of patients. It is also important to note that priorities will differ between institutions due to the variation of patient populations and complement of staff. Each MSO must evaluate the organization to customize priorities.

The MSO is the voice of medication safety in the organization. To build acceptance of the vision and priorities, the MSO should engage various key stakeholders. Key stakeholders could include the patient safety officer, chief executive officer, chief nursing officer, chief operating officer, chief medical officer, director of pharmacy or chief pharmacy officer, and the Pharmacy and Therapeutics (P&T) Committee chair. Often the MSO does not have direct reports; therefore, networking and relationships are essential to ensure the successful implementation of needed changes. The MSO needs to coordinate with senior leadership to develop formal or informal authority to ensure that any unsafe practices are evaluated and immediately addressed if necessary. Developing a mechanism for holding others accountable through committees or senior leaders is essential to the success of medication safety efforts.

Medication Safety Team

Within each health care organization, there will be different committees, teams, and workgroups. The MSO's goal within the organization is central oversight and coordination of all the medication safety activities with local level participation to assist with identification of safety opportunities, action item generation, and implementation of the action plans. One central team dedicated to medication safety is preferred with the following roles and responsibilities:

- Receive and analyze aggregate medication safety data
- Develop action plans and facilitate change in response to data or to proactively prevent error and harm
- Recommend and communicate medication safety priorities
- Set goals and monitor progress toward their achievement
- Make recommendations for resources for areas of need
- Bring visibility to important issues[4]

A team with a safety focus may already exist in the organization, and if it is not possible to have a separate team focused completely on medication safety then the above roles and responsibilities could be incorporated into the existing team's charter.

Ideally, a separate medication safety team that reports to the P&T Committee should be implemented. The P&T Committee's responsibilities include oversight of PPs related to all aspects of medication use and formulary management.[5] For example, this committee ensures that the evaluation of medications for formulary addition identifies and addresses potential safety issues before the product enters the organization. Medication-use evaluation (MUE), monitoring and reporting adverse drug events, preventing medication errors, and developing therapeutic guidelines are also within the scope of the P&T Committee. These responsibilities make the P&T Committee a natural fit for oversight of medication safety. The medication safety team and the P&T Committee should have a strong working relationship.

The medication safety team should include representatives from nursing, medical staff, pharmacy, respiratory therapy, education services, risk management, information technology, data analysis, and the department that sets the organization's metrics and measures. Consider inviting representation from other key departments involved in the medication-use process, such as medical imaging and procedural areas. It is essential to develop a partnership between nursing, physicians, and pharmacists. If possible, identify a single nursing and physician liaison from the team to meet with regularly to create a hard-wired path for immediate review of events and multidisciplinary response.

The frequency and duration of meetings should be sufficient to meet the organization's needs. Typically, teams meet either monthly or quarterly, for 1–2 hours per meeting. A **team charter** is helpful to communicate a consistent mission, vision, and team structure. Developing objective, measurable, and achievable goals for a set time period can be an effective method for the team to facilitate safety changes. Goals can then be incorporated into the team charter on an annual basis. An example of a medication safety team charter is shown in Figure 2-1.

During routine meetings, the medication safety team could include a review of the voluntarily reported events and systemically identified events (e.g., triggers) to monitor ongoing progress and acute events that require action. Voluntarily reported events help to demonstrate the safety culture for the organization but are not appropriate to use for calculating error rates. Identifying a new area of focus or recommending a root cause analysis is also a benefit of voluntarily reported events. Systemically identified events are focused reviews that could provide a measure to identify problems or trend improvements. Valuable lessons can be learned from near misses, and they should be included in the review and action item development during the meeting. In addition, there should be time devoted to follow-up from the previous meeting to ensure that action items are completed and that the actions are resulting in reduction of harm to patients. There should be a process to monitor the implemented action items and to determine whether what was implemented was successful.

Charts and graphs depicting trends can be helpful for the team members to clearly identify areas of opportunity and to determine if improvements are being made. The **balanced scorecard** or **dashboard** approach can be useful to display the identified priorities, summarize the data, and show whether or not goals are being met (see Figure 2-2 for a sample performance improvement report). The Institute for HealthCare Improvement (IHI) has several examples of dashboards to demonstrate the power of aggregating the data in one place to show patterns and trends.[6] It is

Medication Safety Team—"SAFE-MED TEAM"

Vision Statement

Perfect the medication management system to be safe for every patient, every time.

Mission Statement

Prevent patient harm and reduce the potential for medication errors through analysis of internal and external data, literature review, and proactive initiatives to improve the medication management process.

Structure:

- Format:
  - Meetings will be monthly for 1.5 hours
  - Minutes will be recorded and distributed
- Leadership:
  - Medication Safety Officer and Performance Improvement Coordinator will co-chair
- Reporting:
  - Committee will formally report to the Pharmacy & Therapeutics (P&T) Committee, with minutes forwarded to Patient Safety Council
- Membership:
  - Committee will have interdisciplinary representation of staff and leadership involved in the medication management process from a variety of patient care areas.
  - Committee will have representatives from Nursing, Pharmacy, Medical Staff, Risk Management, Informatics, and Respiratory Therapy

Goals:

1. Monitor changes in standards or regulations related to medication use and address or recommend actions as needed.
2. Improve communication, education, awareness of safe medication management by:
   a. Developing a medication safety web page.
   b. Conducting a survey on safe injection practices and developing an action plan based on results.
   c. Offering at least four multidisciplinary educational programs this year.
3. Enhance the review and analysis of risk report data by:
   a. Designing medication-related report modules for new system.
   b. Creating and implementing a report format to evaluate data.
4. Utilize technology to enhance medication safety by:
   a. Decreasing and sustaining automated dispensing cabinet override rate to less than 5% monthly.
   b. Reviewing and revising clinical Alerts (# reviewed/revised/added)
   c. Increasing use of IV infusion pump library to 80% or greater by end of year.

Figure 2-1. Sample medication safety team charter.
Source: Courtesy of D. Saine, Winchester Medical Center.

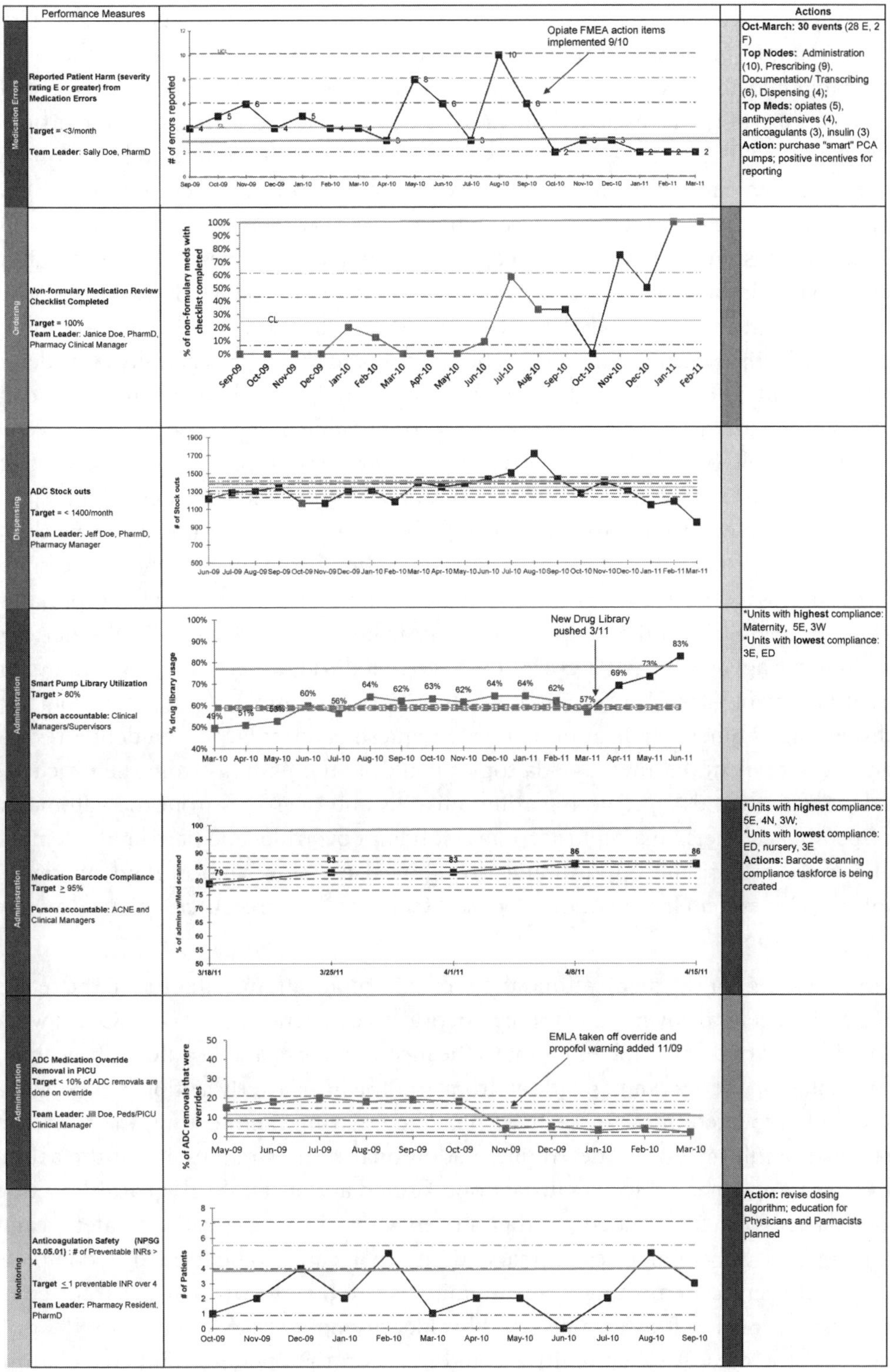

Figure 2-2. Sample improvement performance report: pharmacy.
Source: Used with permission of Karen E. Thompson, Providence Alaska Medical Center.

important during the balanced scorecard development to use the organization's strategic plan as a guide in setting priorities. This is also the opportunity for the MSO to communicate the strategic plan and goals that have been selected specifically for medication safety. As discussed previously, staying focused can be difficult at times for the MSO, but a strong balanced scorecard that is meaningful and based on the strategic plan can aid in the MSO's success. Selection of metrics and meaningful measures can be difficult because sometimes data that are easy to collect may not really demonstrate what was intended. Sometimes, metrics that would be ideal might take several individuals too long to collect, so it is not feasible. Therefore, selecting meaningful metrics is a balance between data collection and the message being conveyed. Finally, denominators can be difficult and should be carefully considered when including in a balanced scorecard. For example, if voluntarily reported data are used as a metric, an overall error rate is not possible to report because the events included would be only those reported and not every single event that has occurred in the institution. When developing a dashboard or balanced scorecard, carefully consider the time needed to collect data, what they really measure, and how these data will be displayed. Reviewing medication safety from many different perspectives ensures a robust review and an unbiased approach. Other potential topics that could be included on the medication safety team's agenda are the ISMP quarterly action item agendas,[7] ISMP newsletters,[8] FDA MedWatch alerts,[9] Joint Commission Sentinel Event Alerts,[10] new initiatives to ensure safe implementation, automated dispensing cabinets medication override requests, and policy or guideline review and development. Further agenda topics could be the findings from the executive safety WalkRounds™,[1] data regarding mis-fills and overrides from the automated dispensing cabinets, smart infusion pump soft limit overrides and hard limit attempts, electronic prescribing opportunities for clinical decision support, and pharmacy information system interventions. Consult Chapter 12 for resources related to these suggested topics.

Preparing for the medication safety team is important in order to use the team's time effectively to cover many topics. An organized agenda is essential. Often work should be started or completed prior to the meeting. For example, information about the status of the recommendations from the ISMP quarterly action item agenda should be updated prior to the meeting. Then, during the meeting, the team can review the information to determine if additional work is required or if the action has been implemented to its satisfaction. A summary of the ISMP quarterly action agenda items can be included and then shared with other organizational safety teams (Figure 2-3). Subcommittees, formal and informal, can also be formed to complete work between team meetings. Subcommittees can be effectively utilized for completing the ISMP self-assessments and for identifying focus areas based on the drill down of the data. A subcommittee could focus on the opiate- or anticoagulation-related events that have been identified by adverse drug event/reaction surveillance, voluntarily reported data, or code response. An interdisciplinary subcommittee with prescribers, nurses, and pharmacists may help to understand why these events are occurring and make recommendations to the medication safety team for actions to

ISMP Quarterly Action Agenda
January–March 2012

Accomplished:

	Topic	Medical Center Action
1	Smart pump custom concentrations without hard "low concentration" alerts	Medical Center uses smart pumps that allow setting limits only for infusion rates and not concentrations. However, drug concentrations are standardized, and for majority of medications, the library does not allow manual entry of concentrations.
2	Prevent counterfeit drugs from reaching patients	Medical Center Pharmacy does not purchase drugs and supplies from unlicensed suppliers. Policy requires pharmacy oversight for any medication procurement at the Medical Center.
3	Adverse events with dabigatran during quarter 1 of 2011	Changed dabigatran name description to include "anticoagulant" in our systems to highlight indication for those unfamiliar with this medication. Provided intensive education to pharmacists, nurses, and physicians. A prescriber letter is planned in 2012.
4	Do not use an insulin pen for multiple patients	Per Medical Center policy, we use one insulin pen for each patient and do not use insulin pens for more than one patient. If we find an insulin pen that is unlabeled in a patient's medication drawer, we remove it from the drawer and discard it. House-wide safety alert sent June 2012.

In progress:

	Topic	Medical Center Action
1	Tubing misconnections self-assessment	This is a goal for SafeMed team to complete in 2012.
2	Medications associated with adverse events that led to hospitalization: warfarin, insulin, oral antiplatelet agents, oral hypoglycemic agents. Recommend specific education to patients discharge on these medications.	Some education for all categories occurs but not consistently. Work with anticoagulation team and diabetes education program. Future planning for discharge process improvement.

Needs work:

	Topic	Medical Center Action
1	New Broselow tape available (2011)	Pediatric resuscitation carts are located on 4A and in resuscitation room in Emergency Department. Broselow tape version on 4A is 2007 Edition B. Plan: Work with dispatch to order new version, and replace on code carts. (Completed June 2012)
2	Eye drop–related infections	Medical Center policy does not allow using eye drops for more than one patient. All eye drops are labeled with patient's identification and placed in patient's medication drawer. Even though we have not heard any issues with eye-drop infections, it is always helpful to remind nursing staff to practice safe eye drop administration for the patients. http://pharmlabs.unc.edu/labs/parenterals/oph_admin.htm

Figure 2-3. ISMP quarterly action agenda summary example.
Source: Courtesy of D. Saine, Winchester Medical Center.

eliminate patient harm. The minutes and summary from the medication safety committee will be reported to the P&T Committee to further ensure the acceptance and implementation of the action items.

If the organization is part of a health system, there should be a corporate or health-system medication safety team. The health-system patient safety officer or MSO can serve as the team's leader. The goal for this team is to review trends and events across the system for opportunities to ensure undesirable occurrences are not repeated at other sites. In addition, there is an opportunity to brainstorm ideas and engage everyone for a root cause analysis or failure mode and effects analysis (FMEA). The team should include the MSOs from each organization, patient safety officers from each organization, directors of pharmacy, and other identified leaders. Coordinating across the health system provides an opportunity for sharing lessons learned to prevent errors and improve care processes.

Participation on Other Teams

The P&T Committee typically reports to the medical staff and executive staff committees, which allows additional medical staff participation in the decision-making process. The MSO should also participate on medical staff committees to collaborate with physicians and ensure understanding of medication safety initiatives. In general, these committees approve what is presented to them, but sometimes meaningful input is generated that changes the process or document to result in a stronger (or weaker) impact to patient safety. In addition, the medical staff review board is made aware of significant and sentinel event medical errors and provides oversight to the performance improvement process along with the organization's safety or patient safety committee. Often the organization will have a patient safety committee that is chaired by the patient safety officer. The MSO should be an active participant on the patient safety committee.

Quality Improvement

Another option for participation by the MSO would include the physician's departmental quality improvement (QI) committees or nursing departmental/service line QI committees. To encourage participation from the local or departmental areas, it is important to discuss medication safety at this level. If medication safety is addressed only at senior level, then it is difficult to gain the acceptance for improvements and the implementation might fail. By designating a physician or nursing representative (e.g., medication safety leader) to lead the local focus on medication safety for his or her area, increased buy-in and teamwork will result. The MSO should work with these local representatives to share findings identified at a hospital level for implementation with their departments and to share improvement ideas that can be implemented among the local departmental committees. Encouraging participation from the local level will enhance acceptance and improve safety solutions, because those who work in a particular area know best how to resolve the issues. Often, the departmental QI committees conduct a peer review of events and could benefit from the expertise of the MSO. Medication safety occurs at all levels throughout an organization, and the MSO can coordinate the sharing among the local departmental committees. The agenda should include lessons learned and action items from across the organization, trends and acute events specific to that department, new initiatives or products being implemented, and a time for feedback from the front line related to areas of concern, near misses, or errors that have occurred.

Surgical Services

Another area for involvement is in peri-operative services. An administrative committee may exist for the operating room (OR), and it is important to ensure that safety is included on this agenda or to create a separate safety team. In the peri-operative setting, new equipment will be introduced and the MSO can help to evaluate the equipment's safety prior to the trial period or implementation. Often, ORs have a different practice than the rest of the organization because the licensed independent provider is present, and the typical double check by a pharmacist may not exist. In addition, a surgical or anesthesia technician may be the one obtaining medications based on the verbal communication from a surgeon or anesthesiologist who is speaking through a surgical mask. It is difficult to understand the words, and often the technicians do not have pharmaceutical training and may not be familiar with all of the different medications that may lead to errors in the OR. Process improvements such "repeat-back" and medication education could be implemented by the peri-operative safety team. The team's agenda may vary based on the products being introduced but should always include a review of the events specific to the peri-operative setting, updates on implemented action items, feedback from frontline staff about concerns, and proactive planning to ensure safety in the OR. The MSO should participate in the design of the peri-operative system to provide the safest outcomes for patients.

Pediatrics

Many hospitals that care for pediatric patients have a separate pediatric medication safety team. The pediatric population has many unique issues that are best addressed by a specialized pediatric team. The team must be both proactive to ensure that events are prevented and reactive to develop strategies for improvement when events do occur. It is important to learn from others proactively rather than wait for harm to occur to the patients. There is often media coverage for the high profile events or ISMP newsletters to help identify the root causes; the pediatric team may use these to develop recommendations to ensure safety. Topics include how to handle patient weights (when to update weights in the electronic systems, which weight is used for dosing, how to communicate a change in weight, when infusion pumps and medication dosing are updated with a change in weight, etc.), standardized concentrations, and decision-making when there is often a lack of controlled trials with evidence for medication use in pediatric patients. The principles for addressing medication safety issues are the same, including a review of the voluntary and surveillance identified events for trends and acute events, following the Joint Commission Sentinel Event Alerts (specifically #39, which is focused on pediatric patients)[11] and listening to feedback from frontline staff. Reviewing these data with a pediatric multidisciplinary team familiar with this patient population will ensure that effective actions are implemented and patient safety is improved.

Clinical Teams

The MSO could also lead or participate in several multidisciplinary teams that focus on the drill down and evaluation of events related to high-alert medications. Review of the individual events related to opiates, anticoagulants, and insulin/hypoglycemic agents can provide insight into why the events are occurring. Often, there is limited information about these events when they are reported by a voluntary system or identified by a surveillance system (e.g., trigger). When a multidisciplinary group reviews each event and identifies key characteristics in a systematic way, data are generated that can be used to develop improvements that are targeted to resolve the issues. These action items can be implemented to improve the safety related to these high-alert medications. The team can meet monthly to review the events of the previous month and monitor the trends to determine if their efforts are making a difference. The MSO can use their skills in project management, root cause analysis, and mistake-proofing to lead the committees.

New Product/Equipment Selection

As a content expert, the MSO may attend various meetings or participate in many discussions to provide a medication safety point of view. The organization may have a standing committee for new product selection or a new committee may be created for each product due to the importance and size of the evaluation. Representation on this committee from across the organization (e.g., inpatient and outpatient) is important to ensure that all areas and roles are represented. It is important to identify equipment that uses medication as part of its operation, or that will be used to deliver medications, so medication safety issues can be identified and addressed prior to equipment selection. Elastomeric infusion devices (balloon pumps) are an example of equipment that may be requested by the OR to a product evaluation committee. The MSO would identify and facilitate compliance with regulations and standards (e.g., USP <797>, The Joint Commission) related to this new equipment before purchase and implementation. Certain devices require use of heparin dilutions to be circulated within the device for proper operation; for example, in delivery of continuous renal replacement therapy. In this situation, the MSO would help design safe practices for preparation and storage of this solution. It is not always obvious which equipment will require the MSO's attention. One method to help a new product selection committee identify products associated with medications is to revise the submission forms to include key questions such as "does this device require use of any IV or irrigation solution for operation or cleaning," and "will this device deliver any medication, IV solution, or irrigation solution to the patient?"

Working with appropriate departments and personnel, the MSO will proactively preserve patient safety.

Technology

It is essential for the MSO to be aware of and participate in selection and implementation of technology used for medication management (e.g., smart infusion pumps, syringe infusion pumps, automated dispensing cabinets, computerized provider order entry [CPOE]). If there is a standing technology committee, consider MSO membership. With experience and expertise in safety principles, human factors engineering concepts, and use of tools such as FMEA, the MSO will offer a unique perspective to the technology team(s). When new technologies are implemented or other new processes are developed, the MSO can recommend metrics to monitor for the introduction of new error types and for reduction of patient harm.

Building/Remodel

When organizations build or remodel facilities, the MSO can provide expert opinion on the design to reduce harm and errors related to medication management. The MSO may draw on his or her knowledge of best practices and standards (e.g., American Society of Health-System Pharmacists, United States Pharmacopeia, The Joint Commission, and Centers for Medicare & Medicaid Services) as well as use of FMEA to help assess design and anticipated workflow for safety. For example, during design of a new patient care unit, the MSO could help with planning of the medication room or medication preparation area by ensuring there is a designated, clean, uncluttered area consistent with Joint Commission standards, if immediate IV product preparation is expected. Placement of sinks, medication storage areas, reference space, task lighting, etc., in relationship to IV product preparation would be part of the MSO review and recommendations.

Patient Safety

The organization should have a patient safety committee chaired by the patient safety officer (PSO). Although PSOs are often physicians or nurses, pharmacists or other disciplines may also fill this role. The patient safety committee should be aware of every aspect of patient safety in the organization. Topics include general awareness of patient safety, patient safety program strategies, transparency and disclosure, just culture, and medication safety. The MSO should be an active participant on this committee to bring forward issues and raise awareness with medication safety. The MSO can also provide expertise in analyzing other events, generating action items, and helping to ensure implementation of these solutions. A summary of teams or committees for MSO participation can be seen in Table 2-1.

Policies, Procedures, and Clinical Care Guidelines

There are many opportunities for the MSO to become involved in the organization by providing expert opinion as the authority on medication safety practices that

Table 2-1. Teams for MSO Participation

Committee/Team	MSO Role
Medication Safety Team, Hospital Level	Review of events across the hospital, development of action items, education, coordination with the local levels.
Medication Safety Team, Health System	Sharing events across the health system.
Medical Staff Executive	Review of sentinel events and provide feedback.
Departmental QI/PI Council, Physician and Nursing	Review of events at a local level, generation of action items, sharing of action items from the medication safety committee for local implementation.
Perioperative	Review of events in the perioperative setting and proactive review of new processes/products/technology in the perioperative setting.
Pediatrics	Review of events in the pediatric setting and proactive review of new processes/products/technology in the pediatric setting.
High-Alert Medications Clinical Teams	Development of new processes or detailed review of events to develop action items specific to opiates, anticoagulants, insulin/glycemic control or other identified topics.
New Products	Proactive review (e.g., FMEA) of new products before a trial or implementation, also consider central supply.
Technology/Information Systems Steering	Proactive review (e.g., FMEA) of new technology before a trial or implementation. Review of existing technology for opportunities for improvement. Examples include CPOE, eMAR, smart infusion pump team, bedside barcode scanning, EHR.
Patient Safety	Integrate medication safety with review of all patient safety activities for overall coordination of the care of patients (e.g., transparency, disclosure, just culture).
Forms Committee	Ensure safety features, prompts, clarity related to medication use.
Order Set Review (Paper and CPOE)	Review all order sets prior to release for safety, clarity, adherence to policy/procedure/protocols/accreditation standards, improvements from RCAs and other performance improvement projects to ensure safety is considered.
P&T	Liaison between the medication safety team and P&T or if no medication safety committee then bring all medication safety information to P&T for review.
Pharmacy Leadership	Coordination with the pharmacy department leadership to ensure that priority areas are being addressed, the urgency is understood, and action items are being developed and implemented.
Nursing Education Council	Education alone is not the strongest method to ensure error prevention, but necessary for successful implementation. Working with nursing to determine the best medium for the various initiatives is important.
Sentinel Event	Medication-use process expert; contributes to identifying the root causes and developing the action items to implement.
Accreditation Steering	Medication management expert; acts as liaison between steering committee and other departments for medication management standards and NPSGs.

CPOE, computerized provider order entry; FMEA, failure mode and effects analysis; EHR, electronic health record; eMAR, electronic medication administration record; NPSGs, National Patient Safety Goals; P&T, Pharmacy and Therapeutics Committee; RCA, root cause analysis, QI, quality improvement; PI, performance improvement.

impact PPs and clinical care guidelines (CCGs). PPs and CCGs often are the result of new findings in the literature but may also be developed as part of an action plan for a medication event if the review identified a gap in a practice or process. The MSO can participate in the development or the review of these documents to ensure that opportunities for patient harm are identified and minimized or eliminated. Successful PP or CCG implementation in an organization requires addressing and resolving any possible safety issues and effectively communicating the new or revised information to the affected staff.

Incorporation of the PP and CCG into order sets or care plans helps to ensure that the processes are followed for all patients in the organization. If the organization uses CPOE to order medications and other care for the patients, then it is important that the MSO participate in the committee that reviews all of the builds into the CPOE system. If the organization does not use CPOE, the MSO should participate in the committee that reviews all paper order sets before they are released for patient use. If an organization does not have a structured review process for order sets and protocols, the MSO should facilitate implementing one to positively impact the patient care.

MSO visibility in the organization will encourage everyone to participate in medication safety. The MSO should be regularly available and easily accessible for questions, comments, or feedback so health care providers will seek out the MSO, resulting in a more robust culture of safety. The MSO should be open and welcoming to encourage a nonpunitive message. If anyone brings forward a safety concern, the MSO should investigate and follow up with the individual to demonstrate the value of participation in the medication safety process. With no or limited direct reports, the MSO must rely on the entire organization's participation, and being accessible and visible will help to elevate the importance of medication safety.

Organizational Education Programs

The MSO will use education to support all efforts and programs. New employee orientation is an excellent place to start, and the MSO should be involved in new employee orientation for those involved in the medication-use process. At a minimum, the MSO should ensure that basic medication safety terminology, process for reporting events, and current safety initiatives are included in the orientation process. Best practices, National Patient Safety Goals, accreditation standards, and safety culture are other key topics. The MSO may be the presenter or may assist in developing the orientation medication safety session(s) for others to lead. Medication safety should be included in the orientation for all new employee pharmacists, pharmacy technicians, nurses, medical staff and residents, and respiratory therapists.

Other educational opportunities include nursing skills days, physician in-services, medical student education, and pharmacy/other department meetings. The MSO may also present at grand rounds or routine educational offerings for medical staff, nurses, pharmacists, or others. Additional educational topics include medication safety fundamentals and feedback on adverse drug events including the root causes, common causes, and actions taken as a result of the event. The medication safety team should include education as part of their agenda. The team should address any immediate educational needs (e.g., sentinel event and root cause analysis lessons learned, new product implementation) and plan long-term foundational education (e.g., what is medication safety, how to participate in medication safety). Staff and faculty will be more likely to participate in medication safety activities if they know that their efforts will result in an action. Therefore, it is important to communicate actions taken as a result of events and voluntary reports. The medication safety team minutes can be emailed or placed in organizational communications as a method for providing this feedback in a consistent format, according to the organization's confidentiality and risk management policies. Lessons learned need to be shared or the error may happen again. Education is part of the MSO's responsibility to become involved in the organization.

Participation in education for learners such as physicians, nurses, pharmacists, physician assistants, physical therapists, etc., will elevate the importance of medication safety from the beginning of their careers. MSOs are encouraged to work with colleges and universities to develop medication safety educational opportunities within existing courses or by creating new ones. If the opportunity arises, teaching all of these students together about medication safety can cultivate a collaborative multidisciplinary approach. Often, between semesters, there is time to conduct a week intersession focused on safety. The week could include an overview of patient safety with specific medication safety topics such as an root cause analysis conducted by the team, safe prescription writing, dangers with sound alike/look alike medications, and mistake-proofing of medication dispensing and administration. MSOs should consider developing or participating in pharmacy student rotations devoted to medication safety. If the organization has a pharmacy residency program, the MSO should strongly encourage mandatory completion of a medication safety rotation and/or integrate medication safety concepts and activities into existing rotations. Encouraging an understanding of safety principles early on will benefit patients and health care teams in the future.

Summary

Organizational involvement is essential for the success of the MSO and for patient safety. Safety is the responsibility of everyone in health care. Engaging the organization in medication safety matters will result in a safer environment for all patients. The MSO needs to set priorities and involve key stakeholders and committees while participating as a content expert for organizational initiatives. Being visible and accessible will help to engage all health care providers, and educational efforts will enhance their skills to be more informed and better participants in improving care for patients. Improving the safety of the medication-use process by getting involved in the organization will result in safer care for patients.

PRACTICE TIPS

1. Develop an MSO "elevator speech" about who you are, what your role is, and how you relate to the group you are addressing. Developing this up front will make you appear more confident and credible.
2. Don't get overwhelmed with data collection and/or analysis. The most important aspect of medication safety is to apply what has been learned to implement changes in the organization to decrease the potential for harm to patients.
3. Develop a strategic plan based on your initial assessment and stay focused on your goals and objectives. Manage your time wisely to address both acute events and proactive initiatives.
4. Become well known in the organization as the medication safety leader. Meet as many individuals as you can, and experience as many processes as possible so that you position yourself as the expert.
5. There is always more to the story with medication safety and events that have occurred. Make sure you gather all the pieces before making decisions on practice changes. Although details may seem obvious, further investigation may reveal many contributing factors that should be addressed.

References

1. Frankel A, Baker EG, Neppl C, et al. Patient safety leadership WalkRounds™. *Jt Comm J Qual Saf.* 2003;29(1):16-26.
2. Institute for Safe Medication Practices. ISMP self-assessments. Available at: http://ismp.org/selfassessments/default.asp Accessed October 8, 2012.
3. Institute for Safe Medication Practices. ISMP's list of high alert medications. Available at: http://ismp.org/Tools/highalertmedications.pdf. Accessed October 8, 2012.
4. Kohn LT, Corrigan JM, Donaldson MS (Institute of Medicine). *To Err Is Human: Building a Safer Health SDystem*. Washington, DC: National Academy Press; 2000.
5. American Society of Health-System Pharmacists. ASHP guidelines on the pharmacy and therapeutics committee and the formulary system. *Am J Health-Syst Pharm.* 2008;65:1272-1283.
6. Martin LA, Nelson EC, Lloyd RC, et al. *Whole System Measures*. IHI Innovation Series white paper. Cambridge, Massachusetts: Institute for Healthcare Improvement; 2007.
7. Institute for Safe Medication Practices. Quarterly action agenda. Available at: http://ismp.org/newsletters/acutecare/actionagendas.asp Accessed February 10, 2013.
8. Institute for Safe Medication Practices. ISMP Medication Safety Alert Newsletters. Available at: http://ismp.org/newsletters/default.asp Accessed February 10, 2013.
9. U.S. Food and Drug Administration. MedWatch safety alerts for human medical products. Available at: http://www.fda.gov/safety/medwatch/safetyinformation/safetyalertsforhuman medicalproducts/default.htm. Accessed February 10, 2013.

10. The Joint Commission. Sentinel event. Available at: http://www.jointcommission.org/sentinel_event.aspx. Accessed February 10, 2013.

11. The Joint Commission. Sentinel event alert. Available at: http://www.jointcommission.org/assets/1/18/SEA_39.PDF Accessed October 8, 2012.

Making Change Happen

L. Hayley Burgess and Karla M. Miller

CHAPTER
3

Key Terms

Change—To transform or guide into a different direction.

Global Trigger Tool—A tool developed by the Institute for Healthcare Improvement that assists with identification of adverse events. This tool's methodology allows for the identification of various "triggers" when reviewing charts in order to determine the presence of adverse events. Examples of triggers include an abnormal lab result, a stop order, or administration of an antidote.

Risk Mitigation Strategies—Tactics utilized to avoid system failures and prevent errors. Risk mitigation strategies may be implemented in response to a recent event or utilized as a proactive strategy. Multiple risk mitigation strategies are often needed to fully address potential failure points. Examples include forcing functions, automation, double checks, and provider education.

Safe Culture—Shared values and beliefs of an organization that result in a common goal among frontline staff and leadership to consistently improve and maintain a safe environment for both its workforce and patients. In a safe culture, the organization is committed to continuous improvement and encourages reporting of potential or actual hazards in this effort.

Walk Round—A tool that assists with discussion between leadership and frontline staff in order to raise awareness of needed system changes, promote accountability for creating a safe environment, and support decisions for future system improvements and resource allocation.

Introduction

One of the greatest challenges a medication safety officer (MSO) faces in an organization is having great responsibility to make **change** happen while having little or no authority. As a system leader, the MSO must understand both the implications of proposed safety changes for the system and the cause-and-effect relationships that such changes may trigger. Accomplished improvement models for medication safety focus on a strong organizational foundation to build the will to achieve results, a process to generate ideas for improvement, and execution strategies that scale across departments and ultimately the institution. Setting the organization's direction can be described as a push-pull strategy to render the status quo uncomfortable and make the future attractive.[1] This concept creates a shared responsibility between hospital administration and all hospital staff for the ultimate goal of reduction in patient harm and improved patient outcomes.

Successful leaders use change models as a framework to improve their organizational performance, culture, and internal leadership strategy.[2-4] Studies of organizations from all industry sectors reveal that failure in reliability and systems performance stems more from inconsistent execution of change rather than from inadequate strategy and planning.[5] Results are achieved when strategies meet the execution of organizational goals. This requires a cadence of accountability and a continuous rhythm of health care workforce engagement—throughout the system.[6]

Transformational change begins with relationships and trust. Building relationships is a critical component of influencing your organization's behaviors. Leaders drive values, values drive behaviors, and the collective behaviors of the individuals in an organization define its culture.[7] MSOs must be involved in creating and sustaining a culture of safety that leads to transformational change.

To make change happen, it is imperative to first identify what "should" change. Einstein stated that if he had an hour to solve a problem, he would spend 55 minutes thinking about the problem and 5 minutes thinking about the solution. All too often, as leaders, especially health care leaders, our first inclination is to fix or "band-aid" an identified problem without thoroughly exploring the root cause.

Gaining momentum for change requires motivating the workforce and creating a revolution from within by activating the heart and mind of health care clinicians and senior leaders. Storytelling is an effective way to leverage the power of the people, human experiences, and our health care network to take on our big challenges.[8] Our organizations' senior leaders can be galvanized by metrics and measures that create a compelling story for change whether focused on heart (harm) or mind (financial) or a combination. Measures can create a constructive tension to rectify unjustified variation.

Once change does occur, creating forcing functions in the system that make it easy to do the right thing and hard to do the wrong thing will lead to sustainability. Designing workflows for daily tasks can establish a consistent behavioral change. We cannot continue to work harder; we must work smarter.

Building Relationships and Creating a Safe Culture

Change does not occur without the support of the people within your organization. Focusing only on the changes themselves and not on the effect to your frontline staff, middle managers, and prescribers will result in a less than favorable response. Gaining the rapport of your hospital teams by continual communication is vital to introducing and sustaining change. In the first several months of your tenure as an MSO, your time should be spent building relationships, inquiring about processes and needs of your teams, and understanding your organization. Offering your clinical expertise in a nonintrusive manner when requested will allow your teams to see you as the subject matter expert for medication safety and system innovations. The MSO should be a leader that clinicians will easily approach to discuss patient care issues.

Identifying What Should Change

While building relationships, the MSO can begin to identify practices that may cause harm to patients. As an MSO, you will be challenged to proactively identify gaps within the medication management system and strategically plan how to close the gaps without prematurely implementing system-wide changes. The saying, "with great power comes great responsibility" is true for many leaders. However, the MSO often has great responsibility with very little enforcement power, creating a unique challenge. The MSO will require an arsenal of tools and methods to identify gaps in the care process, as well as a provision of data to signify strategic gap closure (see Chapter 9, "Medication Error Reporting and Analysis," for additional information).

Gauging the effectiveness of the medication management system will require the review of multiple data sources. Voluntarily reported data, such as near misses or medication errors, should be reviewed with your medication safety committee to guide root cause analysis utilization.[9] Using a multi-method approach is important to detect adverse event occurrence data.[10,11] The use of triggers are helpful in detecting unreported adverse drug events. For example, using naloxone orders as a trigger can help identify a patient chart to review to see if the patient experienced an adverse drug event such as an opioid overdose. The MSO can utilize and tailor the Institute for Healthcare Improvement (IHI) trigger tool to focus solely on medications. The Florida Hospital System utilized the trigger tool and found that 55% of their harm events were related to medications. These results allowed for a targeted effort for organizational improvement to the identified medication management system failures.[12]

Culture surveys and medication management system self-assessments are proactive data collection tools. The Institute for Safe Medication Practices (ISMP) has created the ISMP Medication Safety Self-Assessment™ for Hospitals. This survey provides a comprehensive view of the operational performance of your medication management system and is completed with a multidisciplinary team.[13,14] Multi-hospital systems can cumulate their data and create a large scale medication safety plan to affect process and culture change broadly.

The Safety Attitudes Questionnaire (SAQ) is used to assess safety culture according to frontline staff perception.[15] The SAQ has been used to assess the impact of leadership **walk rounds** on safety climate in two separate institutions. Repeated survey results showed a direct impact on safety climate scores, with improvements in both institutions. According to the study, the implementation of leadership walk rounds not only improved frontline safety culture, but also uncovered safety issues that may not otherwise have been recognized.[16] The MSO can use a pharmacy-centric SAQ to aggregate data on pharmacy microsystem culture conditions.[17]

In general, walk rounds can generate medication management system safety data. One study examining patient safety leadership walk rounds indicated tangible, positive safety outcomes. Various organizational changes occurred, including the expansion of automated dispensing cabinets and the development and review of medication management policies. The process also contributed to a positive impact on senior leadership as one chief executive officer stated, "The walk rounds remind me to pay attention to the day-to-day issues that confront staff, and this awareness is in my head when making bigger decisions."[18] The MSO should engage in regular dialogue during walk rounds with frontline staff, physicians, and patients regarding ways to improve safe medication use.[19] As staff members provide feedback on medication safety issues, the MSO should work diligently to incorporate these ideas and suggestions into actionable plans that are seen by the frontline staff. This builds credibility of the medication safety program and trust for the MSO role as a leader that listens and acts to improve care. Appendix 3-A is an example of a medication safety walk-round tool.

Proactive **risk mitigation strategies** can include learning from external sources and organizations' reported events. Medication safety literature and newsletters highlight timely medication and device adverse events and provide recommended risk mitigation strategies for these harmful events.[20,21]

The MSO can also use the organization's performance measures required by regulatory agencies as a data source to identify suboptimal medication-related performance. A health system in Oklahoma has initiated multiple pharmacy-driven performance improvement projects focused on quality core measures. The community-acquired pneumonia project showcased such a positive impact that the health system received a National Partnership for Immunization Award.[22]

Identifying gaps in the medication management system may seem like a daunting task, but when equipped with the right tools and data the MSO can thoughtfully introduce change ideas. Before initiating a new project, the MSO must understand that change does not come naturally and is a difficult process. Members of an organization will not always share the MSO's eagerness and passion for change. So how do MSOs motivate others to share our change vision?

Gaining Momentum

John Kotter's *Leading Change* outlines an eight-stage process for implementing successful change transformations (see Figure 3-1).[4] The eight stages will be briefly discussed in this section.

1. Establishing a Sense of Urgency
2. Creating the Guiding Coalition
3. Developing a Vision and Strategy
4. Communicating the Change Vision
5. Empowering Broad-Based Action
6. Generating Short-Term Wins
7. Consolidating Gains and Producing More Change
8. Anchoring New Approaches in the Culture

Figure 3-1. Kotter's eight-stage process of creating major change.
Source: Adapted with permission from John P. Kotter, "Why Transformation Efforts Fail," *Harvard Business Review* (March-April 1995): 61.

Establishing a Sense of Urgency

Transformational change requires commitment, motivation, and sacrifices from those involved. Planning for the challenges of pushing people out of their comfort zones into an attitude of change is essential. Organizations can only push staff so far to make these commitments and gain momentum. Individuals have to be personally motivated to drive a change forward. Individuals often become too comfortable in their current work environment and become resistant and unaware of the need for change. A needed change has to be seen as critical before staff will find the time and resources to make the change. An MSO aims to improve an organization by driving the need for change before a harmful or urgent state is reached.

How do we create a sense of urgency before areas in need of change reach critical levels? This requires creating an environment where status quo is not the acceptable norm. Individuals must recognize the harm and dangers of continuing to provide care for patients in their current environment. This will require creative and courageous actions, utilizing proposals that are sensible to the mind and appealing to the heart to activate people. Positioning change as the burning platform takes effort and finesse. Assuming that frontline staff will want to do what has been perceived as the right thing may be a naïve thought process. You must connect to the values of your teams and inspire them to achieve greatness. Make the business case come alive with real experiences and stories to create messages that are simple yet inspiring. Although urgency is imperative in gaining momentum, it is important to avoid creating a sense of hopelessness. The team and staff typically need to focus on their strengths and previous accomplishments to give them the confidence to fulfill the task. They also need to feel that some reward exists that accounts for their sacrifices. Once you have connected to the values and driving forces of your staff, you will be able to construct creative ways to inspire and motivate them to share the same passion and urgency that you possess toward your desired change.

One example is creating a sense of urgency in the ambulatory surgery center setting. As part of large health care organizations where much focus is driven toward acute care, the ambulatory surgery centers have not been a primary focus for medication safety initiatives. Utilizing a self-assessment medication safety tool, a team is able to show a critical need for change in the medication management system. Sharing internal medication event reports and gaining support of the executive, clinical, and physician leadership will enable you to create a local urgency around gaps that need closure to provide safe and effective medications to this population. The goal is for these centers to show their commitment to a safer medication management system and accept the challenges to be at the forefront of change as technology advances, continuity of care is strained, and safety initiatives increase in intensity across the outpatient areas. The centers use competitive tension to share electronic pictures of high-alert and look-alike/sound-alike medication identification and storage with the team for financial incentives and best practice awards within their system.

Creating the Guiding Coalition

Change is difficult and not meant to be driven by a single individual. A strong team is needed to successfully initiate and implement change. There are several considerations when determining the composition of your team. Be sure to include key stakeholders in the process not only to gain their influence, but also to avoid creating barriers that may appear through exclusion of these members. Your team should possess a wide breadth of knowledge and viewpoints to help ensure decisions are well-tested and efficient. The team should be highly respected and consist of individuals not only with strong leadership skills but also gifted with management skills. This will result in both the efficiency and the drive to complete the task. Essential members of health care teams include managers, leaders, multidisciplinary clinicians, and when appropriate, a patient or patient advocate.

The individual make-up of the team is not always determined by the leader. Being a leader of a team that you have not chosen is a common challenge in health care. Many teams are chosen based on an individual's availability to participate; others may be chosen to participate by their managers. Team leaders should respect each person's unique qualities. It is important to observe each member's style, motivation, and ways of thinking and relationship building. Although it may be ideal to develop the perfect team structure or process, that is not always possible. Identifying each member's strengths and empowering him or her to exercise those skills will create a productive team.

A barrier for large health care systems is that the team members are not always in the same location. Many times the members have to meet via teleconference or videoconference. In these situations there may be a tendency for team members to speak up less or multitask during the meeting time. Strategies to encourage active member participation and discourage multitasking during the meeting include:

- Addressing individual members during the teleconference

- Requiring pre-work for the meeting and then requesting each member to present that information to the team
- Utilizing technology that allows the members to actively participate via texting or communication buttons

Developing a Vision and Strategy

A change vision serves as an initial motivator for stakeholder buy-in. When presenting an idea for change to stakeholders, you should be armed with a clear change vision. A change vision is a powerful tool that transforms the details and complexity behind the change process into an easy to understand, desirable picture. Motivating stakeholders is not the only purpose of a change vision. It also sets the course for the duration of the change process and creates a direction and roadmap to ensure the team stays on the right track, which is very important when working with improvement leaders who may have an enthusiastic and passionate flow of new ideas. Keeping these individuals focused on the vision will avoid creating extra work and stretching resources beyond allocation. A vision is also a reminder, in the midst of the hardships and sacrifices that occur with change, of the powerful results that will be achieved from these efforts.

A clear vision simplifies hundreds of details while motivating people to take action. When creating a change vision, there are certain attributes to include. As the name implies, your vision should allow the reader to envision the future state. Consider how the vision will affect the individuals involved. What thoughts will be provoked when visualizing the picture you are painting? Visions must also be realistic to increase the likelihood of buy-in and promote credibility for the team. If the vision seems impossible to achieve, individuals will become overwhelmed at the beginning and become unable to sustain the powerful momentum needed to initiate the change. A vision must also be desirable to achieve stakeholder buy-in and motivation to initiate change. Lastly, the vision must be clear and concise. Individuals must have a clear understanding of the vision to keep their attention and provide guidance in the future. A concise description is important for effective communication of the vision. Listeners should have a clear understanding of the vision and believe that the change process, although difficult, is achievable, and they should leave the meeting feeling excited and motivated.

The leaders of Ascension Health created an example of an exceptional vision statement. Ascension Health created a call to action with the goal of achieving zero preventable injuries or deaths. Their vision, "Health care that works, health care that is safe, and health care that leaves no one behind" was concise yet powerful. In a few short words, this vision covers all strategies and planning behind the change without overburdening the listener. These words create a positive image of the future with the underlying recognition by those in health care that fulfilling these words will be a challenge.[23]

Communicating the Change Vision

A clear vision will lose impact in the absence of strategic communication. Before communicating the vision to others, you should focus on understanding and processing the true impact of the vision on yourself and others. To communicate the vision, a story must be told; not just any story—a story that will engage the stakeholders. An elevator speech is an effective way to accomplish this. An *elevator speech*, often composed of three sentences, is a very short description of the key point you want to make. Consider that the MSO will often meet potential levers of change in short interchange (elevator) situations, where championship can be achieved in moments. Therefore, your vision story should be a thoughtful compilation that grabs attention and persuades your audience that this change improves the safety and satisfaction of patients and staff while being good for business.

To enhance the quality of communication, tailor the message's components based on your audience. Often in health care we must communicate a vision to the organization's various leaders who have varying backgrounds and specialties. The content communicated to the chief medical officer may be different than the material that is communicated to the chief financial officer. Antimicrobial stewardship is a program that affects the entire organization. The results of judicious use of antimicrobials are improved clinical and financial outcomes. This is a clear situation where good quality meets good business. The business case presented to the company's clinical leaders focused on the improvement of patient outcomes and the impact on national antimicrobial resistance. The financial operators certainly expect good clinical outcomes, but also need to clearly understand the cost impact and the potential return on investment to champion programs. An understanding of what motivates your audience is imperative to communicating your vision.

Your vision should not be communicated in just one instance. Look for multiple opportunities and creative ways to remind and include others in your vision. For example, communicate your vision during meetings with multiple stakeholders, with display posters, and during walk rounds. Always remember the most powerful method of communication is your behavior and actions. Ensure that you and your team are living your vision on a day-to-day basis. Your actions will reflect credibility, sincerity, and passion about your vision which will, in turn, encourage stakeholder and staff buy-in.

Empowering Broad-Based Action

Even when equipped with an eager staff, stakeholder buy-in, and a clear vision, difficulties fulfilling a vision can still exist when staff do not have the appropriate tools and resources. Those involved in the change process should receive adequate education, toolkits, resources, and an appropriately structured work environment to initiate the change. If the burden of change is too great because of a lack of resources, individuals will quickly fall back into a less frustrating complacency.

Anticipate areas of resistance and be prepared to defend and influence people, processes, or resources. People resistant to change can be extremely detrimental to a change process. Negative attitudes can quickly destroy any progress that has been achieved. These barriers should be removed swiftly before momentum is lost. There are many reasons for resistance to change including low perceived need, poorly defined processes, doubts of success, unclear expectations, and low involvement. The best approach is to identify the clinicians or leaders who are resisting the change and engage them. Be sure to keep supporters continually engaged and actively involved to empower them to persevere and overcome the negativity of resistant peers. It is important at the forefront to try to anticipate areas of resistance and be prepared to inspire and defend the project. An action plan must be prepared to deal with both anticipated and unforeseen barriers.

A remarkable story of change occurred at the Cincinnati Children's Hospital. A multidisciplinary improvement team initiated a dramatic transformation in the hospital's rounding process by including patients' parents on teaching rounds. This change was initiated as a test period with an attending physician and group of residents. Its success quickly determined the standard of care throughout the hospital. The clinical team reported an enriched learning experience, more efficient use of time, and improved confidence in treatment plans by the patient's family. Physicians, residents, interns, students, and family members were all engaged by assignment of roles and expectations that contributed to the overwhelming success of the experience. This institution successfully performed an innovative change despite initial resistance of hospital staff.[24]

Generating Short-Term Wins

Visible success is essential to change. Individuals will struggle with the continuing sacrifices of change when they feel that there is no end in sight. Establishing intermediate goals or small tests of change will enable staff to see that their efforts are making a difference and contributing to the end goal. The measurement of these goals can result in short-term wins and reward people for making change happen, which in turn will assist individuals in maintaining or regaining much needed momentum to achieve the final goal.

Short-term wins also tend to undermine resistors as well as gain support from the stakeholders. Ultimately, these types of wins have a way of turning resistant people into supporters. Promoting small tests of change may assist in creating a winning team and increase its fan base. The concept is to focus on a small change process that supports the larger goal. As risk issues are identified, the MSO can use this model for rapid change. One example of a small change process was done when the medication safety program was implemented in the ambulatory surgery setting. The plan was to ensure segregation and differentiation of high-alert medication and look-alike/sound-alike medications in medication rooms and anesthesia trays. However, starting with one high-alert medication class, neuromuscular blockers, showed the team that the work was doable and brought attention to the need for safe medication storage. This short-term win led to a long-term commitment for all high-alert medications.

Another example of a short-term win was determining operational inefficiencies in the pharmacy department. The pharmacy team, charged with determining the areas of focus for a process improvement activity, determined that the medication storage areas and pharmacist work space were the greatest areas of concern. During the process, pharmacists and technicians were designated to lead the work. The staff's genuine pride for the organized medication storage and work station changes was apparent. The immediate results in improved efficiency reinforced the excitement for change as the team moved toward a more challenging pharmacy distribution redesign. This event became a grassroots effort for sustained improvement.

Celebrating success is an often forgotten motivator. Celebration can give the team a much needed break from the anxiety associated with the stress of change. Alternatively, short-term wins may create a sense of pressure to fully implement the change when safety issues are thoroughly understood. This sense of urgency can be used as a driving force for continued program success.

Consolidating Gains and Producing More Change

Once the change is occurring, do not let your guard down. Resistors may celebrate with you and then suggest taking a break from the project. Resistors will find it easy to convince tired individuals to take a time out from the change process. If you let up before the job is done, momentum will be lost. Once regression begins, rebuilding momentum is an overwhelming task.

Utilize the short-term wins concept to encourage individuals. Set new goals in order to continue to build momentum. Apply continuous improvement strategies and bring in new change agents and leaders to keep the project fresh and to expand the championship. Encourage staff to lead individual projects. Becoming project leaders will increase their involvement and passion for the change while allowing the leadership team time to initiate more change. Invest time in maintaining and strengthening relationships among your team members and keep the team in alignment with the vision. Continue to keep up a sense of urgency to avoid complacency among team members and staff. An effective way to sustain a sense of urgency is to be publicly transparent with outcome measures. Public awareness of outcome measures will provide a strong motivation for rapid improvement.[1] Visually displaying patient harm events and outcomes with run charts or counting the number of days since a patient was harmed can keep your team and staff connected and striving for greater improvements.

It is easy to celebrate a successful launch of a project and then move on to the next project. However, it is important that once change has been implemented there is a process in place to ensure the project does not lose momentum. For example, in one organization, the launch of electronic barcode medication administration (BCMA) was a monumental step in improving medication safety. The utilization of BCMA was not only a change in process for medication management across the system, but also a change in culture. Once implemented, it was clear that a champion and continuous improvement strategies were needed to sustain the change. To prevent regression, each facility identified a BCMA coordinator. This position was designed to be a rotating position to allow a fresh perspective for the project. The BCMA coordinator was responsible for championing BCMA, orienting new staff to BCMA, and ensuring that continuous improvement strategies were in place at the facility. The role of the corporate BCMA team was to develop continuous improvement strategies. The strategies have evolved with the project. Originally, scanning rates were reviewed across the facilities. Next, the focus moved from scanning rates to medication administration variances between time scheduled and administered. Recently the focus has been on eliminating work-arounds, using a report that identified each time the system was not used appropriately. BCMA now has a continuous improvement strategy to identify needs and maintain a successful program.

Anchoring New Approaches in the Culture

A change process is successful if the results are sustainable. *Sustainability* can be defined as the ability to withstand or maintain throughout a process. Sustaining change in health care can be difficult due to the many challenges encountered when attempting to improve a flawed system. The ability to sustain change can be impacted through every step of the transformation process. As a result, strategic forethought is required at all phases of change. During each phase, careful consideration to the overall structure of the final system and improvement direction is crucial to successfully sustaining change.

Success in the final framework of an improved medication safety system will require implementation of strategies to promote lasting change. Forcing functions, the most effective mitigation strategies, are essential to ensure change is being sustained on a daily basis by those on the frontlines. The value of forcing functions lies in the ability to eliminate choice at specific steps in the medication-use process thereby preventing execution of methods outside of the original design. A few examples of forcing functions include clinical decision support tools, technology solutions, and strategic arrangement and consolidation of medications. These components, when used effectively, can help build a system that guides people to do the right thing and prevents actions that are contradictory to the goal for improvement in safety.[21]

The application of forcing functions and effective communication for the sustainment of change can be illustrated through the safe implementation of a medication-use process for U-500 insulin. At an Indianapolis hospital, a multidisciplinary team was formed to safeguard the use of U-500 insulin in the facility. The need for a policy was based on the obvious safety issues associated with storing and administering two concentrations of insulin (e.g., U-100 and U-500). Forcing functions and other error prevention tools were developed to guide every step of the institution's medication management process including creation of an evidence-based order set (EBOS), verification procedures for home insulin dose, separation of insulin stock, alteration of order entry processes, use of dispensing checklists, implementation of time-out procedures, and standardization of administration methods. In addition to these error prevention tools, certified diabetes educators as well as clinical pharmacists helped manage patient care activities throughout each patient's hospitalization and provided initial and concurrent education to hospital staff. In the 1-year follow-up period following policy implementation, several barriers to safe U-500 insulin usage were encountered. These difficulties were addressed through continued communication, revision of the policy and EBOS, dispensing checklist modification, and further education.[25] This example of a medication safety initiative portrays why careful attention must be maintained throughout each step in the change process design.

Finally, a change in the organization's culture is imperative to sustain change. Tradition is powerful. New practices must be secured in the culture. Although you may focus on changing "behaviors" at the beginning of the process, changing the "culture" is not a quick fix. A culture is transformed over time throughout the change process. It is important to be sensitive to an organization's attachment to its traditions. The team should give recognition to the benefits and successes of the old culture, while explaining why the old culture is no longer sufficient for safe and efficient patient care. Unfortunately, such strong attachments to traditions by individuals may be present that it may require a staff turnover or repositioning for successful culture change. Sustainability of a medication safety effort is possible with appropriate change strategies, effective communication, sensitivity to staff traditions, multi-level collaboration, and commitment to the end goal.

Summary

For the MSO to play a successful role in the change process, the culture of the workplace must embrace the efforts to effectively sustain improvement. Mutual understanding of the direction of improvement requires dedicated communication and collaboration that spans all levels of an organization. In a medication safety system this could include effective documentation methods, new and current employee training, accessible forums for feedback, and prompt attention to voiced concerns. Communication and effective relationships are indispensable elements that are necessary to create a change in culture that will meet an organization's overall goal for improvement and sustainability of change.[26]

CASE EXAMPLE: MAKING CHANGE HAPPEN

Though often scrutinized for the public attention of their journalistic efforts, the true power of a story can create public outcries strong enough to initiate change. This case illustrates a situation where a compelling media release was used as a method to initiate an assessment of the medication management system. A system redesign was identified for neonatal heparin use.

Building Relationships and Creating a Safe Culture

A neonatal clinical pharmacist at a large health care facility had, for numerous years, worked to build a strong relationship and effective communication with the health care providers in her facility. Care was taken during this process to demonstrate professional competency.

Identifying the Problem

In November 2007, Thomas Boone and Zoe Grace were born to parents Dennis and Kimberly Quaid. During a re-admission for staph infections, just days after their discharge, the twins inadvertently received 1000 times the intended dose of the anticoagulant, heparin.[27] National attention was gained by the media uproar that followed; however, this was not the first publicized heparin error in young children. In 2006, six premature infants in an Indianapolis hospital received overdoses of heparin; three of the six infants subsequently died.[28] These catastrophic heparin events led the clinical pharmacist to create a targeted investigation and safety program to protect the infant population in her institution from preventable heparin error.

Gaining Momentum

A sense of urgency is often created by appealing to a person's innermost core values (i.e., "aiming for the heart"). Although news releases may at times seem untimely, they can often aid in public awareness, allowing our efforts in medication-use safety to become a burning platform. Adding performance data and regulatory requirements (i.e., "the head") to patient safety improvement stories can help us to make our business case.

Once the heparin-related problem was identified, the pharmacist and pharmacy buyer began to search product catalogs for pre-filled heparin flush syringes, in addition to initiating discussions with sterile admixing services regarding the manufacture of heparin infusion bags. Once product, cost, and stability information were identified, the pharmacist approached the chief neonatologist, neonatal nurse practitioners (NNPs), and neonatal intensive care unit (NICU) registered nurses with her proposed solution to create a coalition for involvement and championship. The coalition's purpose was to work together to mitigate the risk for harm. From this, a NICU heparin standardization vision was developed. The vision included the removal of heparin-containing vials from the NICU and the purchase of pre-filled heparin flush syringes and heparin-containing intravenous solutions. Red labels with large black print stating "HEPARIN" were attached to the heparin-containing intravenous bags, as a further safety initiative.

As is typical to most change processes, a significant barrier to the change solution was identified during the process. The pre-filled heparin flush syringes were not considered "sterile field ready" by the manufacturer. Knowledge of this information presented a further problem with neonatal intravenous line insertions, as both the neonatologists and NNPs were uncomfortable using this product. Unfortunately, no commercial, sterile-field ready, pre-filled heparin flush products were available. The coalition reconvened and, through engagement of neonatology and pharmacy staff, the barrier was removed and momentum was not lost. A decision was made for the pharmacy department to compound a sterile vial of heparin-flush product to be used only during intravenous line insertions.

With the heparin standardization vision now in motion, education of key staff became a priority. Both NICU and pharmacy staff meetings were utilized to educate and continue to build momentum in this project. Success stories, including the identification of a heparin near-miss, were shared with both departments.

Sustainability of Change

Although a forcing function was utilized in this case to physically remove all heparin vials from stock in the NICU, sustaining the change was yet another project. In this case, the pharmacist routinely participated in NICU walk rounds to monitor heparin storage and utilization and collect nursing feedback. Safety training specific to heparin concentration, storage, and administration was incorporated into the orientation of all new NICU clinicians. The organization's commitment and continued monitoring and feedback proved to be a successful combination for sustainability for heparin standardization.

PRACTICE TIPS

1. Investing time prior to initiating change is important for reflecting on your rationale for change and the implications of your change on the individuals and the health care system.
2. Storytelling is valuable to communicate your change vision and engage stakeholders.
3. Understanding your organization and building relationships and trust among its members are vital to being a successful MSO and change agent.
4. Assessing the culture of safety and the readiness to change is imperative. Evaluate leadership engagement and frontline fatigue before embarking on major initiatives that the team is not ready to pursue.
5. When a medication safety concern is raised by a staff member, engage the team in a thoughtful solution for a "quick win" as appropriate. This will build trust and improve your culture of safety.
6. Identify areas in need of change by using multiple tools including voluntary reporting data, failure mode and effects analysis, root cause analysis, trigger tools, culture surveys, self-assessments, and walk-round scripts.

References

1. Reinertsen JL, Bisognano M, Pugh MD. *Seven Leadership Leverage Points for Organization-Level Improvement in Health Care.* 2nd ed. IHI Innovation Series White Paper. Cambridge, MA: Institute for Healthcare Improvement; 2008.
2. Provost L, Miller D, Reinertsen J. *A Framework for Leadership of Improvement.* Cambridge, MA: Institute for Healthcare Improvement; 2006.
3. Craig TJ, Perlin JB, Fleming BB. Self-reported performance improvement strategies of highly successful Veterans Health Administration facilities. *Am J Med Qual.*2007;22(6):438-444.
4. Kotter J.P. *Leading Change.* Boston: Harvard Business School Press; 1996.
5. Bossidy L, Charan R. *Execution: The Discipline of Getting Things Done.* New York: Crown Business; 2002.
6. Denham CR. Values genetics: who are the real smartest guys in the room? *J Patient Saf.* (2007);3(4):214-226.
7. Rhoades A, Shepherdson N. *Built on Values: Creating an Enviable Culture That Outperforms the Competition.* Hoboken, NJ: Jossey-Bass; 2011.
8. Gantz M. Chapter 19. Leading change leadership, organization, and social movements. In: Nohria N, Khurana R, eds. *Handbook of Leadership Theory and Practice.* Boston: Harvard Business School Publishing; 2010:527-568.

9. Aspden P, Corrigan JM, Wolcott J, et al. Patient safety: achieving a new standard for care. Washington, DC: National Academies Press; 2004. Available at: http://www.nap.edu/openbook.php?record_id=10863&page=R1. Accessed October 3, 2012.

10. Classen DC, Resar R, Griffin F, et al. "Global trigger tool" shows that adverse events in hospitals may be ten times greater than previously measured. *Health Affairs.* 2011;30(4):581-588.

11. Meyer-Massetti C, Cheng CM, Gluglielmo BJ, et al. Systematic review of medication safety assessment methods. *Am J Health-Syst Pharm.* 2011;68:227-240.

12. Griffin FA, Resar RK. *IHI Global Trigger Tool for Measuring Adverse Events.* 2nd ed. IHI Innovation Series white paper. Cambridge, MA: Institute for Healthcare Improvement; 2009. Available on www.IHI.org.

13. 2011 Institute for Safe Medication Practices Medication Self-Assessment for Hospitals. Available at: http://www.ismp.org/selfassessments/Hospital/2011/full.pdf. Accessed October 3, 2012.

14. Lesar T, Mattis A, Anderson E, et al. Using the ISMP Medication Safety Self-Assessment™ to improve medication use processes. *Jt Comm J Qual Patient Saf.* 2003;29(5):211-226.

15. Sexton JB, Helmreich RL, Neilands TB, et al. The Safety Attitudes Questionnaire: Psychometric Properties, Benchmarking Data, and Emerging Research. *BMC Health Services Res.* 2006;6:44.

16. Frankel A, Grillo SP, Pittman M, et al. Revealing and resolving patient safety defects: the impact of leadership walkrounds™ on frontline caregiver assessments of patient safety. *Health Services Res.* 2008;43:6.

17. University of Texas-Memorial Hermann Center for Healthcare Quality and Safety. Safety Attitudes and Safety Climate Questionnaire. Available at: http://www.uth.tmc.edu/schools/med/imed/patient_safety/questionnaires/SAQBibliography.html. Accessed October 3, 2012.

18. Frankel A, Grillo SP, Baker EG, et al. Patient Safety Leadership WalkRounds™ at Partners HealthCare: learning from implementation. *Jt Comm J Qual Patient Saf.* 2005;31(8):423-437.

19. Burgess LH, Cohen MR, Denham CR. A new leadership role for pharmacists: A prescription for change. *J Patient Saf.* 2010;6:31-37.

20. Institute for Safe Medication Practices. ISMP Medication Safety Alert! Acute Care. Available at: http://www.ismp.org/Newsletters/acutecare/default.asp. Accessed October 3, 2012.

21. Institute for Safe Medication Practices. ISMP Medication Safety Alert! Acute Care: Medication Error Prevention Toolbox. Available at: www.ismp.org/newsletters/acutecare/articles/19990602.asp. Accessed October 3, 2012.

22. Smith D. Opportunities for improving core measure performance through pharmacist intervention. Norman Regional Health System. 15 September 2010. Available at: http://www.pharmacyonesource.com/images/sentri7/ImproveCoreMeasures.pdf. Accessed October 3, 2012.

23. Pryor DB, Tolchin SF, Hendrich A, et al. The clinical transformation of Ascension Health: Eliminating all preventable injuries and deaths. *Jt Comm J Qual Patient Saf.* 2006;32(6):299-308.

24. Muething SE, Kotagal UR, Schoettker PJ, et al. Family-centered bedside rounds: A new approach to patient care and teaching. *Pediatrics.* 2007;119;829-832.

25. Samaan KH, Dahlke M, Stover J. Addressing safety concerns about U-500 insulin in a hospital setting. *Am J Health-Syst Pharm.* 2011;68:63-68.

26. Rose JS, Thomas CS, Tersigni A, et al. A leadership framework for culture change in health care. *J Qual Patient Saf.* 2006;32:433-442.

27. Quaid D, Thao J, Denham C. Story power: the secret weapon. *J Patient Saf.* 2010;6(1):5-14.

28. Theodore K, Webber T. Third baby dies after error at Indiana hospital. *USA Today.* 20 Sept 2006. Available at: http://www.usatoday.com/news/nation/2006-09-20-baby-deaths_x.htm. Accessed October 3, 2012.

Appendix 3-A

Example of a Medication Safety Walk-Round Tool

Date:

Participants:

Location:

Conducted by:

Questions	Answers
Quality Processes and Risk Management	
1. Have there been any medication errors or near misses that almost caused patient harm but didn't? What could have been done to prevent it?	
2. When you make a medication error or prevent/intercept an error, do you always report it? If not, why?	
3. If you make or report an error, are you concerned about personal consequences?	
4. Have you developed any personal practices to specifically prevent making a medication error?	
5. Are standardized policies being utilized to reduce/prevent medication errors? If not, where do you think standardization could be implemented?	
6. Are there any instances where technology has contributed or could potentially contribute to medication errors?	
7. What do you predict the next medication error will be?	
8. Are discrepancies with medication counts and waste addressed at the time of discovery?	
Patient Information and Education	
9. How are you ensuring that the patient understands his/her medications before being sent home?	
10. Are patients being asked about over-the-counter medications and supplements they currently take during the medication reconciliation process? Is this information being properly documented?	

Questions	Answers
Drug Standardization, Storage, and Distribution	
11. Are ready-to-use concentrations being utilized? If not, give some examples where ready-to-use concentrations could be used.	
Medication Device Acquisition, Use, and Monitoring	
12. How often are you removing medications from automated dispensing cabinets (ADCs) via the override function? In what situations are you using the override function?	
13. Are override reports routinely reviewed to identify and address the reasons for overrides? (Administration)	
14. Is there a standardized process for loading ADCs?	
Communication of Medication Orders and Other Information	
15. Can you describe how communication between caregivers either enhances or inhibits safe medication use?	
16. In what situations are medication orders not being screened by the pharmacy before administration?	
Environmental Factors, Workflow, and Staffing Patterns	
17. What aspects of your environment are likely to lead to medication errors?	
Miscellaneous	
18. What other medication safety concerns do you have that have not been addressed during this walk round?	

Observations:

Pharmacy	Answers
19. How are look-alike/sound-alike (LASA) medications being identified and differentiated?	
20. How are high-alert medications being identified and differentiated from other medications?	
21. Are medications being stored appropriately? How are you ensuring that they are stored properly?	
22. Are refrigerator temperatures being monitored appropriately?	

Questions	Answers
Nursing	
23. What two patient identifiers are being used to verify that the right patient is being given a medication?	
24. Is the patient's medication administration record (MAR) being reviewed prior to medication administration?	
25. Are patients being counseled on first doses of all of their medications?	
Automated Dispensing Cabinets (ADCs)	
26. Are the ADCs located in areas with minimal distractions?	
27. Is medication for only one patient being removed during a single transaction?	
28. How are LASA medications being differentiated?	
29. How are high-alert medications being differentiated?	
30. Are refrigerator temperatures being monitored appropriately?	

Source: Courtesy H. Burgess, HCA Management Services, L.P.

Accreditation and Regulatory Compliance

Ann E. Wehmeyer

CHAPTER 4

Key Terms

Accreditation—Voluntary process wherein a health care organization meets established standards or criteria as determined through initial and periodic reviews.

Focused Standards Assessment (FSA)—The Joint Commission online tool for subscribers; annual process of performing a gap analysis between practice in your organization and regulatory requirements and correcting deficiencies by developing and completing actions plans with measures of success when indicated.

Regulation—A government-imposed requirement for which compliance is mandatory.

Requirement for Improvement (RFI)—Citation for a standard found that is out of compliance during an accreditation survey. Also referred to as a finding.

Sentinel Event—"An unexpected occurrence involving death or serious physical or psychological injury, or the risk thereof," as defined by The Joint Commission.

Standards—A set of rules or principles established by consensus and approved by a recognized body that describes services, systems, or practices to meet a certain level of quality; in health care to provide safe patient care in a secure environment.

Tracer—An evaluation method that uses the medical record as a guide to follow a patient through transitions in the course of an episode of care to assess compliance with standards. This methodology may also be used to assess the medication management process and other organizational systems to provide or evaluate patient care.

Introduction

The role of the Medication Safety Officer (MSO) in **accreditation** and regulatory compliance varies based on individual job position descriptions and the institution. MSOs are usually responsible for ensuring compliance with accreditation **standards** related to medication use, preparing for accreditation survey and addressing noncompliance identified in the survey,[1] and they may also be responsible for ensuring compliance with federal and state **regulations** related to medication use as well as standards from governmental agencies. The goal is not just to pass the survey, but to ensure safe, quality processes of care for your patients through adherence to regulations and standards.

Accreditation

Accreditation is a method for ensuring an organization achieves and maintains high-quality patient care. Patient safety is a primary driver for all accrediting agencies. Participation in the accreditation process is voluntary, so why do organizations find it important to seek accreditation? The accreditation process helps raise the levels of safety, quality, and value of care provided by the organization. Accrediting agencies present standards reflecting national concerns, helping organizations to stay current and update practices accordingly. Further, because accreditation standards may be cited in determining prevailing standards of care, noncompliance with such standards can influence an organization's potential liability risks.

Another important reason for seeking accreditation is to earn *deemed status*. The Centers for Medicare & Medicaid Services (CMS) requires deemed status or CMS certification as a condition of payment for Medicare and Medicaid services. Deemed status indicates that the healthcare facility meets conditions of participation (CoPs) for CMS.[2,3] The CoPs are minimum standards for health and safety that the provider must meet to be certified for Medicare and Medicaid. As long as a facility is accredited by an organization with "deeming" authority, it is exempt from routine CMS certification surveys to determine compliance with CoPs by the state agency and is eligible to receive reimbursement from CMS for Medicare and Medicaid services.

There are three private accrediting agencies with deeming authority for hospitals:

1. Hospital Accreditation Program—The Joint Commission (TJC), Oakbrook, Illinois
2. Healthcare Facilities Accreditation Program (HFAP)—American Osteopathic Association, Chicago, Illinois
3. National Integrated Accreditation for Healthcare Organizations (NIAHO)—Det Norske Veritas (DNV) Healthcare Inc., Houston, Texas and Cincinnati, Ohio

The standards for all three private accrediting agencies must meet or exceed the CMS CoPs, and surveys must be unannounced.[3-7] Even though this chapter discusses contemporary information, standards are dynamic. Current information on standards, surveys, and scoring should be verified with the accrediting agency's publications or references. TJC is the most widely used accrediting agency in the United States and has had deeming authority since 1965 (see below for a detailed discussion). The strategies for survey preparation are applicable to other accrediting agencies. For all three agencies, there are crosswalk publications for their standards and CMS standards to assist in understanding the differences and assuring compliance for both (see http://www.hcmarketplace.com/prod-9729/Medical-Staff-Standards-Crosswalk.html for additional information). A comparison of these accrediting agencies may be found in Table 4-1.[3,4]

How to Succeed with Accreditation: Focus on TJC

TJC surveys are unannounced to improve the credibility of the survey process, help ensure that the survey represents a more accurate assessment of the quality of care, and encourage organizations to maintain consistent compliance with standards. The concept of continuous survey readiness is that an organization should be ready to host surveyors on any given day for the benefit of patient safety and quality of care. Continuous survey readiness requires an organizational culture change away from the ramping up to get ready for survey and meeting standards purely to satisfy a regulatory body. As the MSO, you must advocate for continuous survey readiness and compliance with standards for the sake of patient safety and quality of care. Although the usual survey is the full triennial survey, there is more than one type of survey:[10]

- A *Full Unannounced Triennial Survey* occurs 18–36 months after the previous full survey. Health care organizations are notified of survey activity by 7:30 a.m. the day of the survey. During the survey, the surveyors are evaluating compliance with standards and National Patient Safety Goals (NPSGs) and issuing a **Requirement for Improvement** (RFI) for each standard found not in compliance.
- An *Evidence of Standards Compliance Validation Survey* may occur around the midpoint of the accreditation cycle. On an annual basis, TJC randomly samples 5% of organizations required to submit evidence of standards compliance (ESC) with or without measures of success. The focus is on areas cited as a RFI and validating that the corrective actions submitted to TJC were implemented.
- A *Survey for Cause* may follow the receipt of a complaint reported to TJC regarding a quality of care issue in an accredited facility. This may be identified by a media event or headlines in the local newspaper. It may also be in response to an event or series of events where there is concern of a continuing threat to patient care or safety, or indication that the organization has not complied with TJC's Information Accuracy and Truthfulness

Table 4-1. Comparison of CMS and Three Private Accrediting Agencies with Deeming Authority for Hospitals

Centers for Medicare & Medicaid Services (CMS) and Accrediting Agencies	Granted Deeming Status	Associations	Central Office Location	Survey Frequency	Survey Methodology	Philosophy	Additional Features
CMS. www.cms.gov State Operations Manual Appendix A: Survey Protocol, Regulations and Interpretive Guidelines for Hospitals http://www.cms.gov/manuals/downloads/som107ap_a_hospitals.pdf	N/A	U.S. Department of Health and Human Services	Baltimore, MD	Annual for certification	Follow interpretive guidelines for CoPs	Medicare CoPs were created to set a minimum requirement for quality in operations of health care facilities.	CMS surveyors do not require an escort, may go anywhere in the organization, and may copy records.
Hospital Accreditation Program (HAP) Joint Commission http://www.jointcommission.org/	1965		Oak Brook, IL	Every 19–36 months	**Tracer**	Joint Commission Vision All people always experience the safest, highest quality, best-value health care across all settings.	National Patient Safety Goals
Healthcare Facilities Accreditation Program (HFAP) http://www.hfap.org/	1965	American Osteopathic Association	Chicago, IL	Every 3 years	Review patient-centered processes	User-friendly standards, an educational and practical approach to survey, and cost-effective accreditation program, straightforward approach.	Standards based on recommendations from IHI, NQF, and AHRQ in addition to CMS CoPs

Table 4-1 (continued).

National Integrated Accreditation for Healthcare Organizations (NIAHO) http://dnvaccreditation.com/pr/dnv/default.aspx Standards available online	2008	DNVHC	Houston, TX, and Cincinnati, OH	Annual survey, accreditation every 3 years	Tracer	Standards less prescriptive and are aligned with CMS quality initiatives. Collaborative approach to survey.	At the first survey, the health care organization receives a gap analysis to ISO 9001, which is an internationally recognized standard for quality management with a plan to achieve within a maximum of 2 years.

AHRQ, Agency for Healthcare Research and Quality; CoPs, Conditions of Participation; DNVHC, DNV Healthcare, Inc.; IHI, Institute for Healthcare Improvement; NQF, National Quality Forum.

Policy. The complaint must be relevant to TJC standards and pertain to performance in last 3 years. If the complaint is considered to be a high priority quality event such as a **sentinel event** or potential for sentinel event, one of the possible actions is a For Cause unannounced survey. The survey may include all areas or only the area where the concern exists.

Prior to the Survey

The accreditation cycle includes pre-survey, survey, and post-survey time periods (see Figure 4-1). The focus of the survey is on improving the safety and quality of care. TJC's mission is "to continuously improve health care for the public, in collaboration with other stakeholders, by evaluating health care organizations, and inspiring them to excel in providing safe and effective care of the highest quality and value."[11]

Prior to an accreditation survey, the MSO should have a firm grasp of:

- the scope of the upcoming survey
- all applicable standards, elements of performance (EPs), and scoring
- ways to prioritize efforts
- current status of compliance with standards
- the process to improve compliance with standards
- the survey process including Tracer Methodology
- survey preparation for the staff

Above all, know the scope of your survey. The accreditation manual that your organization will be surveyed under is determined by the accreditation application.[12]

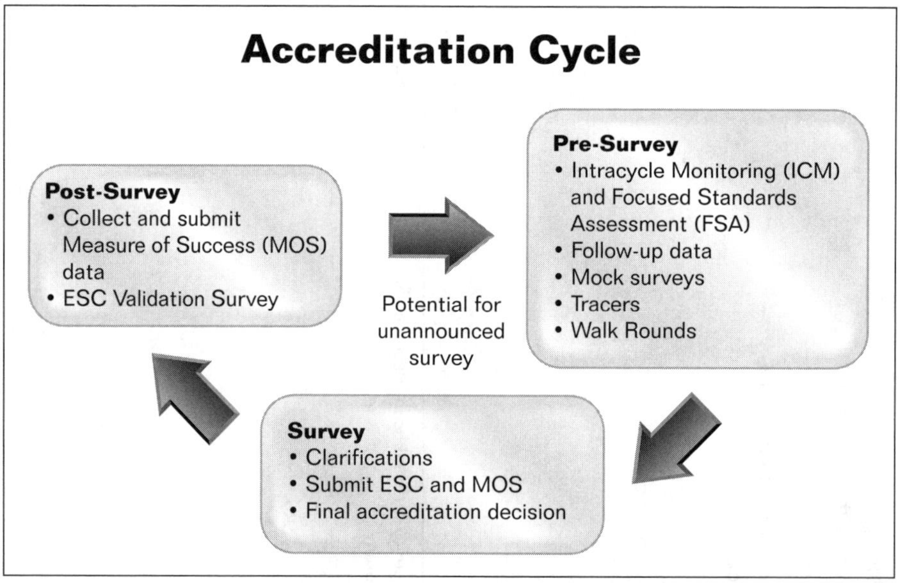

Figure 4-1. Accreditation cycle. ESC, evidence of standards compliance.
Source: Used with permission of Karen L. Tertell.

Areas such as behavior health, ambulatory care, skilled nursing facilities, or rehabilitation units are surveyed as part of the hospital's survey or separately depending on your institution's governance structure and functional integration. Determine which services will be included in your survey by checking with the director/coordinator of accreditation or the department director of performance improvement (PI)/quality improvement (QI) or its equivalent in your organization. For example, if hospital-owned clinics and physician office practices will be included in the hospital survey, you must ensure that those practices are in compliance with hospital standards and national patient safety goals (NPSGs).

Knowledge of Standards and Other Surveyable Material

Standards are organized by chapter, and each standard has a six-digit code preceded by a two- or three-character abbreviation of the chapter. EPs follow each standard and define satisfactory implementation of the standard.[13] Compliance with EPs are determined during the survey through onsite interviews with staff and patients, tracer methodology and documents provided for review.[12] EPs are scored by the surveyor and determine the health care facility's compliance with each standard. Criticality indicates the risk to patient safety. The criticality assigned to an EP for which the organization is found to be noncompliant during a survey impacts accreditation status and the timeframe for corrective action (see Table 4-2 Levels of Criticality).[12]

EPs are assigned one of two scoring categories, A or C.[12] A category "A" EP is usually related to a requirement for a policy or process and is scored as all or none, either a "0" for insufficient compliance or "2" for satisfactory compliance. An "A" EP may also be a CMS or a NPSG requirement that must be fully compliant. A category "C" EP is scored based on the number of times that an EP is not met: score "2," satisfactory compliance, if 0 to one finding of noncompliance; score "1," partial compliance, if two findings of noncompliance; score "0," insufficient compliance, if three or more findings of noncompliance. Any finding other than full compliance will result in an RFI.

The *medication management (MM) standards* are organized by critical processes in the medication-use system.[14] The standards provide a framework for the medication-use process as well as a basis for continuous evaluation and improvement. Although pharmacy leadership is essential, safe and effective medication-use processes require collaboration with other disciplines. Medication management is not just about the department of pharmacy because the medication-use process involves many professions and disciplines such as licensed independent practitioners, nurses, nurse practitioners, respiratory therapists, and radiology technicians. It is common that the MSO is assigned oversight responsibility for the medication management chapter and serves on an organization-wide accreditation committee. To become prepared, you should thoroughly read applicable portions of the most current accreditation standards manual appropriate for your practice site. Additional standards from chapters other than medication management that are applicable to medication safety and the department of pharmacy are summarized in Appendix 4-A. All proposed new

Table 4-2. TJC Levels of Criticality

Criticality Levels	Definition	Application to Elements of Performance	Result of Noncompliance During Survey	Example	Action Required for Resolution
Immediate threat to health and safety	▲1 Patient care impact 1: potential for serious adverse effects on the health or safety of patients.	Not applied to individual EP	Preliminary Denial of Accreditation (PDA) until resolved	Inoperable fire alarm system	Within 72 hours, eliminate immediate threat to health or safety or implement emergency intervention to abate the risk to patients.
Situational decision rule	▲2 Patient care impact 2: situation exists that could pose a significant threat to patient safety and quality of care.	Applied to individual standards–EP with a ▲2 designation	PDA, Contingent Accreditation (CONT), or Accreditation with Follow-up Survey	Unlicensed pharmacist	For CONT, must identify issues and submit Evidence of Standards Compliance (ESC) within 45 days and follow-up site visit.

Table 4-2 (continued).

Direct impact requirement	△3 Patient care impact 3: situations that could directly impact patients by creating an immediate risk to safety or quality of care, treatment, and services.	Applied to individual standards or NPSG–EP with a △3 designation	Requirement for Improvement (RFI)	Medication not properly labeled with required elements	If there are one or more direct impact EPs under a standard found to be partial or insufficient compliance, all noncompliant EPs must be addressed in ESC within 45 days.
Indirect impact requirement	Pose a less immediate risk to patient care and safety but increase risk over time.	Applied to individual EPs without a ▲2 or a △3	RFI	No drug formulary	Submit ESC within 60 days for all partial or insufficient compliance.

NPSG, National Patient Safety Goal. See Reference 12 for more information.

standards, revisions, and changes to surveys are published in the monthly periodical, *Joint Commission Perspectives*, and *Joint Commission Online*, a weekly newsletter, and distributed to all TJC-accredited facilities. Major proposed changes to standards are usually posted online for field review prior to adoption, and MSOs should submit feedback for medication-related standards.[15]

Resources

Any questions regarding interpretation of standards should be identified and clarified prior to the survey. Refer to the Frequently Asked Questions (FAQs) on the TJC website.[13] There are additional resources available through the secure extranet site Joint Commission Connect. Although this site is generally only accessible by the accreditation coordinator and is used to submit secure responses and data to the TJC, a guest log-in is available to access the Lending Practice Library and Core Measure Solutions Exchange. Another resource on the extranet site is TJC BoosterPaks™ that are reference documents on a problematic standard and include implementation suggestions, FAQs, and supporting references. The Standards Interpretation Group (SIG) is the final authority for resolving questions on standards and implementation. Although answers may be obtained over the telephone, it is highly recommended to obtain responses in writing.[10] Written responses may be used to challenge a potential RFI post survey. Alternately, consultants from Joint Commission Resources can provide suggestions on how to comply with a standard or examples of how another organization has been in compliance.

National Patient Safety Goals

The purpose of the NPSGs is to promote specific patient safety improvements in health care identified through extensive literature review and expert consultation.[16] Goals and requirements are developed by the Patient Safety Advisory Group, a multidisciplinary panel of recognized patient safety experts, targeting the highest priority patient safety and quality initiatives. Annual updates are published after an extensive review process that includes public commentary. Requirements for NPSGs focus on systems-wide, evidence-based solutions to problematic areas in health care. The goals and requirements are program specific (e.g., hospital, critical access, ambulatory, behavioral health). Compliance with the requirements for NPSGs is one of the most challenging aspects of continuous survey readiness. Surveyors are required to evaluate compliance with NPSGs during a survey.[17]

As the MSO, you will take the lead in organizational compliance for medication-related NPSGs. You should review any proposed new NPSGs on TJC's website and provide comment on the proposed requirements. Be sure to review each new NPSG for implications to the medication management system. Depending on the goal, it may be appropriate to assemble a multidisciplinary team to develop and activate a plan to achieve and sustain compliance.

Sentinel Event Alerts

TJC has reviewed 9095 sentinel events from January 1995 to June 2012.[18] A *sentinel event*, defined as "any unexpected occurrence involving death or serious physical or psychological injury or risk thereof," may be reported to TJC. The term *sentinel* indicates the need for urgent investigation and response. Refer to TJC's website for a list of reviewable sentinel events. Following occurrence of a sentinel event, organizations are expected to prepare and submit a thorough root cause analysis and action plan to TJC. In addition to reviewing these submissions, TJC maintains a de-identified database of reported events, root causes, and risk reduction strategies.[19]

Since 1995, medication error is the fifth most commonly reported sentinel event.[20] TJC publishes Sentinel Event Alerts periodically in response to a patient safety concern identified from the database or literature source.

Examples of medication-related Sentinel Event Alerts include:

- "Safe use of opioids in hospitals" (Issue 49), August 2012
- "Preventing pediatric medication errors" (Issue 39), April 2008
- "Preventing Errors Related to Commonly Used Anticoagulants" (Issue 41), September 2008

You will also find Issue 42, "Safely Implementing Health Information and Converging Technologies," of interest because it relates to medication management. Sentinel Event Alerts are surveyable material. The expectation is that the organization reviews their processes related to the identified risk, evaluates the recommendations, and makes improvements as indicated under MM.08.01.01 "The hospital evaluates the effectiveness of its medication management system."[21] As the MSO, you should take the lead in preparing a gap analysis to determine the organization's compliance with the recommendations put forth in the Sentinel Event Alert. See Table 4-3 for an example.

Priority Focus Areas and Clinical/Service Groups

The priority focus process is used by surveyors to help focus and customize the survey to organization-specific issues and patient populations. The process is based on data from a variety of sources including the organization's application for accreditation, prior survey findings, complaints, and other publically reported data and identifies the organization's priority focus areas (PFAs) and clinical/service groups (CSGs).[10] A *PFA* is a process, system, or structure that significantly impacts patient safety and quality of care such as communication, infection control, or orientation and training. A *CSG* is a group of patients or a patient population, such as cardiac surgery, HIV infection, or neonatology. The surveyors have access to these data prior to survey and use this as a starting point for their tracer activities. If Orthopedics is identified as one of your CSGs, then it is likely that a tracer patient on Orthopedics service will be selected from an active patient list. This information is updated quarterly and is available on the organization's Joint Commission extranet site. Definitions for the PFAs can be found online or in the *Hospital Accreditation Standards* manual.[12] Although the names are similar, a PFA is not the same as TJC's chapter. The

Table 4-3. Example Format for Sentinel Event Alert Gap Analysis

Sentinel Event Alert: Preventing Pediatric Medication Errors

Risk Reduction Strategies	Organization Assessment	Action Requirement	Responsibility	Target Completion Date
Establish and maintain a functional pediatric formulary system with policies for drug evaluation, selection, and therapeutic use.	Currently in place.	No action required.	N/A	N/A
Limit the number of concentrations and dose strengths of high-alert medications to the minimum needed to provide safe care.	Currently in place—we have a standard concentration list.	As new medications are introduced, standard concentrations are developed for dispensing.	Pediatrics Pharmacist	Ongoing
Provide ready access, including website access, to up-to-date pediatric-specific information for all hospital staff.	Hospital-wide access to electronic drug information resource—includes pediatric information. Also available in main Rx and satellite: *The Pediatric Dose Handbook* for doses, growth charts, and normal lab/vital sign ranges; *Neofax* for NICU dosing; and *Teddy Bear Book* for Pediatric IV information. Pharmacy access to University resources, which include journal search engines.	Continue subscriptions to our online resources, which update regularly. Monitor for new editions of stated references, evaluate for replacement.	Pharmacy Clinical Manager	Ongoing

continued

Table 4-3 (continued).

Orient all pharmacy staff to specialized neonatal/pediatric pharmacy services in your organization.	Currently in progress; orientation includes time in each area of the pharmacy, with one-on-one training with the specialist in each area. We have a new training manual, in which NICU/Pediatrics is covered by pediatric pharmacist.	We are in the process of re-training all existing employees on the services provided to NICU and Pediatrics.	Pediatrics Pharmacist	December 2008
Develop preprinted medication order forms and clinical pathways or protocols to reflect a standardized approach to care. Include reminders and information about monitoring parameters.	We have many paper NICU order sets and protocols.	Assure all protocols are up to date.	Informatics Pharmacist	September 2008
	Currently we don't have standard order sets for pediatrics.	Develop standard pediatric admission order sets for most common admissions.	Pediatrics/NICU Performance Improvement Team	February 2009
		Transition to electronic when software available.	Clinical Transformation	Future state

NICU, neonatal intensive care unit.
Source: Courtesy, Deb Saine, Winchester Medical Center.

medication management PFA includes MM standards as well as standards from other chapters. Of the 14 possible PFAs, all but 2 include MM standards. Become familiar with your organization's PFAs and which MM standards are included in those PFAs.

How to Prioritize Survey Preparation Activity

When preparing for a TJC survey, the job seems overwhelming. A targeted approach is suggested in Figure 4-2. Obtain the previous survey report from your accreditation coordinator to get a sense of the survey's focus. Start with the most critical issues:

- *Any prior RFIs:* Any RFI must be addressed prior to the next survey. A finding from a previous survey found to be deficient may be cited under the chapter of origin as well as under the Leadership standards.
- *NPSGs:* These goals are a significant focus of a TJC survey and must be reviewed to ensure compliance. Prioritize any medication-related NPSGs.[17]
- *Top 10 Issues:* The top compliance issues resulting in RFIs are periodically published in *Joint Commission Perspectives* and provide an indication of the hot topics for surveyors. The most common MM standard resulting in an RFI is consistently MM.03.01.01 involving safe storage of medication.[22] Key issues include expired medications and medication labeling.
- *PFAs:* These are the four PFAs based on your organization's data that surveyors use to focus their survey efforts. The organization's PFAs are posted on the extranet site and may change quarterly.[12]

A Targeted Approach to Achieving a Successful Survey Outcome

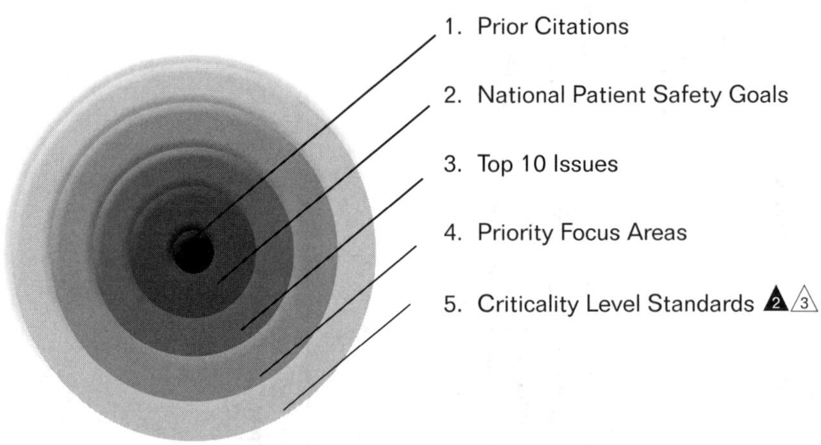

Figure 4-2. A targeted approach to achieving a successful survey outcome.
Source: Used with permission of Karen L. Tertell.

- *Criticality Level 2 and 3 Standards:* Criticality level 2 and 3 standards have the largest direct impact on your accreditation decision. Level 2 standards (Situational Decision Rules apply) and level 3 standards (Direct Impact Rules apply) indicate an increased risk to patient safety.[12]

How Do You Monitor and Assess Compliance with Standards?

Focused standards assessment (FSA) is an online tool that is included in the Intracycle Monitoring Process and assists your organization with continuous standards compliance efforts and promotes ongoing quality improvement.[12,23] To help provide focus, TJC has designated standards that minimize risk and improve safety as risk-related standards within the FSA. In many organizations, the MSO would take the lead on completing the FSA for the MM chapter. You will need input from other disciplines, especially nursing, to assess compliance with many of the standards. The process involves reviewing compliance with applicable standards, identifying areas of noncompliance, developing and implementing action plans, and tracking progress toward compliance using measures when required. There are several options for completing the FSA process. Most organizations evaluate compliance with all standards and elements of performance and submit the evaluation electronically to TJC annually at 12 and 24 months after the last survey. For every noncompliant standard, the organization must submit a plan of action (POA) to achieve compliance for each applicable EP. On receipt of the evaluation and POAs, the SIG works with the hospital to come to consensus on the POA. During a phone conference, the SIG reviews the POA and may make revisions. The POA is approved by the conclusion of the call. The organization has 45 days from the date of submission of the POA to achieve compliance. The FSA offers the additional advantage that if during a survey a surveyor identifies a compliance issue identical to that contained in the FSA, the SIG will review the accreditation report. As long as the POA is appropriate and the implementation date is not exceeded, the RFI will remain on the accreditation report but not count toward the accreditation decision.

How to Write a Plan of Action

The *POA* is a detailed description of the steps that the organization has taken to achieve compliance with an element of performance either as part of a FSA or post-survey.[12] The POA should include the following elements:

- Description and a list of each action to be taken to address the EP
- Target date for completion of each action
- The person responsible for each action
- Description of how the action was implemented
- Documentation tracking the progress made toward POA implementation
- Methods for preventing future recurrence

If a measure of success (MOS) is required for the EP, this must be included in your POA. The MOS must be quantifiable and demonstrate successful implementation of your POA. Define the numerator and denominator of the measure (expressed as a percentage), as well as sample size, sampling methodology, and audit frequency. The sample size for the MOS is defined in Table 4-4.[12] For category "C" standards, the results of the MOS over a 4-month period must average at least 90% for satisfactory compliance. During a survey, the surveyor may ask for the MOS data from your FSA.

Multidisciplinary Review of Standards. To complete your organization's FSA, it is essential to understand how the MM standards and related NPSGs are implemented in every surveyable area of the organization. This includes not just in an inpatient nursing unit, but also the operating room (OR), procedural areas, outpatient areas, and hospital-owned physician practices. Sample questions include:

- How is the temperature monitored for refrigerators containing vaccines in off-site clinics?
- Is the patient education distributed from physician offices consistent with what is given to patients while in house?
- How is narcotic waste documented in procedural areas?
- How are medications labeled in the OR?
- What is the allergy-checking or medication-administration process in Interventional Radiology?
- Is access to automated dispensing cabinets (ADCs) terminated when employees leave your organization?
- Who has access to areas where medications are stored?
- Where in the organization are sterile parenteral admixtures prepared outside of the pharmacy?
- Do staff follow the Centers for Disease Control and Prevention (CDC) guidelines for safe injection practices?

Although it is manpower intensive, it is highly recommended for the MSO to assemble a multidisciplinary group that can represent the application of the MM standards in all areas of your organization. FSA quality increases with broader participation from across the organization. This group needs to take ownership of the application of these standards in their area. You should pay special attention to new

Table 4-4. Sample Size for Compliance Measurement

Number of Applicable Cases	Sample Size
<30	100% of cases
30–100	30 cases
101–500	50 cases
>500	70 cases

See Reference 12 for more information.

standards or NPSGs, standards that have been recently revised, and new services within your organization. Also consider that compliance with standards is not static and that more than one assessment may be required to determine compliance. Prior to the survey, it is invaluable to identify any variation in practice that exists within your organization.

Leadership Walk Rounds. Many organizations will organize leadership walk rounds. Administrators and hospital leadership make rounds in patient care areas according to a schedule. Often these include the use of a checklist and/or script. The purpose is both to identify deficiencies as well as opportunities for staff education. In addition, involvement of top leadership in walk rounds sends a message to staff that that issues of quality and safety are a priority. Managers of the area surveyed are notified of findings, and results are aggregated and distributed through the performance improvement structure to determine corrective actions and to then monitor compliance over time. As the MSO, you can attend or participate in walk rounds and contribute questions to a walk rounds checklist. Alternately, you can organize medication safety rounds.

Sample Questions to Be Incorporated. These include:

- What is the process for removing a medication from an ADC on override?
- How do you clarify an issue regarding a medication order with the prescriber?
- Are there any medications at a patient's bedside?
- How do you monitor the effects of medications?
- What do you do to ensure safe use of high-risk medications?
- How do you document narcotic waste?
- How and what do you report as a medication error? When is the prescriber notified?

Medication Storage Inspections. All medication storage areas are inspected regularly, and the inspection is documented for the past year. Monthly inspections are recommended and required by some states.[10] All areas where medications are stored, dispensed, or administered are inspected by a pharmacist or other qualified health care professional, such as a nurse or pharmacy technician, with pharmacist oversight. Remember to include OR, procedural areas, or anywhere that sedation is administered, and outpatient areas in which medications are administered. The primary focus is to evaluate the safe and secure storage of medication and to check for expired or compromised medications and supplies. Inspections in procedural areas and ambulatory care clinics can be an opportunity to evaluate safe medication practices including procedural labeling of medications and also to ensure medication administration processes in these areas are consistent with inpatient practices.

In addition to reviewing monthly inspections data, you should take at least an annual visit to the ORs, post-anesthesia recovery areas, Emergency Department, Radiology, Dialysis, and outpatient infusion areas. These critical areas warrant special attention from the MSO. You should use this opportunity to query the staff on critical issues affecting these unique areas and make sure they know how an error or near miss is reported. Any identified deficiencies or patterns of noncompliance must be addressed in a timely manner. The MSO must make sure that the inspectors have an appropriate tool to identify and document deficiencies. Appendix 4-B is an example of a medication inspection form. There are also commercially available checklist management systems to assist in data collection and compilation.

Pharmacy Inspections. Perform at least monthly inspections of the pharmacy and pharmacy satellites using a checklist. The inspection form tool noted above could be modified to target the pharmacy areas. Findings should be compiled and identified deficiencies addressed.

Examples of inspection points include:

- There is beyond-use dating of vials in laminar flow hood
- Staff working in laminar flow hood are appropriately gowned and gloved
- Refrigerator temperature logs and logs documenting cleaning of laminar flow hoods are complete
- High-risk medications and look-alike/sound-alike drugs are identifiable and stored according to policy
- Surfaces are clean and uncluttered
- No expired medications are identified
- Current drug references are available
- No unsecured controlled substances are present

Mock Surveys. Ideally, mock surveys using Tracer methodology are conducted throughout the accreditation cycle to support continuous survey readiness. The purpose is to assist the organization in identifying areas of noncompliance prior to the survey and to prepare staff for the survey. Surveyors for a mock survey may be hired as external consultants or internal consultants. External consultants have the advantage of being unbiased and objective toward the organization. However, internal consultants using a data-driven approach focusing on the standards identified in RFIs from last two surveys, FSA findings, and PFAs can provide a valuable mock survey.

Develop Quality Plans to Support Accreditation

Compliance with accreditation standards should be integrated with your medication safety and quality program to optimize continuous readiness. Gearing up for a survey from an accrediting agency is challenging at best and if it is left to the last moment it can be grueling. The goal is not just to pass the survey but to ensure safe processes and quality care for your patients. A sample quality improvement plan is presented in Table 4-5.

Table 4-5. Sample Quality Improvement Plan: Evaluation of Medication Management System

Stage in Medication Use Process/Standard	Process on Site	Measure	Frequency
Planning			
MM.01.01.03 EP 3 The hospital implements its process for high-alert and hazardous medications.	High-alert and hazardous medications are stored separately or labeled.	Inspect pharmacy for location and labeling of high-alert and hazardous medications.	Quarterly inspection
Selection and Procurement			
MM.02.01.01 EP 8 The hospital implements its process to select, approve, and procure medications that are not on its formulary.	Non-formulary medications requests are reviewed by a pharmacist and attending physician before obtaining.	Evaluate non-formulary requests for pharmacist and physician review.	Quarterly
MM.02.01.01 EP 11 The hospital implements its process to communicate medication shortages and outages to LIPs and staff who participate in medication management.	A checklist is utilized to ensure that all the steps are taken and personnel notified to safely manage a drug shortage.	Evaluate compliance with checklist.	Monthly
Storage			
MM.03.01.01 EP 8 The hospital removes all expired, damaged, and/or contaminated medications and stores them separately from medications available for administration.	Expired medications are removed and segregated.	Inspect medication storage areas for expired medications.	Monthly
MM.03.01.01 EP 18 The hospital periodically inspects all medication storage areas.	All medication storage areas in the medical center are inspected monthly.	Review compliance with inspections.	Monthly
MM.03.01.05 EP 2 Before use or administration of a medication brought into the hospital by a patient, his or her family, or a licensed independent practitioner, the hospital identifies the medication and visually evaluates the medication's integrity.	The pharmacist visually inspects patient's medication, determines if it meets criteria for use, and places note in medical record prior to medication administration.	Review a sample of orders for use of patient's medication to ensure inspection and note placed prior to first administration.	Quarterly

continued

Table 4-5 (continued).

Ordering			
MM.04.01.01 EP 9 A diagnosis, condition, or indication for use exists for each medication ordered.	A distinct prn reason is included in each as-needed order.	Review a sample of medication profiles to evaluate the prn reasons included in the orders for a given patient to identify if there are cases of ambiguous or duplicate prn reasons.	Quarterly
Preparing and Dispensing			
MM.05.01.01 EP 4 All medication orders are reviewed for the following: patient allergies or potential sensitivities.	Medication allergies or "no known allergies" are documented in the medical record prior to prescribing medication except in cases of emergency.	Review a sample of prescriptions to ensure allergy documentation occurred prior to prescribing.	Quarterly
MM.05.01.11 EP 3 The hospital dispenses medication within the time frames it defines to meet patients' needs.	Stat medication orders are dispensed within 15 minutes of receipt.	Study a sample of stat medication orders to evaluate turnaround time.	Quarterly
Administration			
MM.06.01.01 EP 3 Before administration, the individual administering the medication does the following: verifies that the medication selected matches the medication order and product label.	Prior to medication administration, the patient wristband and the medication are scanned using barcode technology to ensure that the medication is correct for that patient.	Evaluate compliance with bar code scan of medication prior to administration.	Monthly
Monitoring			
MM.02.01.01 EP 3 Before using a medication new to the hospital, the hospital determines a method to monitor the response of the patient.	For medications recently added to the formulary, the required monitoring is performed.	Select a new medication added to formulary in the last 6 months with monitoring that is required and evaluate cases to see if required monitoring is performed.	Quarterly

continued

Table 4-5 (continued).

MM.07.01.03 EP 3 The hospital complies with internal and external reporting requirements for actual or potential adverse drug events, significant adverse drug reactions, and medication errors.	All severe adverse drug reactions are reported to FDA MedWatch.	Review severe Adverse Drug Reaction reports and forward any cases that have not been sent to MedWatch.	Quarterly
Evaluation			
MM.08.01.01 EP 7 The hospital evaluates its actions to confirm that they resulted in improvements for its medication management system.	Newly implemented improvements and corrective actions are evaluated to determine if the desired effect was achieved.	Select an improvement/action and study effectiveness by reviewing cases.	Quarterly

PRN, as needed.
For more information and standards, please see The Joint Commission. *2012 Hospital Accreditation Standards* (HAS). Oak Brook, IL: Joint Commission on Accreditation of Healthcare Organizations; 2012.

Become Familiar with the Survey Process. The goal of the survey in addition to accreditation is to offer education and guidance to assist the staff in improving the hospital's performance. Review a sample survey agenda and Program Specific Survey Activity List for your survey type.[24] The survey agenda will include survey planning session, opening conference, leadership session, medical staff credentialing and privileging, visits to patient care areas using tracer methodology, Life Safety Code building assessment, environment of care rounds, emergency management, special issue resolution, and survey report preparation. The duration of the survey and number of surveyors is determined by the organization's size and scope. The survey team is made up of one or more health care professionals including a physician, nurse, life safety code specialist, or hospital administrator. Surveyors expect that you have been in compliance with standards since your last survey but require a 12-month documentation of history.

Tracer Methodology

Tracer Methodology was launched with the new Joint Commission survey process in 2004. Instead of reviewing a policy or discussing how care is performed with management staff, the surveyor sees the policy/procedure in action or as described by the health care providers involved, how it is applied to an individual patient's care, and the results. At a minimum, an organization should practice tracer methodology prior to the survey to familiarize the staff with the process. In addition to being a fundamental component of TJC onsite surveys, tracer methodology has evolved into a continuous improvement tool. Routine use of tracer methodology is a means of assessing and ensuring compliance with standards. The organization gets an accurate pragmatic assessment of day-to-day performance in carrying out processes of care using an actual case and determines if reality meets the standards. Conducting tracer methodology requires thorough knowledge of organizational policies and accreditation standards. The surveyors expect that the organization's policies are consistent with accreditation standards and are followed by staff.

Tracer methodology is performed by selecting a patient and, using that patient's medical record as a guide, following that patient's experience of care. Tracer methodology carried out in a non-confrontational, non-punitive manner provides education for staff. Some additional tips for conducting tracers include asking open-ended questions, involving a variety of disciplines, taking notes, and providing feedback to the staff. MSOs can conduct tracers evaluating MM as preparation for the survey, as performance improvement, or both. Because the MM standards are organized by processes making up the medication-use system, the tracer follows application of the standards for a given therapy. A variety of tracer tools are available, or you can develop your own to include standards that are problematic in your own organization (see Appendix 4-C for a sample Tracer tool).

During the survey, the number of tracers performed depends on the length of the survey and number of surveyors. During an average three-day survey with three surveyors, 11 tracers will be completed.[25] There are different types of program-specific tracers such as Patient Flow, Laboratory Integration, and Suicide Prevention system tracers, but the two types of tracers that you should be most familiar with are the individual tracer and the system tracer.

Individual Tracer Activity

Individual tracer activity begins with the selection of a patient who is in one of the top CSGs and who has received complex services (surgery, critical care) or has transitioned across different programs or departments.[12,24] The tracer begins at the patient's current location, and the patient is followed through the processes of care. The tracer evaluates individual processes as well as how well processes are coordinated or integrated. If the surveyor arrives in the patient care area and is required to wait for staff to assemble, the surveyor will begin to evaluate environment of care and record observations. During the evaluation of the patient's care, questions are asked of individual staff members regarding the tracer patient's care. Any standard may be evaluated. The surveyor may observe the medication-use process and may ask questions of frontline staff regarding communication, use of data, NPSGs, patient education, and staff orientation and training. For example, patients may be selected who are receiving a high-risk medication, anticoagulation therapy, a medication recently added to formulary, or a medication that requires a weight or laboratory result to calculate dosing.

System Tracer

System tracers follow a patient's care through the course of the visit or hospital stay and analyze one system or process of care. There are three types of system tracers:

data management, infection control, and MM.[12,24] The purposes of the MM system tracer are to assess compliance with standards, evaluate continuity of the medication-use process, identify risk points in the medication-use system, and educate staff. In addition to tracing a patient who has received medication while under the organization's care and inspecting pharmacy locations, the MM systems tracer may include a multidisciplinary group discussion that typically lasts approximately 1 hour. Prior to the survey, the MSO should identify the key disciplines whose participation at this meeting is essential. The team should include representation from medical staff, Nursing, Pharmacy, Outpatient Services, Respiratory Therapy, Radiology, Patient Safety/Risk Management, Dietary Services, and Performance Improvement. This team likely includes many of the same individuals who were initially involved in assessing compliance to the MM standards for the FSA. Assemble the team and provide guidance for the session including the meeting's format and likely content. Possible topics for discussion during this tracer include medications brought into the organization by the patient, access to medications and medication security, addition of new medications to formulary, high-alert medication strategies, process for reporting errors, and performance improvement activities. The MSO will likely be involved in the data management session tracer preparation session as well.

Be Prepared

Prepare yourself professionally for survey by becoming fully informed. Attend lectures or seminars on accreditation at professional meetings or TJC programs. MSOs should read TJC publications and standards manuals. Network with colleagues and sign up for applicable professional listserves. It is a great idea to get to know your counterparts at other local hospitals or facilities so that you have peers to ask questions and share solutions.

Another recommended strategy is to collaborate with your institution's department that is responsible for quality improvement, accreditation, and regulatory compliance. Forming a working and collaborative relationship prior to survey will be beneficial for both parties. You should work out a communication plan for survey day in advance and plan to share quality and performance improvement data. The MSO can serve as a resource for the quality department with regard to MM. You can help ensure that a consistent and accurate message is delivered across the organization by contributing to or reviewing annual competencies related to accreditation, educational materials prepared for staff education pre-survey, checklists designed for walk rounds, quality newsletters, etc. Your organization's accreditation staff can be a great source of information regarding compliance in remote areas. The accreditation staff may also provide access to TJC publications, updates, manuals, and other regulatory resources. This department has access to TJC's secure extranet site where data, such as the organization's priority focus areas, reside.

It is essential to prepare your staff to verbalize processes that are consistent with both TJC standards and your own policies. The surveyors expect to see evidence that your policies have been fully implemented. Don't wait until the last minute as there is too much information to be absorbed. Your staff should be familiar with participating in a tracer. The surveyor most likely will ask to speak to a staff member who has been involved in the care of a tracer patient or an alternate staff member who performs the same job functions. Surveyors expect that staff will step up and participate.

Some suggestions to help prepare staff include:

- Conduct mock tracers to familiarize staff with accreditation concepts
- Contribute to or develop an annual competency for accreditation issues
- Display a departmental bulletin board that highlights the department's performance improvement data and medication safety initiatives as well as a standard and "NPSG of the Month"
- Have staff participate in departmental inspections
- During staff meetings, ask staff questions that a surveyor might ask
- Distribute a question-and-answer document for important standards
- Keep staff informed of updates to medication-related hospital policy
- Develop flyers for facility-wide distribution (e.g., when to report a medication error)
- Post information where is it needed (e.g., a list of beyond-use dating posted on the IV hood)
- Organize essential documents for the staff on an intranet site or shared drive
- Utilize staff to clean and organize the pharmacy dispensing areas and refrigerators
- Remove outdated references, pre-printed forms, drugs, etc.

You should assemble in advance any documents that you may need during the survey. It is recommended that the MSO take the lead in assembling a binder of necessary documents and keeping it updated.

Required documents for the Preliminary Planning and Surveyor Planning sessions during the first few hours of survey include:[24]

- Performance improvement data for last 12 months
- Documentation of PI projects including the rationale and progress to date (can be contained in minutes)
  - Last 12 months of Pharmacy and Therapeutics Committee minutes
  - Last 12 months of Medication Safety Committee minutes
- MOS data from most recent FSA
- Analysis from a high-risk process—include if a MM failure mode and effects analysis (FMEA) has been completed
- List of sites where deep or moderate sedation is used
- List of unapproved abbreviations

If the required documents are not available at the time the surveyors arrive on the first day, the surveyors will go directly to patient care areas and begin tracers, and the organization loses the ability to ready frontline staff.

Here are some examples of additional data to have readily available at time of survey:[10]

- Turnaround time from when medication is ordered to when it is administered
- Adverse Drug Event reporting
- ADC overrides
- Approved drug formulary and non-formulary drug requests
- Notification of drug recall and actions taken
- Narcotic wastage audits
- Documentation of required education and competencies
- PI data
- Policies required by MM standards and NPSGs
- Employee files with updated licensing and documentation of orientation and training information

Day of Survey

On the first day of the survey, TJC posts the survey notice as well as copies of biographies and pictures of the assigned surveyors by 7:30 a.m. local time on the organization's secure Joint Commission Connect extranet site. Many hospitals have systems in place for communicating survey information with staff (e.g., group e-mails and/or paging, phone trees). Signs are posted at hospital entrances to notify the public that TJC is on site.[24]

Surveyors evaluate compliance with accreditation standards by reviewing medical records, policies, and other documents provided by the organization, on-site observations and interviews, and tracing the care of patients through the organization. Surveyors are looking for consistency in how the solutions are applied across the organization, multidisciplinary collaboration, and for examples that you have improved your processes, even if not perfect. During the survey, the surveyors not only evaluate compliance with standards but also teach and provide suggestions to improve performance. Some tips for how to work with surveyors include being respectful, polite, truthful, interactive, and open to suggestions. Although it is permitted to ask questions, never argue with a surveyor. Staff should be ready to answer a surveyor's questions but should not volunteer unnecessary information or mention past surveys or departmental problems.

Daily Briefing sessions occur each morning of the survey except the first day and typically last for approximately 30 minutes.[24] At Daily Briefings, surveyors present their findings from the previous day and may comment on significant issues or patterns which may lead to an RFI. The organization clarifies anything that they do not understand and has the opportunity to provide additional available data to demonstrate compliance or to present written documentation of standards clarification from SIG. The accreditation consultant or designee should alert the MSO if an issue is identified with a MM standard so that you are prepared with policies and data to support compliance at the Daily Briefing the following morning or other session designated for issue resolution. It is preferable to resolve any identified issues with the surveyors while they are on site. If possible, the MSO and/or the director of pharmacy should attend Daily Briefings. If this is not possible, the MSO can provide their administrator with supporting documentation.

At the conclusion of the survey, the survey team compiles and analyzes findings that have been entered into a software program in a laptop computer throughout the survey.[24] During the Exit Briefing, the survey team leader meets with the chief executive officer (CEO) prior to the exit conference to discuss any concerns and to provide the CEO with the preliminary Summary of Survey Findings Report. The report does not include an accreditation decision or an overall score, but the report includes a listing of the preliminary RFIs as well as any CMS standard and condition-level findings. Finally, an exit conference is held at the discretion of the CEO. During the exit conference the surveyors review the Summary of Survey Findings Report with invited senior leaders and discuss any patterns identified in performance.

Post Survey

Following the survey, the Report of Survey Findings is posted on the organization's extranet site and includes any RFIs.[12] If there are no RFIs, the accreditation decision is available at this time. For each EP found not fully compliant, an RFI is generated and requires that an electronic ESC report be submitted on the extranet site within 45 days for direct findings and within 60 days for indirect findings. All corrective actions must be completed at the time the ESC is submitted. If you have data supporting compliance for any EP listed as an RFI, it is highly desirable to submit the supporting data as a clarification for possible removal of the RFI. Following acceptance of an ESC report, the final accreditation decision is delivered.

If there are RFIs for any MM or other medication-related standards, you will likely be involved in creating a corrective action plan for submission to TJC as well as ESC and MOS if required. If the ESC is accepted, the organization audits data for at least 4 consecutive months and submits the average compliance rate for the 4-month period. At 4 months, if the MOS demonstrates acceptable and sustained improvement, no further monitoring is required. If the MOS results are not acceptable, the organization goes under Provisional Accreditation and has another 4 months to demonstrate sustained improvement. The MSO generally partners with the accreditation coordinator to assist with assessing progress toward the corrective action plan, data collection, and staff education. In addition, any compliance issues identified at the survey, but not recognized by the surveyors, should also be addressed at this time. You should refer to the TJC manual for information on submitting a clarifying ESC in the event that an organization believes that it was compliant with a particular standard at the time of survey. Also refer to the TJC manual for all possible accreditation decisions and the appeal process.

How to Prepare for a CMS Survey

CMS contract with a state agency, usually the state department of health, to perform the survey of a health care facility. The successful outcome of a CMS survey is an organization's *certification* to participate in the Medicare program. A CMS survey is unannounced and may result from a complaint being filed with the state department of health. Validation surveys are performed on a small percentage of accredited hospitals to ensure the quality of accreditation surveys.[10] Also, a hospital that loses or discontinues accreditation from a private agency is considered not *deemed* to meet CMS CoPs and is scheduled for a CMS survey. The survey team's makeup, interpretation, rigor, and duration may vary somewhat from state to state.

CMS CoPs for Pharmaceutical Services are organized by the condition that must be met, followed by the standard (e.g., expected performance) and the interpretive guideline for meeting the standard. CMS has established Survey Protocols and Interpretive Guidelines to provide guidance to surveyors and to clarify the intent of the regulations. Both can be found online in the *State Operations Manual*, Appendix A: Survey Protocol Regulations and Interpretive Guidelines for Hospitals.[26] Updates are published in the *Federal Register* and can be searched and viewed on the CMS website under Regulations and Guidance/Transmittals.[27] To receive updates via e-mail, subscribe to CMS Quarterly Provider Updates. It is important to become familiar with the CoPs and Interpretive Guidelines related to pharmacy services and medication because there is generally no warning that a CMS visit will occur. Similar to TJC preparation, it is useful to assemble a binder containing the relevant standards and evidence of compliance such as policies or audits. Identify your risk points for a CMS survey and develop an action plan to address deficiencies. Share this information with your staff and have the material readily available. Surveys notoriously occur when the most knowledgeable personnel are on vacation.

During a CMS survey, surveyors are evaluating hospital compliance with the CoPs for all services that receive reimbursement for patient care services under a provider name, through observation, interviews with staff and patients, and document review. Surveyors look for a well-designed QI plan and evidence of data and reporting. CMS surveys tend to focus on documented evidence of compliance with the CoP. In addition, emphasis is placed on storage and administration of medications.[10] Important topics include expired medications, refrigerator temperature logs, narcotic record keeping, and compliance with medication administration time policies. Of note, in November 2011 CMS updated its requirement for the medication administration "30-minute rule" (administration within 30 minutes before or after a scheduled time) to allow organizations the flexibility to design safer processes to avoid dangerous work-arounds taking place to meet the short timeframes. Organizations may customize medication administration policies within a 1- to 4-hour window (30–120 minutes before or after scheduled time) according to specific elements stated by CMS. Measurement of adherence to the policy is required. From the CMS manual, key differences between TJC and a CMS survey include surveyors who do not require an escort; can go anywhere in the hospital, at any time of day, evenings, and weekends; and can photocopy records and information to demonstrate noncompliance.

Surveyors are also looking for indications of *Immediate Jeopardy*, defined as "a situation in which the provider's noncompliance with one or more requirements of participation has caused, or is likely to cause, serious injury, harm, impairment, or death to a resident."[28] Medication-related examples of Immediate Jeopardy may include failure to protect a patient from adverse medication events or to provide the medication as ordered, such as administration of a medication to a patient with a known allergy or contraindication to the medication, or lack of required monitoring for efficacy or safety.

The hospital is informed of preliminary findings including citations and recommendations for noncompliance at the time of the exit conference.[26] How the deficiency is cited is based on the nature and extent of noncompliance. The State Department of Health mails a statement of deficiencies within 10 working days of the survey. A written plan of correction must be submitted within 10 working days of receipt of the statement of deficiencies. The statement of deficiencies along with the plan or correction is made public not later than 90 days after it is received by the hospital. If the hospital does not demonstrate compliance within a reasonable period of time, the state department of health certifies noncompliance and Medicare and Medicaid participation is terminated. There are outside agencies available for hire to help navigate a CMS survey and Immediate Jeopardy and to advise on the development of action plans.

CMS Quality Initiatives

The quality indicators known as core measures were initially developed by TJC and were later revised and adopted by CMS. Core measures relate to disease states such as pneumonia and heart failure, as well as processes such as the Surgical Care Improvement Project (SCIP).[29] Because performance for selected core measures is publicly reported, annual hospital PI goals may commonly include a goal to improve a core measure. Although an MSO is generally not responsible for performance on core measures, you will have a role in collaborating on strategies to improve performance. You may participate in teams working on a set of core measures or ensure that there is a pharmacist appointed to the team. MSOs can assist by reviewing order sets and guidelines for compliance with core measures and by educating pharmacy staff on requirements for meeting core measures.

In addition to core measures, CMS has developed other quality initiatives that are of interest to an MSO. The value-based purchasing (VBP) initiative applies to CMS payments in FY 13 for hospital discharges occurring on or after October 1, 2012. *VBP* refers to an incentive payment structure that rewards hospitals based on performance or improvement on quality measures. VBP offers opportunities for the MSO to support their organization through awareness of how their hospital is performing on publically reported quality measures and patient satisfaction measures. One of the patient satisfaction measures is related to patients receiving information about their medications prior to administration. The MSO can collaborate on gap analysis and improvement projects to help meet organizational goals.[30] *Hospital-acquired conditions* (HAC) or "never events" are severe, largely preventable occurrences that should "never" happen; CMS will not reimburse the health care facility for treatment of that condition. Selected HACs have medication safety implications such as falls, manifestations of poor glycemic control, and deep vein thrombosis/pulmonary embolism. As the MSO, you can participate by developing and monitoring guidelines and protocols to prevent these conditions. You can also review cases identified as HACs to identify opportunities for improvement.[31] Through funding from the Affordable Care Act, the CMS Innovation Center created hospital engagement networks (HENs) for collaboration on patient safety initiatives including reduction of adverse drug events. Although hospital participation in HENs is voluntary, they offer access to federally funded resources and an opportunity for MSOs to participate in the development of safety measures and offer leadership both locally and regionally.[32]

Other Regulatory Agencies

The Occupational Safety and Health Act of 1970 created both the Occupational Safety and Health Administration (OSHA) and the National Institute for Occupational Safety and Health (NIOSH). OSHA is under the U.S. Department of Labor and is responsible for development and enforcement of workplace safety and health regulation. Their website includes resources for health care facilities and Hospital eTool, which focuses on hazards found in the health care settings including the pharmacy, and describes standard requirements as well as recommended safe work practices for employee safety and health.[33,34] Additional topics include emergency preparedness and first responders' exposure to hazardous chemicals and latex allergies. OSHA enforces a number of standards that apply to pharmacies in health care facilities:[35]

- Employee Exposure and Medical Records Standard: 1910.1020
- Bloodborne Pathogens Standard: 1910.1030
- Hazard Communication Standard: 1910.1200
- Personal Protective Equipment: 1910.132(a)
- Eye and Face Protection: 1910.133
- Respiratory Protection Standard: 1910.134
- Hand Protection: 1910.138(a)
- Medical Services and First Aid: 1910.151(c)
- General Requirements—Walking/Working Surfaces: 1910.22

The Hazard Communication Standard requires that pharmacy staff know where to find and how to use the pharmacy's hazard communication program, a list of hazardous substances in the facility, material safety data sheets (MSDS), personal protective equipment, and spill kits.[10,36] OSHA responds to complaints filed against an employer with phone investigations or on-site investigations depending on the severity of the hazard.

NIOSH is part of the CDC under the Department of Health and Human Services and is the federal agency responsible for conducting research, providing education and training, and making recommendations for the prevention of work-related injury and illness. NIOSH serves in an advisory capacity and does not survey health care organizations. It offers information on occupational exposure and safe handling of chemotherapy and hazardous medications.[37] The NIOSH List of Antineoplastic and Other Hazardous Drugs in Health Care Settings 2012 is an important reference for the MSO for creating policies and procedures on handling of hazardous medication.[38,39]

The Environmental Protection Agency (EPA) develops and enforces regulations related to protecting human health and the environment. Under the Resource Conservation and Recovery Act (RCRA), the EPA has the authority to regulate hazardous waste including hazardous pharmaceutical waste from generation to disposal.[40] Approximately 5% of marketed drugs are considered hazardous including warfarin, nitroglycerin, and certain chemotherapy medications. Health care facilities currently are required to dispose of hazardous pharmaceutical waste separately from general waste, but proposed changes have been sent out for public comment and are forthcoming.[41,42]

The United States Pharmacopeia (USP) is a not-for-profit public health organization that sets standards for prescription and over-the-counter medications manufactured or sold in the United States. In September 2009, they published a *White Paper on USP's Role in Patient Safety* to promote patient safety through setting standards related to labeling and nomenclature.[43] TJC and other accrediting agencies expect hospitals to comply with USP <797> Standards on Pharmaceutical Compounding of Sterile Preparations.[44] Although USP does not survey, standards can be enforced by state boards of pharmacy as defined in the individual state's regulations.

Some state departments of health, notably the state of California, have taken a leadership role in furthering patient safety standards. The California Department of Public Health requires hospitals to develop a Medication Error Reduction Plan (MERP) and surveys hospitals for implementation of the plan as well as state regulations.[45] You should become familiar with your state's requirements.

State Boards of Pharmacy grant licenses for pharmacies and professionals and enforce the Pharmacy Practice Act as well as other laws including both federal and state Food, Drug and Cosmetic Acts, federal and state Controlled Substances Acts, and the Poison Prevention Packaging Act of 1970.

Summary

The MSO plays an important role in leading accreditation and regulatory compliance efforts. Opportunities include assessing compliance with accreditation and regulatory standards, developing action plans, educating staff, setting a tone of compliance for patient safety, and leading by example. When the opportunity arises to review proposed standard changes, you should take advantage of this to make sure the expectation is sound from a patient/medication safety and pharmacy perspective. Consider potential strategies to ensure compliance with the proposed new or revised standard to ensure a practical action plan is feasible.

Medication standards and regulations are not always easy to interpret, and designing practical strategies to ensure compliance and, more importantly, patient and medication safety, can be challenging. As an MSO, you must develop and maintain expertise on current accreditation and regulatory compliance information to fulfill your leadership and consultative organizational role in this area.

PRACTICE TIPS

1. Document performance improvement activities and actions taken *clearly and specifically* in committee minutes or through attachments in sufficient detail to serve as evidence of standard compliance activities during survey.
2. For policies required by accreditation standards, keep abreast of updates by requiring Pharmacy and Therapeutics Committee (or equivalent) review, as policy committees may inadvertently edit out policy and procedure statements required for accreditation.
3. Evaluate your organization's compliance honestly. Identifying, acknowledging, and correcting your problems up front will make the survey process more successful.
4. Highlight a Standard and "NPSG of the Month" via bulletin board, website, screen-saver, newsletter, or posters to assist with staff survey readiness.
5. For compliance challenges, use listserves to identify new strategies that work for other organizations.

Resources

CMS Conditions of Participation. Available at: http://www.cms.hhs.gov/manuals/downloads/som107ap_a_hospitals.pdf

CMS Quarterly provider updates by email (subscription)

Controlled Substances Act. Available at: http://www.deadiversion.usdoj.gov/21cfr/21usc/index.html Accessed October 8, 2012

http://www.cms.gov/AboutWebsite/EmailUpdates/itemdetail.asp?itemID=CMS1205639. Accessed October 8, 2012.

http://www.hospitalcompare.hhs.gov/ Accessed October 8, 2012.

http://www.osha.gov/SLTC/etools/hospital/expert/ex_pharmacy.html Accessed October 8, 2012.

Joint Commission on Accreditation of Healthcare Organizations (The Joint Commission). www.jointcommision.org

Joint Commission on Accreditation of Healthcare Organizations. Applied tracer methodology: tips and strategies for continuous systems improvement. Joint Commission Resources. 2007.

Joint Commission BoosterPak on Medication Storage.

Joint Commission Connect. Guest log-ins are available.

Joint Commission Hospital Accreditation Standards (HAS). *2012 Hospital Accreditation Standards*. Oakbrook Terrace, IL: Joint Commission Resources; 2012.

Joint Commission International. www.jointcommissioninternational.org

Joint Commission on Accreditation of Healthcare Organizations. *The Handbook on Storing and Securing Medications*. 2nd ed. Oakbrook Terrace, IL: Joint Commission Resources. 2009.

Joint Commission Perspectives. www.jcrinc.com/The-Joint-Commission-Perspectives/

Joint Commission Resources. www.jcrinc.com

Medicare Hospital Compare. Available at: www.hospitalcompare.hhs.gov Accessed November 17, 2012.

NIOSH list of antineoplastic and other hazardous drugs in healthcare settings 2012. Available at: http://www.cdc.gov/niosh/docs/2012-150/pdfs/2012-150.pdf. Accessed October 8, 2012.

OSHA Hospital eTool Expert Systems-Pharmacy. Available at: www.osha.gov/SLTC/etools/hospital/pharmacy/pharmacy.html Accessed November 17, 2012.

Safe Injection Practices to Prevent Transmission of Infections to Patients. Available at: http://www.cdc.gov/injectionsafety/ip07_standardprecaution.html Accessed November 17, 2012.

Standards Interpretation Group. http://www.jointcommission.org/standards_information/online_question_form.aspx Accessed November 17, 2012.

Uselton, JP, Kienle, Patricia C, Murdaugh, LB. *Assuring Continuous Compliance with Joint Commission Standards: A Pharmacy Guide*. 8th ed. Bethesda, MD: American Society of Health-System Pharmacists; 2010.

References

1. American Society of Health-System Pharmacists. Sample job descriptions. Available at: http://www.ashp.org/menu/PracticePolicy/ResourceCenters/PatientSafety/SampleJobDescriptions.aspx Accessed October 1, 2012.
2. Centers for Medicare & Medicaid Services. Hospitals. Available at: http://www.cms.gov/Medicare/Provider-Enrollment-and-Certification/CertificationandComplianc/Hospitals.html Accessed October 8, 2012.
3. The Joint Commission. Facts about federal deemed status and state recognition. Available at: http://www.jointcommission.org/assets/1/18/Facts_about_Federal_Deemed_Status.pdf Accessed October 8, 2012.
4. Vallejo BC, Flies LA, Fine DJ. A comparison of hospital accreditation programs. *J Clin Engineer.* 2011;32-38.
5. Meldi D, Rhoades F, Gippe A. The big three: A side by side matrix comparing hospital accrediting agencies. *Synergy.* 2009;12-14.
6. HFAP. Overview. Available at: http://www.hfap.org/about/overview.aspx. Assessed October 8, 2012.
7. DNV. Introduction to DNV Healthcare and NIAHO^{SM}: A new choice for hospital accreditation. Available at: http://dnvaccreditation.com/pr/dnv/document/introduction_to_dnv_healthcare_and_niaho-a_new_choice_for_hospital_accreditation-overview_tcm4-331352.pdf Accessed October 8, 2012.
8. DNV. Comparison of accreditation organizations. Available at: http://dnvaccreditation.com/pr/dnv/document/comparison-dnvhc_to_tjc_tcm4-358498.pdf Accessed October 8, 2012.
9. DerGurahian J. DNV setting new standard. *Mod Healthc.* 2008;October 27:2-4. Available at: http://www.nxtbook.com/ygsreprints/ygs/modh-1-25337720/#/2 Accessed October 8, 2012.
10. Uselton JP, Kienle PC, Murdaugh LB. *Assuring Continuous Compliance with Joint Commission Standards: A Pharmacy Guide.* Bethesda, MD: American Society of Health-System Pharmacists; 2010.
11. The Joint Commission. About the Joint Commission. Available at: http://www.jointcommission.org/assets/1/18/Mission_Statement_8_09.pdf Accessed October 8, 2012.
12. The Joint Commission. The accreditation process. In: *2012 Hospital Accreditation Standards (HAS).* Oak Brook, IL: Joint Commission on Accreditation of Healthcare Organizations; 2012.
13. The Joint Commission. How to use this book. In: *2012 Hospital Accreditation Standards (HAS).* Oak Brook, IL: Joint Commission on Accreditation of Healthcare Organizations; 2012.
14. The Joint Commission. Medication management. In: *2012 Hospital Accreditation Standards (HAS).* Oak Brook, IL: Joint Commission on Accreditation of Healthcare Organizations; 2012.
15. The Joint Commission. Facts about Joint Commission accreditation standards. Available at: http://www.jointcommission.org/assets/1/18/Standards1.PDF Accessed October 8, 2012.
16. The Joint Commission. Facts about national patient safety goals. Available at: http://www.jointcommission.org/assets/1/18/Facts_about_National_Patient_Safety_Goals.pdf Accessed October 8, 2012.
17. The Joint Commission. Hospital 2012 national patient safety goals. Available at: http://www.jointcommission.org/assets/1/6/2012_NPSG_HAP.pdf Accessed October 8, 2012.
18. The Joint Commission. Summary data of sentinel events reviewed by The Joint Commission. Available at: http://www.jointcommission.org/sentinel_event.aspx Accessed October 22, 2012.
19. The Joint Commission. Sentinel event statistics for 2011. *Jt Comm Perspect.* 2012;32(5):5.
20. The Joint Commission. Facts about the sentinel event policy. Available at: http://www.jointcommission.org/assets/1/18/Sentinel_Event_Policy_3_2011.pdf Accessed on October 8, 2012.

21. The Joint Commission. Sentinel events. Available at: http://www.jointcommission.org/assets/1/6/2011_CAMH_SE.pdf Accessed on October 8, 2012.
22. The Joint Commission. Top standards compliance issues for first half of 2012. *Jt Comm Perspect.* 2012;32(11):1,13-19.
23. The Joint Commission. Joint Commission to launch new intracycle monitoring process. *Jt Comm Perspect.* 2012;32(10):10-11.
24. The Joint Commission. Survey activity guide for healthcare organizations. 2012. Available at: http://www.jointcommission.org/assets/1/18/2012_Organization_SAG.pdf Accessed September 30, 2012.
25. Joint Commission Resources. Applied tracer methodology: tips and strategies for continuous systems improvement. Oakbrook IL: Joint Commission on Accreditation of Healthcare Organizations; 2007.
26. Centers for Medicare & Medicaid Services, Department of Health and Human Services. *State Operations Manual*, Appendix A: Survey protocol, regulations, and interpretive guidelines for hospitals, Rev 78 (12-22-11). Washington DC: Government Printing Office; 2008. Available at: http://www.cms.hhs.gov/manuals/downloads/som107ap_a_hospitals.pdf Accessed on October 8, 2012.
27. Centers for Medicare & Medicaid Services, Department of Health and Human Services. Regulations and guidance: Transmittals. Available at: http://www.cms.gov/Transmittals/2012Trans/list.asp Accessed on October 8, 2012.
28. Centers for Medicare & Medicaid Services, Department of Health and Human Services. *State Operations Manual*, Appendix Q-Guidelines for determining immediate jeopardy, Rev 1 (05-21-04). Washington DC: Government Printing Office; 2008. Available at: http://cms.gov/manuals/Downloads/som107ap_q_immedjeopardy.pdf Accessed October 8, 2012.
29. Chassin MR, Loeb JM, Schmaltz SP, Wachter RM. Accountability measures: Using measurement to promote quality improvement. *N Engl J Med.* 2010;363(7):683-688.
30. Centers for Medicare & Medicaid Services, Department of Health and Human Services. Medicare Program; Hospital Inpatient Value-Based Purchasing Program. http://www.gpo.gov/fdsys/pkg/FR-2011-05-06/pdf/2011-10568.pdf Accessed October 8, 2012.
31. Centers for Medicare & Medicaid Services, Department of Health and Human Services. Hospital acquired conditions. Available at http://www.cms.gov/HospitalAcqCond/06_Hospital-Acquired_Conditions.asp#TopOfPage Accessed on October 8, 2012.
32. Centers for Medicare & Medicaid Services. Partnerships for Patients. Available at: http://www.innovations.cms.gov/initiatives/Partnership-for-Patients/index.html Accessed November 4, 2012.
33. Occupational Safety & Health Administration (OSHA). Hospital E-tool. Available at: http://www.osha.gov/SLTC/etools/hospital/index.html Accessed October 8, 2012.
34. Occupational Safety & Health Administration (OSHA). Healthcare facilities-OSHA standards. Available at: http://www.osha.gov/SLTC/healthcarefacilities/index.html Accessed October 8, 2012.
35. Occupational Safety & Health Administration (OSHA). Regulations. Available at: http://www.osha.gov/pls/oshaweb/owasrch.search_form?p_doc_type=STANDARDS&p_toc_level=1&p_keyvalue=1910 Accessed October 8, 2012.
36. Occupational Safety & Health Administration (OSHA). Hazard communication. Available at: http://www.osha.gov/pls/oshaweb/owadisp.show_document?p_table=STANDARDS&p_id=10099 Accessed October 8, 2012.
37. National Institute for Occupational Safety and Health [NIOSH]. NIOSH alert: preventing occupational exposure to antineoplastic and other hazardous drugs in health care settings. Available at: http://www.cdc.gov/niosh/docs/2004-165/ Accessed October 8, 2012.

38. National Institute for Occupational Safety and Health [NIOSH]. NIOSH list of antineoplastic and other hazardous drugs in healthcare settings 2012. Available at: http://www.cdc.gov/niosh/docs/2012-150/pdfs/2012-150.pdf Accessed October 8, 2012.

39. National Institute for Occupational Safety and Health [NIOSH]. NIOSH workplace safety and health topics. Available at: http://www.cdc.gov/niosh/topics/healthcare/ Accessed September 30, 2012.

40. United States Environmental Protection Agency. Summary of the Resource Conservation and Recovery Act. Available at: http://www.epa.gov/lawsregs/laws/rcra.html Accessed October 8, 2012.

41. United States Environmental Protection Agency. Management of Hazardous Waste Pharmaceuticals. Available at: http://www.epa.gov/wastes/hazard/generation/pharmaceuticals.htm Accessed October 8,2012.

42. United States Environmental Protection Agency. Draft document: best management practices for unused pharmaceuticals at health care facilities. Available at: http://water.epa.gov/scitech/wastetech/guide/upload/unuseddraft.pdf Accessed October 8, 2012.

43. The United States Pharmacopeial Convention [USPC]. White paper USP's role in patient safety. Available at: http://www.usp.org/sites/default/files/usp_pdf/EN/members/patientSafety.pdf Accessed October 8, 2012.

44. The United States Pharmacopeial Convention [USPC]. General Chapter <797>: Pharmaceutical compounding—sterile preparations. In: *The United States Pharmacopeia*, 32nd rev. ed., and the National Formulary, 27th ed. Rockville, MD: USPC; 2009.

45. California Department of Public Health. Medication Error Reduction Plan (MERP) Program. Available at: http://www.cdph.ca.gov/programs/LnC/Pages/MERP.aspx. Accessed November 4, 2012.

Appendix 4-A

Selected Standards from TJC Chapters Other Than Medication Management Relevant for MSOs

Chapter	Standard	Content
Environment of Care (EC)	**EC.02.02.01** The hospital manages risks related to hazardous materials and waste.	Implements procedures for response to hazardous material or waste spill or exposure which include precautions and personal protective equipment. Minimize risk associated with disposal of hazardous mediations, chemicals, and radioactive materials. The hospital labels and maintains a list of hazardous materials and waste, and has access to material safety data sheets (MSDS).
Emergency Management (EM)	**EM.02.02.03** As part of its Emergency Operations Plan, the hospital prepares for how it will manage resources and assets during emergencies.	Emergency operations plan includes how to obtain and restock medications required throughout emergency response and recovery including access to and distribution of stockpiles.
Human Resources (HR)	**HR.01.02.05** The hospital verifies staff qualifications	Verify licensure, education, criminal background check and health screening at time of hire. Primary source verification for license renewal.
	HR.01.04.01 The hospital provides orientation to staff.	Requirements for orientation and ongoing training.
	HR.01.05.03 Staff participate in ongoing education and training.	
	HR.01.06.01 Staff are competent to perform their responsibilities.	Define competency, initially assess competency and re-assess every 3 years at minimum.
	HR.01.07.01 The hospital evaluates staff performance.	Staff performance is evaluated at minimum every 3 years.
Infection Control (IC)	**IC.02.04.01** The hospital offers vaccination against influenza to LIPs and staff.	Annual program to vaccinate staff against influenza and provide education. The hospital improves its vaccination rates.

continued

Information Management (IM)	**IM.01.01.03** The hospital plans for continuity of its information management process.	Plan for managing interruptions to information processes and back-up systems.
	IM.02.01.01 The hospital protects the privacy of health information.	Use protected health information only for purposes allowed by law and regulation or authorized by the patient.
	IM.02.02.01 The hospital effectively manages the collection of health information.	The hospital designates a list of abbreviations that are prohibited from use.
Leadership (LD)	**LD.04.01.01** The hospital complies with law and regulation.	Controlled substance record keeping.
	LD.04.03.09 Care, treatment, and services provided through contractual agreement are provided safely and effectively.	Applies to medication procurement, such as "outsourcing" medications. Written contracts are reviewed by leaders. Monitor services provided and take steps when expectations are not met.
	LD.04.04.03 New or modified services or processes are well designed.	Incorporates an assessment of risks to patients and evidence-based best practice.
	LD.04.04.05 The hospital has an organization-wide, integrated patient safety program within its performance improvement activities.	Organization-wide, integrated patient safety program includes review of potential events, blame-free reporting of errors, root cause analysis for sentinel events, proactive risk assessment of one high-risk process at least every 18 months, and external reporting of significant adverse events.
Medical Staff (MS)	**MS.05.01.01** The organized medical staff has a leadership role in organization performance improvement activities to improve quality of care, treatment, and services and patient safety.	Provides leadership in measurement, assessment, and improvement of use of medications.
	MS.08.01.03 Ongoing professional practice evaluation information is factored into the decision to maintain, revise, or revoke existing privileges prior to or at the time of renewal.	Professional practice evaluation may include patterns of medication use as it relates to patient safety and quality of care.

continued

Provision of Care, Treatment, and Services (PC)	**PC.01.02.07** The hospital assesses and manages the patient's pain.	Comprehensive pain assessment and response to the patient's pain.
	PC.01.02.08 The hospital assesses and manages the patient's risk for falls.	Implement interventions to prevent patient falls.
	PC.02.01.03 The hospital provides care, treatment, and services as ordered or prescribed, and in accordance with law and regulation.	Scope of practice issues regarding prn medication orders or titration orders. "Read back" process for verbal orders.
	PC.02.03.01 The hospital provides patient education and training based on the patient's needs and abilities.	Provide patient with information on the safe and effective use of medications and pain management.
	PC.03.01.01 The hospital plans operative or other high-risk procedures, including those that require the administration of moderate or deep sedation or anesthesia.	Staff credentialed to administer sedation and rescue patients from whatever level of sedation is achieved, adequate personnel to monitor sedation, and availability of emergency resuscitation equipment
Performance Improvement (PI)	**PI.01.01.01** The hospital collects data to monitor its performance.	The hospital collects data on: ▪ adverse events related to moderate or deep sedation or anesthesia; ▪ significant medication errors; ▪ significant adverse drug reactions.
	PI.03.01.01 The hospital improves performance on an ongoing basis.	The hospital takes action and evaluates that actions taken have achieved desired improvement.
Record of Care, Treatment, and Services (RC)	**RC.02.01.01** The medical record contains information that reflects the patient's care, treatment, and services.	The medical record contains: ▪ any allergies to medication, ▪ any medications ordered or administered, ▪ any adverse drug reactions, ▪ any medication prescribed on discharge.
	RC.02.01.07 The medical record contains a summary list for each patient who receives continuing ambulatory care services.	The summary list contains any adverse or allergic drug reactions and any current medications. The list is updated whenever there is a change.

continued

Rights and Responsibilities of the Individual (RI)	**RI.01.01.03** The hospital respects the patient's right to receive information in a manner he or she understands.	Drug information is provided in an appropriate manner for the patient's age, language, and ability to understand.
	RI. 01.03.05 The hospital protects the patient and respects his or her rights during research, investigation, and clinical trials	Information is provided to the patient to assist in making the decision to participate in research or clinical trials.
Waived Testing (WT)	**WT.03.01.01** Staff and LIP performing waived tests are competent.	Staff and LIP have been trained for each test that they are authorized to perform. The training and competency for each waived test are documented. Applies to point-of-care testing.

For more information and standards, please see The Joint Commission. *2012 Hospital Accreditation Standards* (HAS). Oak Brook, IL: Joint Commission on Accreditation of Healthcare Organizations; 2012.

Appendix 4-B

Medication Areas Inspection Form

Area	Date			Comments
	Yes	No	N/A	
Automated Medication Cabinet Storage Area				
1. Medications are in approved storage area				
2. Medication area clear of food/drink				
3. Potentially hazardous drugs labeled with special labels				
4. Patient's medications are labeled properly				
5. Automated medication cabinet area is secured				
6. Saline bags are NOT being used as multidose bags for flushing				
7. No unsecured drugs on top of carts, counters, or patient bedsides				
8. No samples or non-formulary drugs in unit stock				
9. Multi-dose vials dated and initialed in conformance with policy				
10. All single-use vials discarded after use				
11. Syringes/needles stored securely from public access				
12. Automated medication station functions properly				
13. Medications stored in medication server not expired and still active				
14. Patient medication drawers clean and organized				
15. Patient-specific medications stored separate from stock meds				
16. Cytotoxic and biohazard waste disposed of properly				

continued

17. All medications have clean, legible labels				
18. Sharps disposed of properly				
19. Medication storage area is locked and secure				
Crash Cart				
20. Crash cart has a backboard				
21. Crash cart has RPH's initials				
22. Crash cart lock number matches the appropriate documented number				
23. Crash cart expiration date is >1 month from date of inspection				
24. Crash carts locked and secure and in assigned area				
Emergency Drug Box				
25. Emergency drug boxes locked and secure				
26. Emergency drug box has (RPH/TECH) initials				
27. Emergency drug box expiration date is >1 month from date of inspection				
28. Emergency drug box lock number matches the appropriate documented number				
Medication Refrigerator				
29. Medication refrigerator temperature between 4–8 degrees Celsius or 36–46 degrees Fahrenheit				
30. Daily temperature log being maintained, actions noted				
31. Medication refrigerator clean and organized				
32. No food or unauthorized medications in medication refrigerator				
33. Medication refrigerator is labeled with "No Food: Medications Only"				

continued

Patient's Home Medications				
34. Discharged patient's home medications have been removed				
35. Patient's medications from home cabinet checked				
Miscellaneous				
36. Is the pharmacy's phone number posted?				
37. Poison control number available				
38. Appropriate tablet crusher available (no mortar and pestle)				
Documentation Reminder				
39. If applicable, drug box/crash cart lock number(s) and expiration date(s) are noted on inspection form				

Source: Adapted with permission from Uselton JP, Kienle PC, Murdaugh LB. *Assuring Continuous Compliance with Joint Commission Standards: A Pharmacy Guide.* Bethesda, MD: American Society of Health-System Pharmacists, Inc; 2010:385–386.

Appendix 4-C

Medication Management Mock Survey Tracer

Follow Administered Medication Through Medication-Use Process

Element/Question	Resource	Yes	No	If No, Explanation	Action Plan
Prescribing					
Authorized prescriber?	P/P				
Ordering criteria followed?	P/P				
Complete order, no abbreviations					
If order set, approved and in-date					
If verbal order, meets criteria for use					
High-alert requirements followed if applies	P/P				
Patient information accessed used for medication, e.g., INR for warfarin	P/P, medical record				
Diagnosis, condition, or indication for use documented	medical record				
Procurement/Storage					
Medication on formulary?	formulary				
If not on formulary, NF policy followed	P/P				
If medication shortage: Evidence of communication Policy followed	documents, P/P				
Medication stored at proper temperature/light	mfr, P/P				
Medication storage is secure	P/P				
Most ready-to-administer dosage form?	mfr, formulary				

continued

Element/Question	Resource	Yes	No	If No, Explanation	Action Plan
If patient's own medication, stored per P/P	P/P				
If high alert, requirements followed	P/P				
Pharmacist Review					
Review completed prior to dispensing or removal from ADC If not, exception criteria met?	PIS, P/P				
Any concerns re: allergy, interactions, dose/route/frequency, duplications, contraindications, lab values	reviewer, PIS				
If order was clarified, documentation exists Clarified directly w/prescriber if appropriate	PIS, medical record, P/P				
If manual entry, transcription accurate	PIS, medical record				
If manual entry, two patient identifiers used	observation				
Scheduled appropriately	P/P, eMAR				
Dispensing/Medication Preparation					
If ADC, fill process per P/P	P/P				
If sterile product, follows all standards	USP <797>, NIOSH, P/P, CDC Safe Injection Practice				
If high alert, P/P followed	P/P				
If on hazardous substance list, P/P followed	P/P				
Product labeled appropriately	P/P, TJC				

continued

Element/Question	Resource	Yes	No	If No, Explanation	Action Plan
Unit dose?	product				
Ready-to-use form?	product				
Administration					
Administered by authorized person?	P/P				
MAR accurate?	MAR				
Administered according to schedule or PRN indication	MAR				
Observed administration process follows established process, including: ■ Two patient identifiers ■ Bar code drug, patient wrist band ■ Correct medication verified prior to administration ■ Correct medication preparation, if required (for example, dilution) ■ Hold parameters followed if applicable	observation, P/P, MAR				
Patient education completed	observation, medical record, P/P				
Monitoring					
Documentation of patient response	medical record				
If error occurred during process, was it reported?	P/P, risk report system				

continued

Element/Question	Resource	Yes	No	If No, Explanation	Action Plan
If ADR occurred, was it reported?	P/P, risk report system				

ADC, automated dispensing cabinets ; CDC, Centers for Disease Control and Prevention; eMAR, electronic medication administration record; MAR, medication administration record; mfr, manufacturer; NIOSH, National Institute for Occupational Safety and Health; NF, non-formulary; PIS, pharmacy information system; P/P, policy and procedure; PRN, as needed; TJC, The Joint Commission.

Source: Courtesy of Deb Saine, Winchester Medical Center.

An Overview of Human Errors and Culture of Safety

Sarah Hein

CHAPTER 5

Key Terms

Blame and Train Culture—A culture in which the person is assumed to be able to perform without error, if properly educated and motivated. Latent failures are not considered. Errors are attributed to laziness, negligence, or incompetence, resulting in blaming and/or retraining the person that made the error.

Hindsight Bias—The tendency for those evaluating an error to overestimate what they would have known, and what others should have known at the time of the error.

Human Error—The failure of planned actions to achieve their desired ends, without the intervention of some unforeseeable event. Human errors can be further divided into slips, lapses, and mistakes.

Just Culture—A culture that recognizes the contribution of systems in error along with a focus on behavioral choices and accountability. Just Culture distinguishes between acceptable and unacceptable behavior, between unsafe acts and the blatant disregard of safety procedures with which most peers would comply. Just Culture is one component of an overarching safety culture.

Slips and Lapses—A human error whereby the action deviates from the intention. A slip is when an action is carried forth, but deviated from the intention. A lapse is when there was an intention of an action, but the action was forgotten.

Symmetry Bias—The tendency to assign blame for an error in a manner that is proportional to the severity of the outcome (also called *Severity Bias*).

Systems Thinking—Evaluating the whole process rather than a particular single part, since all parts are inter-related. This approach includes consideration of everyone who could potentially influence the process.

Violation—The action of bypassing a rule, standard, or safe operating procedure. Violations can be further divided into optimizing violations, necessary violations, and routine violations.

Introduction

This chapter is designed to introduce the medication safety officer (MSO) to the theory behind **human errors**, and entice him or her to learn more. It provides a foundation for understanding the importance of this information, and how it can be utilized to improve organizational culture and system-wide safety. The historical **"blame and train"** model for error management needs to be permanently abandoned. Understanding human error theory helps an MSO evaluate, improve, and design processes to reduce the risk of error. Even more importantly, human error theory recognizes that when humans are involved in a system, the risk of error can be reduced, but not eliminated. With that in mind, human error theory also helps an MSO to design processes to capture and mitigate the effects of those ever-present human errors, thus reducing the potential for harm. The discussion begins with *How We Think* and *How We Err*. Then the human error is merged with the concepts of culture, which discusses the progression of human error management in health care over time. A discussion of strategies the MSO may use to influence culture follows. Finally, the review of adverse outcome events, and some related tools are discussed.

This chapter serves as an introduction to a broad and complicated subject. It is highly recommended that the reader add two books by James Reason to their reference library, *Managing the Risks of Organizational Accidents*[1] and *Human Error*.[2] These books take chapters to describe, eloquently and in detail, what might be described here in a paragraph. In particular, the sections How We Think and How We Err are derived from these books.

How We Think[1,2]

Skill-Rule-Knowledge Model

The skill-rule-knowledge model assists in the understanding of the types of human errors that can occur during cognitive processing by outlining how the mind is working during different types of tasks. A thorough understanding of this model is essential for the MSO in procedure design and evaluation, during which the goals are to minimize the number of errors that occur, and maximize the likelihood that they are captured before causing harm.

- **Skill-based processing.** Skill-based processing is used when performing routine tasks and is sometimes referred to as *automatic processing*. It is routine, automatic, and requires no real focus, only occasional checks to see that the task is progressing as usual. Skill-based processing allows for multitasking, and without it, humans would be unable to function. An example of skill-based processing would be the process of an experienced driver encountering a stop sign. An experienced driver does not need to carefully consider when to begin pressing the brake pedal; it happens automatically. Braking at a stop sign can even occur safely during a conversation with a fellow passenger, because it is automatic for experienced drivers. In health care, skill-based processing occurs while an experienced pharmacist is performing one of his or her usual daily tasks, such as entering medication orders into the computer, or while an experienced nurse is performing one of his or her usual daily tasks, such as administering medications. The error rate during skill-based processing is a low percentage of the number of tasks that are being done, because the processes are familiar. However, because humans are so often using skill-based processing, the overall number of errors is high. Thankfully, the recognition and correction of skill-based processing errors is also high.

- **Rule-based processing.** Rule-based processing is used when, in the course of skill-based processing, a person becomes aware that there is a problem. The conditions of the problem are matched with the conditions of past problems. When a match with a past problem is found, a past solution is applied, using an "if–then do" rule. *If* a process is not progressing as usual because of a problem *then do* this, as this is what solved the problem last time. Rule-based processing is also described as *intuitive processing*. Continuing with the driving example above, an experienced driver may be on the way home from work when it begins to rain heavily. From experience, the driver knows that deep puddles quickly accumulate at certain street corners during a heavy rain. From experience, the driver knows which alternate route avoids the deep puddles, and the driver sets off on the non-puddle-encountering route. *If* it is raining heavily *then* take the alternate route. In health care, consider the example of the experienced pharmacist entering a medication order into the computer. During order entry, the pharmacist receives an allergy flag, indicating that the patient has an allergy to the medication being entered. The pharmacist recognized that a problem has occurred and applies the usual procedure to solve it—halting the order entry and telephoning the physician with an alternate recommendation. *If* a patient has an allergy to an ordered medication, *then* call the physician to discuss alternatives. As with skill-based processing, rule-based processing has a low error rate compared to the number of rule-matches being done. But, because it is a level of processing that is often used, rule-based errors are seen frequently, although not as frequently as skill-based errors.
- **Knowledge-based processing.** Knowledge-based processing is focused problem solving and is sometimes called *analytical processing*. As with rule-based processing, there is awareness that a problem has been encountered, but with this problem, there is an inability to find a match with a previous problem, so

there is no rule to apply. Knowledge-based processing is entered very reluctantly due to its requirement of focus and attention. Only after every possible rule has been exhausted will a person move to knowledge-based processing. For novices, knowledge-based processing is encountered frequently, until expertise (in the shape of rules) is developed. The potential for a solution, or new rule, increases with time and with the ability to test potential solutions through trial and error. In emergency situations or situations with time constraints and no opportunity to test solutions, there is a high risk of failure, in the form of an incorrect solution. The medical professions recognize the value of experience and the risk of knowledge-based processing and require extensive observed training as part of licensure. Automobile insurance companies recognize the risk of knowledge-based processing as well, as evidenced by the insurance premiums for new drivers. Although the risk of error is very high, knowledge-based processing is not encountered very often. As a result, knowledge-based processing results in a low contribution to the overall number of errors occurring or being reported in most systems.

Interestingly, all three levels of processing may occur at once. Consider a person getting dressed (skill-based), finding shoes to match (rule-based), and thinking about a problem that needs resolution at work (knowledge-based).

How We Err[1,2]

For the purposes of this chapter, we will use Reason's definition of human error: "The failure of planned actions to achieve their desired ends—without the intervention of some unforeseeable event."[2] Human errors can occur in the planning, storage, or execution of a process. Failures in storage and execution of a process are called **slips and lapses** and occur during skill-based processing. Mistakes—failures in planning or choosing a course of action—occur during rule-based or knowledge-based processing. The skill-rule-knowledge model and associated errors are outlined in Table 5-1.

Skill-Based Slips and Lapses

A *slip* is an action that was not carried out, or executed, according to plan. Slips are attention failures, so it follows that the risk of slips is increased with mental states that may affect a person's attention, like stress, preoccupation, depression, or distraction. Slips can also be perception failures, as with look-alike or sound-alike medication names or packaging that results in the wrong medication being picked from the shelf for dispensing. Because skill-based processing involves only occasional cursory checks, the human mind will "fill in the blanks" frequently, so that the mental check appears to confirm that the action is being carried out correctly, when in fact, it is not. A *lapse* is an action or step in the process that was forgotten. Lapses are memory failures, so it follows that the risk of lapses increases with interruption during the action (causing a person to forget their place in a series of actions) or if there is a delay between the time the action is decided and the time it is actually carried out (causing the person to forget the action altogether). An example of a lapse would

Table 5-1. Skill-Rule-Knowledge Model and Associated Errors

Processing	Description	Error Types
Skill-based (Automatic)	Routine tasks with occasional checks	Slip (execution/action failure) Lapse (storage/memory failure)
Rule-based (Intuitive)	Problem encountered, use experience to solve (refer to previously used rules)	Mistake (planning failure), rule-based ■ Good rule/wrong time ■ Bad rule
	Bypassing of rules or safety procedures	Violation ■ Optimizing (thrill-seeking) ■ Necessary (impossible to follow rule) ■ Routine (corner-cutting)
Knowledge-based (Analytical)	Problem encountered, no experience, create solution	Mistake (planning failure), knowledge-based ■ Created solution incorrect

be forgetting to place an auxiliary label on a medication before dispensing, resulting in a call from the nurse to inquire about food-drug interactions.

A more dramatic example of a lapse is reported all too frequently in the newspaper: the story of a child forgotten in a car on a hot summer day. Typically, the person driving the child does not routinely drive the child. The child is in the back of the vehicle, and the driver begins a routine route, such as driving to work or driving home. Once the process of driving the routine route has begun, the driver enters skill-based processing. Because taking the child out of the car is not part of this normal routine, and because the child is often sleeping quietly and out of sight, there is nothing to alert the driver at the end of the process, and the sleeping child is forgotten. Story after story tells of a parent calling the person who drove the child—the other parent, grandparent, or friend—hours later, to ask why the child is not at daycare. It is at that moment that the person who drove the child realizes that the child is still in the car.

What is interesting about these two lapses—forgetting an auxiliary label on a medication leading to a nurse's phone call, or forgetting a child in the back of a car leading to death—is that they are the same human error, even if the consequences are tragically different. Why does the death of a child make that lapse seem so much more blameworthy? It is because there is a tendency for humans to assign blame for an error in a manner or amount that is roughly proportional to the severity of the outcome. To illustrate this **symmetry bias**, Reason refers to the writings of Sir Frances Bacon in 1620, "The human mind is prone to suppose the existence of more order and regularity in the world than it finds."[3] This tendency has also been referred to as severity bias.[4] Recognizing the tendency to incorrectly balance the blameworthiness of an error to the severity of the outcome is extremely important when evaluating medication errors as part of a medication safety system.

Rule-Based Mistakes

Rule-based processing requires application of rules to solve problems. *Rule-based mistakes* can occur if the current problem is assessed incorrectly, and therefore incorrectly "matched" to a previous problem, so that a usually good rule is applied at the wrong time. This misapplication of a rule occurs for a number of reasons such as the need to review a large number of factors to assess the current problem for matching, the similarity of the current problem to past problems in which the rule would be correctly applied, and the good rule's previous frequency of success. An example of a good rule/wrong time error would be a technician mistakenly sending a fragile, protein-based medication through the jarring tube transport system to a nursing unit. Many hospitals use tube systems to deliver first doses of medications or medications that are needed emergently. The technician knows that *if* the medication needs to be delivered emergently *then* it is sent via the tube system. This rule typically results in success. However, this rule does not apply to a very small subset of fragile, protein-based medications.

A *violation* is another rule-based mistake that involves a good rule. A violation is a good rule that is not used when it should be, when a standard or safe operating procedure is bypassed. Violations are discussed in detail later.

There are also rule-based mistakes that involve the use of a bad rule. Bad rules are usually due to procedures that are incomplete or misunderstood, which results in an informal method for carrying out the task. The informal method may, unbeknown to the users, introduce safety risks. An example of a bad rule would be the use of intravenous syringes to deliver a dose of oral medication, when oral syringes are available for use but there is no procedure dictating that they must be used. It may be that a nurse observed this bad rule in training: *if* an oral medication must be administered *then* these intravenous syringes will accomplish the task. Without an understanding of the danger in the use of intravenous syringes to administer oral medications, or a policy outlining the appropriate use of oral syringes, the availability of oral syringes does not cause the nurse to change this dangerous practice and use them.

Knowledge-Based Mistakes

Knowledge-based mistakes are those that occur during focused problem solving. Because there is no experience with the problem and no rule that can be used to manage it, there is a high likelihood that the devised plan will be incorrect. Most pharmacists remember many knowledge-based mistakes from early in their practice and remember how thankful they were to be working under the oversight of an experienced pharmacist.

Violations

As stated earlier, a violation occurs when a good rule, standard, or safe operating procedure is bypassed. Violations are further divided into three types: optimizing, routine, and necessary.

- **Optimizing violations.** *Optimizing violations* are the bypassing of a good rule because it is fun or exciting. An example of an optimizing violation would be driving at excessive speeds while test driving a sports car. Optimizing violations are well recognized in the common aviation expression: *There are old pilots, and there are bold pilots, but there are no old bold pilots.* An optimizing violation is difficult to imagine in the medication-use process, aside from riding a delivery cart down a hospital hallway. Although there are violations that clearly lead to a shorter pathway from point A to point B, these should not be confused with optimizing violations because those are not the result of thrill-seeking behavior.
- **Necessary violations.** *Necessary violations* are the bypassing of a good rule because it is impossible or inadvisable to follow the good rule at that time. An example of a necessary violation would be the requirement for a nursing double check of subcutaneous insulin doses. This requirement might work well on most days, but be difficult to meet on a shift in an outlying clinic when one of the two nurses working must leave suddenly for a family emergency. The remaining nurse may deem it necessary to administer the insulin to a hyperglycemic patient without the double check, which is a necessary violation. In the absence of an adverse outcome, the nurse may choose to again bypass the double check of a subcutaneous insulin dose on a day when both nurses are present, but really busy. With continued absence of adverse outcomes, the nurse may adopt the bypassing of the double check into the routine insulin administration process. This is no longer a necessary violation; it has become a routine violation.
- **Routine violations.** *Routine violations* can also be called corner-cutting. Routine violations may be due to clumsy procedures, or those that seem clumsy because of an inadequate understanding of the need for the procedure's additional safety steps. As humans will naturally gravitate toward the processes that require the least effort, or the shortest route from point A to point B, routine violations can always be found in an organization. An example of a routine violation is the bypass of double checks of subcutaneous insulin doses when two nurses are present, as above. The most effective way to manage routine violations is to reward those complying with the safety procedures, rather than punishing those who do not.

Migration: Production Versus Protection

Within an organization, there will be fluctuations in the balance between production goals and protection goals, which can affect the frequency of necessary and routine violations. Production refers to output—things like the number of patients seen, paperwork completed, orders entered, surgeries done, etc. Production keeps the bills paid and the organization open for business. Protection refers to safety procedures that prevent error and harm but can also slow production. Production pressure is increased when practitioners are encouraged to do more with less resources, time, or staff. To keep up with the load, the staff may begin to bypass safety procedures. Without a visible adverse outcome, the staff will be rewarded by their managers for meeting the production goals. Ironically, the managers are also unknowingly rewarding the staff for bypassing safety procedures.

This might go on for some time without an adverse outcome. Eventually, the bypassed safety procedures will undermine protection, and processes will migrate to beyond the edge of safe practice. Suddenly, the organization is faced with a catastrophic event due to an error. In response to the event, the original safety procedures are judged inadequate, even if they would have prevented the event had they not been bypassed. Additional, unnecessary defenses might be added to enhance the safety procedures, increasing protection, but decreasing production. The cycle continues after some time passes, and production comes back into focus, as is necessary to keep the bills paid and the organization open for business.

It is important to realize that there will always be this fluctuation in the balance between production and protection, and there will always be migration toward the violation of safety procedures. The best course of action is to investigate the system-based sources of the migration.[2,5,6] Consider the need for updating of safety procedures that may no longer apply or could be streamlined. Also, review what is being rewarded by management and whether both production and protection rewards are included.

Culture of Safety

Culture is the collection of values and practices shared by people and groups in an organization. These shared beliefs and attitudes determine the way people and groups interact with each other and with stakeholders outside the organization. Simply put, the culture is "the way we do things here." Patient safety culture is often thought of as a subset of the overall organizational culture. Reason describes five components of a safety culture: flexible, informed, learning, reporting, and Just Cultures (see Figure 5-1).[7]

Evolution of Cultural Perspectives in Patient Safety

Adverse outcome events are comprised of both active failures and latent failures. Active failures are the human errors and violations. Latent failures are at-risk situations that have set the stage for an active failure to become an adverse event, by either increasing the likelihood of the active failure, or by allowing the active failure to go unnoticed. Latent failures occur through the allocation of resources, hiring practices, training, scheduling, layout of workspaces, etc. Latent failures will always be present in a system.[2,8]

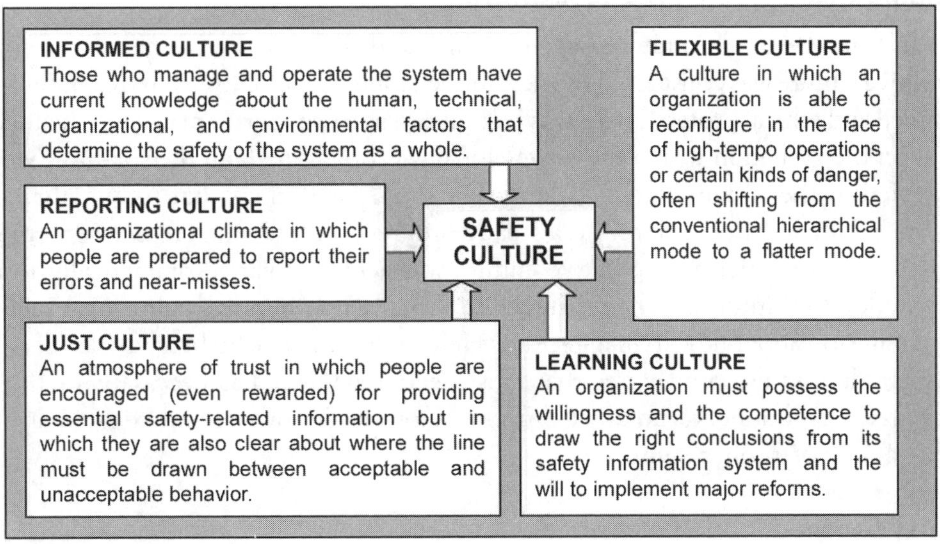

Figure 5-1. Five components of a safety culture.
Source: Reprinted by permission from the Global Aviation Information Network.

Blame and Train/Punitive Culture

Before the 1990s, only the active failures were recognized in medicine. As a result, the culture of medicine was punitive and addressed only the fault of the people who committed the active failures, regardless of the setting in which the errors occurred. This outcome-based approach meant that reckless behavior was unpunished, provided there was no adverse outcome. At that time, it was generally believed that perfect human performance could be achieved through education. Those who did not exhibit perfect human performance needed further education to attain perfection, thus the blame and train model for error management.[9] If the error resulted in a catastrophic outcome, training could be bypassed in favor of termination. It was mistakenly thought that the threat of this type of discipline would encourage those who had not yet erred to continue to exhibit perfect human performance. The result appeared to be almost perfect human performance, but underneath this illusion were countless errors that were unreported, buried out of fear. Buried with them was information that might have advanced patient safety through learning and devising useful risk-reduction strategies. Patient safety no doubt suffered during this time. The blame and train model still survives today, although it has been weakened somewhat. The model is still the focus of many state boards of nursing, pharmacy, and medicine, who continue to respond to errors with discipline and additional educational requirements.

Blame-Free/Non-Punitive Culture

By the mid-1990s, the culture began to shift, and the idea of a blame-free or non-punitive culture was considered the new model. Human fallibility, even that of highly trained and ethical professionals, was recognized as a risk to patient safety. The focus was on the system in which the professional was operating, and the solutions were directed to the systems' latent failures. For those institutions that truly embraced a non-punitive culture, there was a steady progression toward increased reporting. The extent to which non-punitive culture was accepted varied dramatically from institution to institution. The resistance to a totally non-punitive culture was fueled by confusion about how to manage those few practitioners who behaved recklessly, disregarding safety procedures that most peers recognized as necessary, or those very rare practitioners who acted with malicious intent or were intoxicated at the time of a catastrophic event.[10]

Just Culture

The **Just Culture** recognizes the contribution of both latent failures and active failures. It also recognizes that punishment for most active failures—unsafe acts or honest mistakes to which we are all vulnerable—is counter-productive to reporting, learning, and the advancement of safety. However, the Just Culture also recognizes that there must be a clear line between acceptable and unacceptable behavior, between unsafe acts and the blatant disregard of safety procedures with which most peers would comply.

The Just Culture represents a combined, balanced approach: consideration is given to the role of systems in error, along with a focus on behavioral choices and accountability. It is a way of safety thinking that:

- Promotes a questioning attitude,
- Is resistant to complacency,
- Is committed to excellence, and
- Fosters both personal accountability and corporate self-regulation in safety matters.[7]

A Just Culture is considered a component of an overall safety culture.

MSO Role and Culture

Attainment of a safety culture depends on individual and organizational attitudes and behaviors. These values and practices (i.e., culture) can enable or facilitate the unsafe acts and conditions that lead to errors and adverse outcomes. By affecting culture change, therefore, the MSO can promote active identification of safety issues and respond with appropriate action.

The MSO must understand the patient safety culture of their organization. Suggestions for assessment of culture are reviewed in Chapter 3. Does the current culture support medication safety? What improvements are necessary? Before embarking on any change, you must know what you want it to look like in the future. The MSO should be able to articulate the future vision of the desired culture. Culture change is a difficult task; however, it is fundamental to the success of the MSO's work in medication safety. As the MSO, you must win not only the minds, but also the hearts of the people you work with. This will take innovation and persuasion, using strategies discussed further in Chapter 3.

To make broad changes in culture, the MSO should work to overcome four barriers:

1. *Cognition*—people need to understand why culture change is necessary. (Example: why is medication safety error/risk reporting essential to a safe culture?)
2. *Limited resources*—as culture changes, resources may shift away from some areas to other areas. (Example: implementing technology safely may shift resources from implementation phase to maintenance.)
3. *Motivation*—ultimately, workers will have to want to make the change.
4. *Institutional politics*—just as with culture, each organization has its own political strengths and weaknesses.[11]

What can the MSO do to facilitate or improve the culture of safety? A combination of strategies is often the most effective approach. Consider using some of the following options.

Build Influence

Consider the *tipping point idea*: recognize that it is not possible to convert everyone at once. Target those who have increased influence in the organization—formal as well as informal leaders. Build coalitions across disciplines to devise strategies for culture change. Work to get them committed to a safe culture and highlight their accomplishments toward this goal. If safety is not a topic of leadership walk-arounds, campaign to have it added. Or, collaborate with others to begin safety walk-arounds. Having trouble gaining momentum? Consider a pilot program and share successes to expand the initiative.

Encourage Involvement

At the same time, look for ways to have people experience the realities that make it necessary for culture change. For example, where possible, consider engaging staff members and management in event report follow-up. This often provides a greater insight for the participants than just having the MSO report on the event, its contributing causes, and preach the need for culture change. The MSO can provide real-time education on culture of safety and allow the participants to present their findings and further spread the culture change ideas.

Provide Education

Include patient safety culture in orientation when employees are integrated into your organization. This is best done from an organizational perspective, for example, through organizational values and behavioral expectations. If you are not able to influence this, include it in your section on medication safety. No orientation to practitioners on medication safety? Take the opportunity to initiate one! Identify the coordinator of pharmacy, nursing, medical staff, and other departmental organizers of training and orientation. You may need to convince them of the importance for this section and the relationship to their work and impact on patient safety. There are many methods to achieve your goal, from personal presentations (you might choose this for regularly scheduled large groups), self-study, or a "canned" presentation for others to deliver.

Take advantage of your educational presentations to include a section on safety culture. This can be incorporated into orientation sessions, continuing education, and even creatively into routine reporting to teams and committees on safety-related topics. Strive to involve all those who participate in medication management processes, including those often forgotten populations such as pharmacy technicians, procedural area staff, operating room staff, or respiratory therapists. Awareness of safety culture is a first step toward change!

Create an Environment That Supports Reporting

As your safety culture evolves toward the desired state, you will notice a progression in types of reporting. Initially, people will report events related to equipment failures. When comfort level increases, you will note reports on other people's errors, followed by reporting of one's own human error, then finally, reporting on one's own violation of policy.[4] As noted earlier, reporting is a critical component of a culture of safety.

The MSO should strive to make the organizational reporting system user-friendly and accessible to all employees, students, and teaching staff (if not employees). Consider system design changes to make it easy and meaningful to report; for example, minimize the number of screens or paper pages required for reporting, balance the need for detail with ease of use, and utilize check-boxes or drop-downs. If your organization is considering a revised or new reporting system, MSO participation is essential for building the medication-related reporting modules (see Chapter 9). Ensure all users are educated on the access and use of the reporting system or forms.

The goal is a culture that rewards reporting. The MSO should encourage reporting of near miss and actual events, as well as situations that represent risk for error or harm. Take advantage of any opportunity to do so—educational presentations, meeting updates, personal encounters, etc. However, as the MSO, you should be fully aware of the organizational culture toward reporting and may need to adjust your zest for this education if the leadership is not sufficiently supportive or ready for this change. In this event, concentrate your efforts toward the organizational and leadership change to support a reporting culture and improved culture of safety.

Say Thank-You!

Take opportunities to publicly highlight positive accomplishments toward culture of safety. For example, share a practice change that directly resulted from a risk or event report. Make the connection clear. Communication methods can include e-mail, newsletter, bulletin board, or meeting updates. Try beginning team meetings with a "good-catch" story, being sure to invite participation from members. If you find little participation at first, be prepared to provide your own examples and continue to provide encouragement (or rewards) to others until the practice catches on.

Use Data to Drive Improvement

As you may already realize, this is a recurrent theme in this book: Using data collection and analysis as important elements for continuous quality improvement (Chapter 6), enhancing safety of the medication-use system (Chapter 7), using technology to improve safety (Chapter 8), and applying medication error information to identify opportunities for change (Chapter 9). Practitioners are more likely to report if they know the information is used to improve practice. If they perceive the report is used only for numbers and is never evaluated, they will cease reporting. The only way for them to know the information is valued is reinforcement. The MSO must ensure that this occurs. Again, many communication methods are available. The information does not necessarily need to come directly from the MSO, but it does need to occur!

Clarify Expectation

Relevant to safe culture, what are the expectations of the staff, management, and leadership? This is an area where the MSO must generally use influence to support culture change, as they rarely have direct authority over performance expectations. Goals for a Just Culture include valuing questioning and continuous learning. The MSO can look for opportunities to encourage these behaviors by working with organizational and department leadership. Depending on your reporting structure, start within your department to develop or enhance these values. Be a role model when interacting with other departments—consider asking questions to engage leaders or staff during discussion of safety concerns.

Integrate Safety Culture into Daily Work

Working together with management, hardwire teamwork and communications into everyday tasks. Shift-to-shift communication via use of checklists, huddles, or SBAR (situation, background, assessment, recommendation) structures is helpful. Encourage active questioning as a component of shift reports if something doesn't seem quite right. The MSO can provide visible leadership through walk rounds, role modeling, and mentoring. Expectations may be delineated through clear policy and procedures, when needed. These written documents serve as references for expected behaviors and can be used as teaching resources. As a member of technology teams and projects (as well as other types of process building), the MSO has opportunity to educate on and integrate human factors engineering concepts into system design. Just Culture includes consideration of both systems design and human behavior.

Incorporate Safety Culture into Teams

By incorporating safety culture into team and committee efforts, the MSO helps to broaden the base for safety culture change. Encourage leaders to place safety at the top of the agenda. Take a look at where safety falls (if at all) on meeting agendas: is it present at the Board of Trustees level? How about Pharmacy and Therapeutics Committee, Equipment Evaluation, Medical Staff, or Pharmacy Department meetings? Lack of safety as an agenda topic or where it is placed on the agenda is very telling of an organization's culture of safety. Work with leaders to include safety as a standing agenda item to highlight its importance. The MSO can spread the idea of pairing *cost* questions with *safety* questions during evaluation of any new service, equipment purchase, or building project.

Evaluation of an Adverse Outcome Error

The MSO has an important role in the evaluation of adverse outcome errors with risk management and/or other hospital leadership. In addition to helping identify system risks, the MSO can use the review meetings as an opportunity to educate about and promote a Just Culture.

Hudson's Evolution of Culture

Hudson describes an evolution of culture based on how the culture responds to errors.[7,12] The evolution begins with "pathological" that blames and hides errors, to "generative," which is a true safety culture. As the organization evolves from pathological to generative, trust increases, and the organization becomes more informed. Hudson's evolution of a safety culture, along with the possible implications for the MSO, is outlined in Table 5-2.

Because the tendency to blame is so strong, evaluation of adverse outcome errors can undermine a Just Culture if those doing the evaluation do not have an adequate understanding of the concepts discussed earlier—levels of performance, human errors, routine violations, and the like. Without this understanding, there is significant risk of assigning inappropriate blame, regardless of what method or tool is used for review of an adverse outcome error. So how does one identify those behaviors in the gray area between obviously unacceptable (malicious intent or reckless behavior) and honest mistake (simple human error)? A brief overview of some methods is provided here, but the reader is encouraged to investigate these in more detail.

Reason[1] and Marx[4] describe two approaches. A detailed outline of both can also be found online.[7] The National Patient Safety Agency (NPSA) for the National Health Service (NHS) of the United Kingdom later developed and tested another method[13] based on Reason's work. All are intended for use in evaluating an error with an adverse outcome or a near miss, not behaviors in general. Note that with

Table 5-2. Hudson's Evolution of a Safety Culture and Implications for the MSO

Prevailing Culture	Focus	Response to Error/ Activities	Implication for Medication Safety Officer
Pathological Culture (not a safety culture)	Cheaper and faster targets	Blame/denial that adverse outcome errors exist.	Professionals dismissed inappropriately, regardless of circumstances. Lack of access to information, including error reports. Frontline workers reluctant to share information about true practice patterns in the use of medications, so evaluation of true practices is impossible. (The illusion of perfection.)
Reactive Culture (not a safety culture)	Prevent adverse publicity and ranking	React to adverse outcome errors by looking for solutions to only those problems identified in adverse outcome errors.	All actions after an event are driven by fear of headlines and bad publicity. All safety improvements are the result of adverse outcome, so there is no ability to prioritize safety actions. MSO becomes medication safety "fire fighter." Safety improvements recommended as a result of adverse outcomes from outside organizations are met with "That's never happened here," and "If it ain't broke, don't fix it."
Calculative Culture (common to large organizations, not a safety culture)	Systems to manage hazards as a result of regulatory pressures	Based on current regulations/ accreditation agencies	MSO will be focused on regulations and standards only. Error evaluation still hindered by trust/input from those working in the systems.
Proactive Culture (safety culture with potential for improvement)	Systems to manage hazards; staff and management begin to believe there is value to safety systems outside of regulatory pressures.	Attempt to identify and eliminate latent failures prior to events. Incorporate frontline workers in evaluations.	MSO able to evaluate errors and systems more readily, with input from frontline workers who speak freely regarding procedures. MSO able to receive support from management to implement safety systems even if they are not required by regulation or standard. MSO provides support for management in the understanding of human error theory, to promote a Just Culture.
Generative Culture (true safety culture)	Safety behavior fully integrated into everything the organization does. Value system associated with safety.	Strives for resilience—recognizing that system will never be error free, focus is on capture and mitigation of errors.	Potential for errors brought to the MSO from the front lines, which has developed an awareness and level of trust. MSO involved in process design that anticipates and is designed to capture and mitigate errors. Processes are evaluated for error risks prior to implementation. MSO provides support for management in the understanding of human error theory, to promote a Just Culture.

most adverse outcome errors or near misses, there will be more than one associated unsafe act, and each is evaluated separately.

Reason developed the Culpability Decision Tree (see Figure 5-2), an evaluation technique, which assesses factors to determine the level of culpability of a person involved with an error (see Chapter 10 for more discussion and techniques). The factors include the intention of the person committing the unsafe act, the influence of alcohol or medications (prescribed or otherwise), abnormal safety procedure violations (procedures typically followed by peers), and determining whether the person has a history of unsafe acts. Marx breaks it down a little differently.[4] He divides behaviors and unsafe acts into four distinct types, which he calls the "four evils." These are human errors, negligent conduct (unaware of risk that peers would recognize), reckless conduct (intentionally taking risks), and intentional rule violations (not tied to risk taking). Any one or combination of these can apply to the adverse outcome error or near miss and help to assess culpability. Reason and Marx both argue against discipline with negligence, as those who were negligent did not recognize they were taking risks. There is much to be learned about why they were unaware of the risk, and this information could lead to system improvements to capture errors before they cause harm.

The NPSA for the NHS of the United Kingdom developed the Incident Decision Tree, based on Reason's Culpability Decision Tree.[13] The Incident Decision Tree was tested and refined in 2003 and guides the user through a series of structured questions or tests about a behavior or unsafe act that resulted in an adverse outcome or near miss. The tests include:

- *Deliberate harm test:* Identifies those rare cases in which harm was intended.
- *Incapacity test:* If deliberate harm is discounted, the incapacity test identifies the contribution of ill health or substance abuse. Questions are related to awareness of condition, realization of the implications of working in the condition, and if there were any safeguards to protect the patient.
- *Foresight test:* If intent to harm and incapacity are discounted, the foresight test identifies compliance with safe working practices. Questions are related to the existence of good procedures, conflicting protocols, routine violations, and intention with regard to following the protocol. Additionally, emergency settings, situational motivations and a lack of information are also evaluated, and guidance for slips in perception is provided.
- *Substitution test:* The substitution test is applied to further clarify foresight. Questions are related to how a peer from the same domain of activity and level of experience might behave given the same circumstances. Deficiencies in training, experience, and supervision are addressed.

In the testing and refinement of the tool in 2003, there were some interesting observations:

- The tool was considered helpful, fair, and a good framework for dialog about the event.

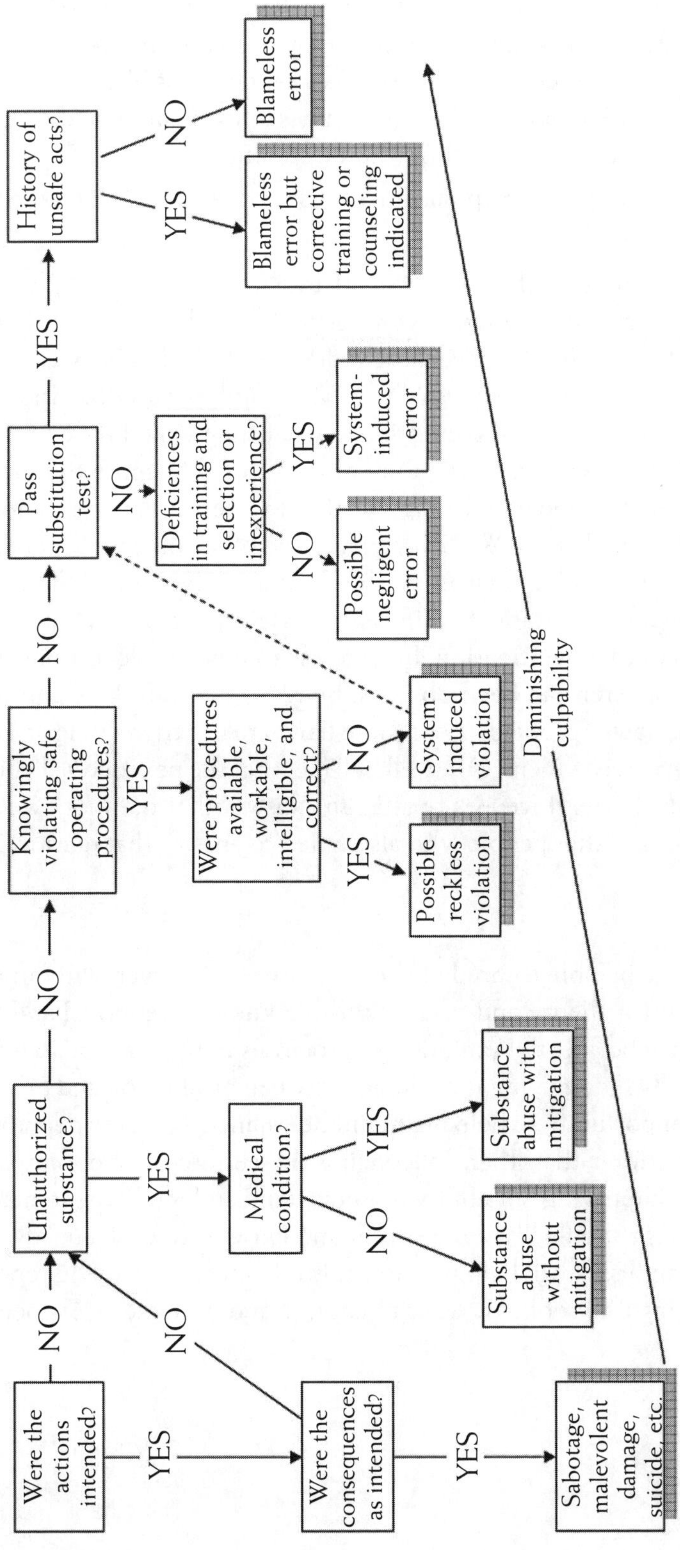

Figure 5-2. Reason's Culpability Decision Tree.
Source: Reprinted by permission from the Global Aviation Information Network.

- Younger or inexperienced managers tended to assign more blame, especially if they were evaluating a person in a profession that was not their own.
- There was a tendency to assign blame to those whose routine violations resulted in an adverse outcome so that others would be less likely to commit the same routine violations. This undermines a Just Culture and is not a good approach to the management of routine violations.
- Some managers decided on the punishment first and used the tool to justify the punishment.

A word of caution with the use of these types of tools—some of the outcomes discussed above demonstrate the need for an understanding of human error theory for them to be useful. The results also reveal the influence of **hindsight bias** in the evaluation of an adverse event error or near miss. *Hindsight bias* describes the tendency for those evaluating an error to overestimate what they would have known, and what others should have known, at the time of the error. The more significant the outcome, the greater the tendency to suggest that the person involved should have seen it coming.[2] Admiral Harold W. Gehman Jr., head of the independent board investigating the shuttle Columbia breakup in the skies over the United States on February 1, 2003, grew quite frustrated by hindsight bias during a press conference discussing the progress of the investigation. In response to reporters' questions suggesting the risk of the disaster had been obvious, he responded, "In hindsight, it's really easy to find these flaws." He said, "So if these flaws are out there lying around and everybody should have seen them, OK, well, tell me what the next one is if you're so smart. Tell me the next one. If we as a board can't answer that question, we are very slow to sling spears at other people who also failed to answer that question."[14]

Summary

In the end, we will never be able to predict the "next one." However, with an understanding of human error theory and of the skill-rule-knowledge model and the associated errors, we may be able to better design processes to prevent and identify errors to prevent harm. By recognizing the conflict between production and protection, we have a better opportunity to help maintain the balance when the pendulum swings too far toward one or the other. Influencing the culture of safety impacts attitudes and practices, improving our ability to understand and modify system and behavioral vulnerabilities. And finally, a consistent and fair way to evaluate adverse outcome errors and near misses will help promote a Just Culture, improving reporting, learning, and the possibility of new ways to capture and mitigate errors before they cause harm.

PRACTICE TIPS

1. A culture of safety is foundational for MSO success. Use your role to enhance or move your organization toward a Just Culture. MSOs *can* influence change!
2. Medication errors are multidisciplinary and multifactorial. Our lessons lie in the analysis of how the systems failed, the contribution of human behaviors, and initiating actions for prevention.
3. Educate staff (all disciplines) that errors *will* occur, and that's why we spend so much time designing our systems, using technology tools, and building in redundancy to avoid errors. Stress the importance of *using* the system as designed in order to keep patients safe.
4. Work with vendors to improve systems for patient safety. Share your identification of system weaknesses and ideas for improvement through collaboration with informatics colleagues, vendor user groups, and direct vendor contact.

References

1. Reason J. *Managing the Risks of Organizational Accidents.* Burlington, VT: Ashgate Publishing Company; 1997.
2. Reason J. *Human Error.* Cambridge, U.K.: Cambridge University Press; 1990.
3. Reason J. Foreword. In: Bogner M, ed. *Human Error in Medicine.* Hillsdale, NJ: Lawrence Erlbaum Associates; 1994:vii-xv.
4. Marx D. *Patient safety and the "Just Culture": A primer for health care executives.* Funded by a grant from the National Heart, Lung and Blood Institute, National Institutes of Health. New York: Trustees of Columbia University; 2001.
5. Amalberti R. Normal and abnormal violations. Paper presented at: The Third Halifax Symposium on Healthcare Safety; October 17, 2003. Halifax, Nova Scotia, Canada.
6. The Institute for Safe Medication Practices. ISMP Medication Safety Alert! Reducing "at-risk behaviors" part II of patient safety should not be a priority in healthcare! October 7, 2004. Available at: http://www.ismp.org/newsletters/acutecare/articles/20041007.asp. Accessed April 13, 2011.
7. GAIN Working Group E, Flight Ops/ATC Ops Safety Information Sharing. A roadmap to a Just Culture: enhancing the safety environment. 1st ed. September 2004. Available at: http://flightsafety.org/files/just_culture.pdf. Accessed September 11, 2012.
8. Cook R, Woods D. Operating at the sharp end: the complexity of human error. In: Bogner M, ed. *Human Error in Medicine.* Hillsdale, NJ: Lawrence Erlbaum Associates; 1994:255-301.
9. The Institute for Safe Medication Practices. ISMP Medication Safety Alert! Our long journey towards a safety-minded Just Culture. Part I: Where we've been. September 7, 2006. Available at: http://www.ismp.org/Newsletters/acutecare/articles/20060907.asp. Accessed April 13, 2011.
10. Reason J. Overview: unsafe acts and the 'person'. Paper presented at: The Third Halifax Symposium on Healthcare Safety; October 17, 2003. Halifax, Nova Scotia, Canada.

11. Kim WC, Mauborgne R. Blue Ocean Strategy: *How to Create Uncontested Market Space and Make the Competition Irrelevant*. Boston, MA: Harvard Business School Publishing Corporation, 2005.

12. Hudson, P. Safety culture: the ultimate goal. *Flight Safety Australia*. September-October 2001:29-31. Available at: http://www.casa.gov.au/fsa/2001/sep/29-31.pdf. Accessed April 13, 2011.

13. Meadows, S., Baker K., Butler, J. The incident decision tree: guidelines for action following patient safety incidents. *Advances in Patient Safety: From Research to Implementation*, Volumes 1–4, AHRQ Publication Nos. 050021. February 2005. Agency for Healthcare Research and Quality, Rockville, MD. Available at: http://www.ahrq.gov/qual/advances. Accessed April 13, 2011.

14. Harwood, W. Demonstration flight not likely for space shuttle. *Spaceflight Now*. May 28, 2003. Available at: http://spaceflightnow.com/shuttle/sts107/030528requal/. Accessed April 13, 2011.

Continuous Quality Improvement Principles

Susan J. Skledar

CHAPTER 6

Key Terms

Continuous Quality Improvement—A systematic, organized approach for continually improving processes to deliver quality services and products.

Error Trap—Component of failure mode and effects analysis that seeks to prevent error through mechanisms aimed at detecting the error; elimination of alternatives or choices that may lead to error or potential mix-up/confusion; preventing actions that would result in or contribute to the error; and/or minimizing error consequence should it occur.

Failure Mode and Effects Analysis—Problem-solving tool used to analyze a process or system to identify possible modes of failure, and potential consequences of those failures.

FOCUS-PDCA Cycle—A nine-step process (Find-Organize-Clarify-Understand-Select-Plan-Do-Check-Act) that emphasizes work teams, data-driven analysis, careful planning, organized implementation, and measurement of results.

PDCA Cycle—A quality improvement methodology involving Plan-Do-Check-Act steps for planning, implementing, evaluating, and changing a process or system.

Stakeholder—A person, group, or organization that will be affected by or can themselves affect a process.

Statistical Process Control Chart—A statistical graph that helps to detect process variation over time and is a tool for monitoring the ongoing stability of a process, distinguishing variation due to causes common to the process versus special (potentially actionable) causes.

Introduction

The medication safety officer (MSO) should have a working knowledge of **continuous quality improvement** (CQI) principles. Health care resources, information, and external regulatory influences are constantly changing, and the MSO needs to understand CQI methodology to provide guidance or facilitate process change.[1] A critical element is knowing how to assess baseline practices and identify trends pointing to processes needing improvement to meet a new external quality measure or regulation. Additionally, facilitating problem-solving sessions is necessary to gather appropriate input, especially with interdisciplinary work teams. The MSO must understand potential process breakdowns to ensure safety. Despite advances in health care and medicine, reports continue to show that the U.S. health care system has much opportunity for improvement.[2] The chasm or gap between what we should do in health care for our patients and what is actually done accounts for billions of dollars per year in lost productivity and hospital costs.[3] The framework for organizational performance improvement includes a thorough understanding and ability to apply CQI principles, and there is much opportunity for measurement and improvement.

A formal definition of CQI is "a systematic, organizational approach for continually improving all processes that deliver quality services and products."[4] More recently, it has been defined as a "structured, organizational process for involving personnel in planning and executing a continuous flow of improvements to provide quality health care that meets or exceeds expectations."[5] There are many different CQI methodologies and models in practice today, including industry-based and clinically oriented approaches. There is a common set of elements or characteristics for CQI as it is used to improve organizational performance:[4-7]

- A definition of CQI for the organization and link to the strategic plan
- A quality council comprised of organizational leadership
- Strong patient and customer focus
- Employee process improvement work teams
- Education and training programs for personnel on CQI methodology
- Structured processes for identifying and selecting problems (opportunities) and solutions
- Staff support and resource for process redesign
- Atmosphere that supports employee ideas for change and motivates staff for participation in CQI efforts
- Belief that the front-line staff is the most knowledgeable about the work or problem to be solved

Key structural elements used to support CQI processes are shown in Figure 6-1.[5] Overall, essential components of CQI problem-solving include interdisciplinary work teams, a structured CQI methodology to identify and solve the problem, data-driven development and analysis, and evaluation of the impact of the change. This chapter describes CQI tools for process improvement and analysis, **failure**

mode and effects analysis (FMEA), identification of problems, problem-solving tools, and development of action plans.

Medication Safety Officer's Role in CQI

The MSOs, as part of their work in ensuring safe use of medications, consistent processes for medication use, and compliance with regulatory and safety standards, must have a good understanding of CQI principles. It has been shown that safety organizing—collecting, analyzing, and disseminating information from errors as well as proactive checks on the organization's vital signs—helps to promote safe care of patients.[8-10] In addition, the safety leader should help to ensure processes and procedures for safety are supported and staff feel empowered to identify and report unsafe practices and help to generate ideas and solutions for change. Trusted leaders can foster

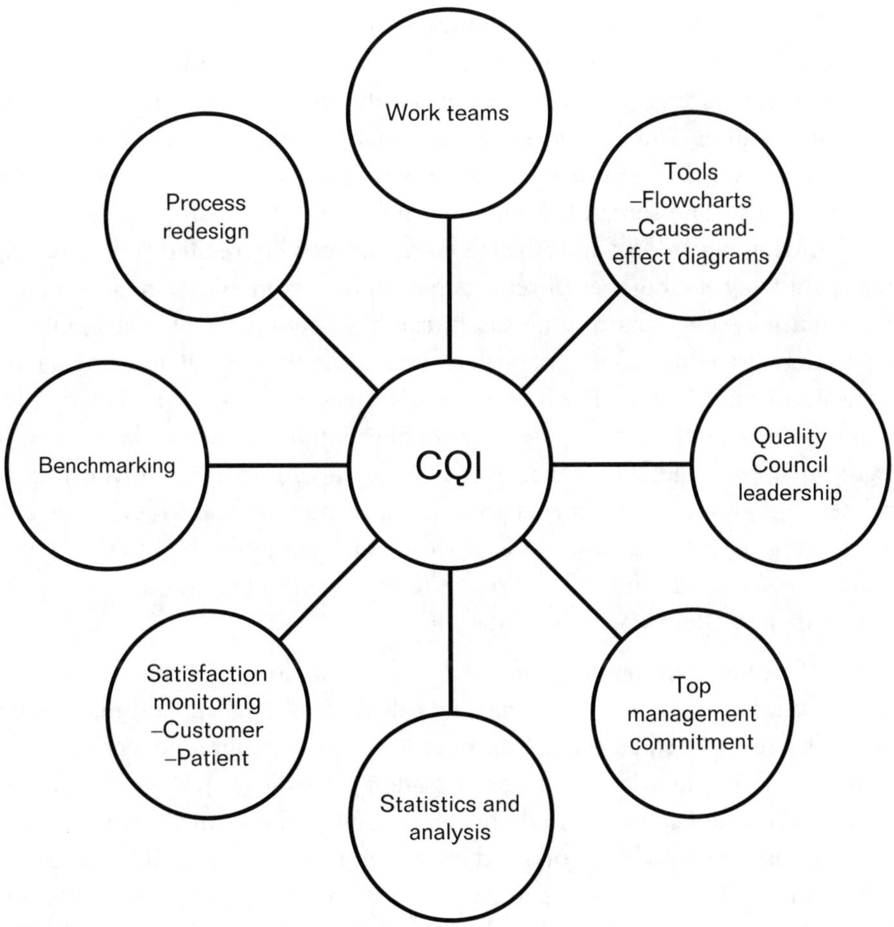

Figure 6-1. Key structural elements of CQI.
Source: Adapted from Reference 5.

safety culture and promote engagement of staff in health care improvements.[8,11,12] The MSO should team with organizational leadership to promote a culture of safety.

The MSO needs to be aware of The Joint Commission (TJC) national patient safety goals (NPSGs) and medication management standards (or other accreditation standards) and lead the efforts to work with interdisciplinary teams to do the sample tracers and Focused Standards Assessments as ongoing policy and practice assessments. These mechanisms provide an ongoing evaluation of performance and activity, to identify process gaps and create action to change policy or practice, to meet the spirit of the NPSGs or accreditation standard. Additionally, the required measures of success involve data collection and assessment, with action plans for change. These audits, or snapshots of performance, are quick data-driven practice assessments, which also are grounded in continual improvement of process based on data.

The medication management standards denote that the effectiveness of the complete medication management system and process be evaluated, including risk points, technology, best practices, safety and operational priorities, and trends in practice. These trends can be identified through process measures, outcome measures, or even economic measures of monitoring. Exact measures or indicators of the medication management program can be defined by the site; TJC expects sites to identify the indicator, gather data to reflect practice, analyze the practice in comparison to established site-specific and/or national targets, and then take action to improve performance or sustain/spread the change. This is the CQI change cycle at its basic roots. Medication error data and adverse event data can be trended and reported, for example, showing the number of reports per high-alert medication class, and then showing harm events. Smart pump safety catches and impact of smart pump drug library changes to reduce unnecessary alerts is another newer CQI measure that many sites are adopting. If the facility is at a computerized provider order entry (CPOE) site, CQI indicators can include measures of alert fatigue, actions taken in response to decision-support rules, and impact of CPOE on targeted medication dosing safety guidelines (e.g., limits on daily acetaminophen amounts). The MSO needs a deep understanding of the medication-use process steps to see the big picture[13] of how accreditation standards and NPSGs relate to the health care practitioners' roles in ensuring safe and effective use of medications.

The TJC leadership standards apply globally to the organization, and the MSO should be familiar with them. These standards discuss creating and maintaining a culture of safety, as well as evaluating practices and providing educational efforts to promote safety. The MSO is the ambassador of medication safety for the organization, and is often called on to do presentations on medication error trends, top medications associated with errors, and efforts to prevent harm and adverse events. A standard discusses that the organization's patient safety program is integrated, so the MSO must be connected to hospital patient safety committees and risk management teams that evaluate safe practices related to medication management. The safety program, according to TJC, includes the full range of prevented errors to sentinel events. The MSO must be integrated into and perhaps lead site-specific root-cause analyses and sentinel event discussions, as well as proactive mechanisms to prevent error and harm. A proactive risk assessment on a high-risk process must be completed every 18 months, and if this involves medications in any way, the MSO should be a part of the risk assessment team, inviting additional pharmacy and other health care practitioner content experts to participate. The MSO does not have to have in-depth knowledge of every aspect of medication use, but should be the broad-content expert for medication management practice in the hospital and its associated hospital-based clinics and departments. The MSO should be comfortable and confident to draw in clinical, informatics, or automation experts to help solve issues. The MSO often is the facilitator of change and is expected to see the improvement solution through to completion.

Origins of Quality and CQI Methodologies

In the 1930s, Walter Shewart, a statistician, studied the quality of work and process in industry. His thinking was that if a process had variation, the cause of the variation had to be determined and eliminated.[5] He is best known for two important CQI tools: (1) the **statistical process control chart**, which helps to detect process variation over time and is a tool for monitoring the ongoing stability of a process; and (2) the **Plan-Do-Check-Act** (PDCA) cycle, which allows process change planning, implementation, study of change, and action to spread or modify the change.[5,6] W. Edwards Deming was responsible for building on the PDCA concepts of Shewart (his colleague) and introducing this to the Japanese in the post-World War II automobile industry.[14] According to Deming's approach, problems should be identified as opportunities for improvement, the causes of the problem that are within the organization/team's control should be identified, and then actions should be tested and implemented that can reduce or eliminate those causes.

Avedis Donabedian, a physician and scholar, who is known for asking the question "How can you tell if you have good quality health care?" defined the foundational principles of measuring quality in health care—structure-process-outcome—meaning simply that good organizational infrastructure plus defined processes equals good outcomes.[15] Structure can be measured in terms of resources that are available to deliver or provide necessary care. Process measures are designed to analyze activities of health care providers to see if the work is being done according to established standards or guidelines. Outcome measures, often called clinical measures, are broad measures of patient conditions as a result of the care; for example, morbidity, mortality, or patient satisfaction.[3-5] Donabedian also expanded management of quality beyond the process logistics to include people (relationships), access to care, and continuity of care.[5] Donabedian is known for the Seven Pillars of Quality to characterize quality care provision: efficacy, effectiveness, efficiency, acceptability, optimality, equity, and legitimacy.[16] These principles are very similar to the Institute of Medicine's statement that health care should be "safe, effective, patient-centered, timely, efficient, and equitable," indicating that external influences on quality management (e.g., economics, regulatory) should also be evaluated.[2]

There are many CQI methodologies available to the MSO. These include but are not limited to:

- Lean Production System
- Six Sigma
- FOCUS-PDCA

- The *Lean Production System* or *Just-in-Time Process* focuses on the optimal way or process to do the work, with the output desired as identical every time, aiming for zero defects. Unnecessary or wasteful steps are undesirable, and processes of work are very well defined by using observation methodology.[17,18] This process uses direct observations of the work, identification of value-added and non-value-added steps, and rapid cycle changes. Rules-in-use and the 5S (sort, straighten, shine, standardize, sustain) strategy are outlined in Figure 6-2.
- *Six Sigma* is a rigorous, systematic, and disciplined data-driven process that focuses on customer expectations and considers a defect anything outside of customer requirements. Companies or organizations embracing this philosophy strive to achieve near perfection, or "six standard deviations from the mean and the nearest specification limit," specifically no more than 3.4 defects per one million opportunities.[19] Two specific improvement process tools that are part of this methodology are listed in Figure 6-3. The Lean Production and Six Sigma methodologies are newer approaches to CQI in health care, and you should be familiar with these approaches for detection of error if they are used at your facility.

Rules-In-Use	
1	All work shall be highly specified as to content, sequence, timing, and outcome.
2	Every customer-supplier connection must be direct, and there must be an unambiguous yes-or-no way to send requests and receive responses.
3	The pathway for every product and service must be simple and direct.
4	Any improvement must be made in accordance with the scientific method, under the guidance of a teacher, at the lowest possible level of the organization.

5S Principles	
Sort	Keep only important items. Tools are easier to find.
Straighten (set order)	Keep essential items nearby and in same location.
Shine (scrub)	Keep everything clean. Clean often.
Standardize	Make sorting, straightening, and shining the routine.
Sustain	Audit and keep other steps occurring.

Figure 6-2. Lean Production tools.[3,17,18]

DMADV: used for designing new processes and products	
D	Define
M	Measure
A	Analyze
D	Design
V	Verify

DMAIC: used for incrementally improving processes	
D	Define
M	Measure
A	Analyze
I	Improve
C	Control

Figure 6-3. Six Sigma tools.[19]

A more common approach to CQI, the FOCUS-PDCA methodology, is described below in step-wise fashion.

The FOCUS-PDCA Cycle

The Deming **FOCUS-PDCA** Methodology encompasses a systematic approach to CQI that incorporates his approach to measurement and the Donabedian focus on people and environment. The Hospital Corporation of America adopted this methodology, and it is widely used in hospitals across the country. Figure 6-4 displays the basic steps of this model.[5,20] The most commonly used CQI approach in health care delivery systems today is this cycle or its adaptations.[3] This method emphasizes work teams, data-driven analysis, careful planning and implementation, and measuring results. It focuses on prevention of harm and allows flexibility of process and approach for the complex patient care environment.

F	Find the process to improve
O	Organize an interdisciplinary team
C	Clarify the current (or baseline) problem
U	Understand variation in the current process
S	Select the process for change
P	Plan the change
D	Do (implement) the change
C	Check the results of change
A	Act to spread or sustain the change

Figure 6-4. The FOCUS-PDCA cycle.[5,20]

F (Find the Problem)

Identification of the problem and focusing it to an accomplishable task is the first step in using this CQI methodology. For today's MSO and patient safety officer, example key focus areas are high-alert medications and national patient safety goals. High-alert medications are defined by the Institute for Safe Medication Practices (ISMP) as "drugs that bear a heightened risk of causing significant patient harm when they are used in error."[21] These include agents such as anticoagulants, opioids, sedatives, insulin, and inotropic agents. The Institute for Healthcare Improvement (IHI), as part of its "5 Million Lives Campaign," assembled a high-alert medication how-to guide to assist clinicians to understand why focusing on medication safety for these error-prone agents is important.[3] Evidence-based findings of adverse events and risk of harm are provided for the end-user.[22] Additionally, a global risk assessment was performed, and, similar to ISMP recommendations, the IHI denotes that opiates (narcotics), insulin, anticoagulants, and sedatives are the agents where safety efforts should be targeted. Regarding medication safety, TJC also focuses on high-alert medications as the foundation for its NPSGs.[23] The Institute of Medicine studies showed that adverse drug events (ADE) result in over three billion dollars in hospital costs, affecting 400,000 hospitalized patients.[24] The recommendations of these major national patient safety advocacy groups provide a focused, evidence-based approach to identifying medication safety opportunities.

To identify the problem on a hospital level, several approaches can be taken. A review of voluntarily reported medication errors (MEs) and ADEs can be done. This may, however, be only a small reflection of the problem, as it is must be acknowledged that MEs and ADEs are often under-reported. A prevalence study, or snapshot audit of practices related to anticoagulation, for example, can identify real-time opportunities for improvement (see Figure 6-5). As an example, the anticoagulation NPSG delineates elements related to safety with anticoagulants, such as unfractionated heparin (UFH), low molecular weight heparin (LMWH), and warfarin.[25] Any or all of these medications, and how they are prescribed, transcribed, dispensed, administered, or monitored in patients receiving them could be a topic for investigation and improvement.

Data from clinical information systems or charge records can also be used to identify and focus the problem. Published literature and other reporting sources can be used for evaluating your local hospital practices and noting if the problem has occurred on a national level. Using the actual medication error or adverse event rate as an assessment of overall safety of the organization is not recommended since events are typically underreported and there is too much variation within and across organizations. These data can be helpful to show trends in medication classes or processes to focus safety improvement and also show that the problem at a particular facility is also a problem at a regional or national level.

Drug Use and Disease State Management Program

Anticoagulation Monitoring Form

Patient Name: ______________________ MRN: ______________ Date of Audit: _________

Attending Physician: _________________ Service: ___________ Date of Admission: _______

Target Anticoagulant: ☐ Heparin ☐ Enoxaparin ☐ Dalteparin ☐ Warfarin

Start date: ________________ Prescriber: ____________________

Indication for use:

- ☐ Deep vein thrombosis
- ☐ Pulmonary embolism
- ☐ Unstable angina
- ☐ NSTEMI
- ☐ Non Q-wave MI
- ☐ A fib/flutter
- ☐ Other: ________________________

National Patient Safety Goals Element Evaluation

Enoxaparin/Dalteparin	**Heparin** *(received heparin for >48 hours)*	**Warfarin**
Unit-dose product ☐ YES ☐ NO Dosing ☐ Initiation ☐ Maintenance	Unit-dose product ☐ YES (premix) ☐ NO Used programmable pump ☐ YES ☐ NO	Unit-dose product ☐ YES ☐ NO Dosing ☐ Initiation ☐ Maintenance
Documented use of approved protocol/order set for LMWH initiation ☐ YES ☐ NO ☐ N/A	Documented use of approved protocol/order set for heparin initiation ☐ YES ☐ NO Used order set for correct indication (or was valid exception) ☐ YES ☐ NO	Documented use of approved protocol/order set for warfarin initiation ☐ YES ☐ NO ☐ N/A
Baseline Monitoring: CBC with platelets: ☐ YES ☐ NO SCr ☐ YES ☐ NO aPTT: ☐ YES ☐ NO	Baseline Monitoring: CBC with platelets: ☐ YES ☐ NO aPTT: ☐ YES ☐ NO	Baseline Monitoring: CBC with platelets: ☐ YES ☐ NO PT/INR: ☐ YES ☐ NO

Figure 6-5 (continued).

Enoxaparin/Dalteparin	**Heparin** *(received heparin for >48 hours)*	**Warfarin**
Ongoing Monitoring: CBC with platelets at least every 7 days during first 2 weeks then every 2 to 4 weeks thereafter ☐ YES ☐ NO ☐ N/A SCr at least every 7 days during first two weeks then every 2 to 4 weeks thereafter (more frequent monitoring is desired if lab values are not within normal range at any time on LMWH) ☐ YES ☐ NO ☐ N/A Patient refused labs ☐ YES ☐ NO	**Ongoing Monitoring:** Obtain an aPTT level or heparin assay 6 hours after the initiation of IV heparin infusion ☐ YES ☐ NO aPTT if spontaneous bleeding occurs from any site at any time ☐ YES ☐ NO ☐ N/A aPTT every 6 hours (from rate change) until goal aPTT is reached for two consecutive times ☐ YES ☐ NO ☐ N/A aPTT daily once stabilized in target aPTT ☐ YES ☐ NO ☐ N/A Guaiac stools routine once ☐ YES ☐ NO CBC and platelets at a minimum of every other day until discontinuation of heparin ☐ YES ☐ NO Patient refused labs ☐ YES ☐ NO	**Ongoing Monitoring:** Daily PT/INR until patient therapeutic (two consecutive PT/INR values within range at least 24 hours apart) ☐ YES ☐ NO ☐ N/A PT/INR every 72 hours once patient at therapeutic goal ☐ YES ☐ NO ☐ N/A PT/INR every 7 days once patient has been therapeutic on warfarin for a period of 2 weeks or longer ☐ YES ☐ NO ☐ N/A Patient refused labs ☐ YES ☐ NO
Dosed correctly based on LMWH Reference Table for LMWH initiation ☐ YES ☐ NO ☐ N/A	Infusion rate/bolus properly dosed based on approved order set/nomogram ☐ YES ☐ NO ☐ N/A	Dosed correctly based on approved protocol for warfarin initiation and continuation ☐ YES ☐ NO ☐ N/A

Education provided regarding anticoagulant therapy to patients and/or families:

☐ YES ☐ NO ☐ Attempted

If yes, education provided by: ☐ Dietary ☐ Pharmacy ☐ Nursing

Adverse event: ☐ YES ☐ NO

☐ Protamine Administered ☐ Phytonadione Administered ☐ FFP Administered

Event reported in Riskmaster: ☐ YES ☐ NO ☐ N/A

Other notes:______________________________

Overall Assessment:

☐ Meets all of the elements of NPSG

☐ Meets all of the elements of NPSG except for lab monitoring

☐ Does not meet Explain: ______________________________

Figure 6-5. Drug use and disease state management program anticoagulation monitoring form.
LMWH: Low molecular weight heparin, aPTT: partial thromboplastin time; PT; prothrombin time.
Source: Courtesy of Drug Use and Disease State Management, Susan Skledar.

- *Failure Modes and Effects Analysis.* FMEA is a complex, yet informative and revealing process for identifying problems. The FMEA process, simply defined, is a problem-solving tool that can help to analyze a process (or system) to identify possible modes of failure in that process, and the consequences of those failures. It identifies what could happen when something goes wrong. Cohen further defines FMEA as a technique that "looks at a given process, identifies possible errors, and gauges what their effects could be, even before they take place."[26] This methodology has been used by the airline, aerospace, and transportation industry as a whole, as they realize that although systems can be made as fail-safe as possible, the honest accidents and mishaps cannot be eliminated.[27] The FMEA process recognizes that errors may occur, but seeks to prevent the error from becoming an accident, through the use of a safety system, or **error trap**.[26,28] These traps can include actions such as (1) improving detection of the error; (2) eliminating alternatives; (3) preventing completion of actions that would result in error; and (4) minimizing consequences of errors if they do occur.[29] As errors traps are identified, they are incorporated into the implementation of the process change.

Like CQI, FMEA is best carried out using a multidisciplinary team of pharmacists, nurses, physicians, and other health care providers and/or administrators who are the major **stakeholders** for the process in question. It is important to also have front-line staff participate in the FMEA (and overall CQI) process, as they can cite the true workflow involved in the process being studied, versus what should be happening. Figure 6-6 delineates a step-by-step process for conducting FMEA. Additional details and a case example of using FMEA to improve the timeliness of medication delivery are provided in the FMEA case study later in this chapter.[29-31]

FMEA Steps

1. Assemble a multidisciplinary team
2. Define the specific focus of the FMEA topic
3. Process Flow Diagram
   - Describe the process with a process flow diagram
   - Identify all sub-processes
   - Create a flow diagram of identified sub-process
4. Hazard Analysis
   - List possible/potential failure modes under the sub-process
     - Use brainstorming or cause-and-effect analysis charts
     - List root cause(s) of each failure mode
   - Determine possibility (frequency), severity, and probability of detection of the potential failure mode
   - Calculate the criticality index (CI)
5. Actions
   - Determine which causes you can eliminate, control, or accept
   - Decide on actions to reduce the CI
   - Assign responsibility for completing each action
   - Take action!
6. Follow-Up
   - Create process or outcome indicators that can be measured for the improved/changed process

Figure 6-6. Stepwise approach to failure mode and effects analysis.[30-32]

O (Organize an Interdisciplinary Team)

As described above, the importance of the interdisciplinary work team is very important to CQI effort development and implementation. Continuing with the FOCUS-PDCA steps, the team's function is to help find, or identify and focus, the problem and then take part in subsequent steps such as determining quality indicator measures, gathering and analyzing baseline compliance data, reviewing the literature for best practices, benchmarking other facility approaches to the problem, and determining the implementation plan. Having the team comprised of the process's major stakeholders, for example, the content experts, as well as front-line staff who do the work each day, is critical to ensure discussion of all improvement possibilities. For the CQI effort, it is important to have a guidance person or persons to provide general oversight to the team's decisions and plan to ensure efforts align with organizational priorities.

The guidance team, usually hospital or department administration, can help to eliminate barriers to improvement that the work team identifies during planning or implementation. Remaining team members include content experts, front-line staff, and others involved in regulatory and/or quality improvement. The team's exact composition depends on the CQI effort, but typically includes members of nursing, pharmacy, medical staff, and other clinicians as appropriate such as respiratory therapists and dietitians. It may also be important to have information technology experts on the team. The team members will learn from each other and share perspectives on the problem causes, especially during the brainstorming sessions, which are explained in the next step of the FOCUS-PDCA process. The project team will do the work to develop the improvement, implement it, and monitor successes and failures. It is very important at the start of the CQI effort to designate the team members' roles, for example, team leader (or co-leaders), recorder (minutes, plans meetings), and timekeeper (keeps meetings running smoothly, sends reminders to team). Meetings can be held with the team together in person, or by using innovative technology such as teleconferences, video conferencing, or electronic discussions. It is recommended that the first meeting be one where everyone can attend to get the effort started in the right direction and lay the groundwork for the steps moving forward.

C (Clarify the Current Problem)

The team has responsibility to clarify the current problem, which includes creating a flowchart or process map of the current process, defining customers and their expectations, reviewing the literature, and defining the quality indicators that will measure the impact of the improvement. Drawing out the process from the start to the finish, with steps in the process defined and discussed, will help the team understand the current, or baseline, work. Observation of the process is helpful, as it will create a flowchart that represents the *actual* steps in the process, not what *should* be occurring. Figure 6-7 displays a sample flowchart. The flowchart should be a realistic representation of the process, including decision points that can lead to problems.

The flowchart is a visual representation of the process delineating each activity or step. The inclusion of front-line staff on the team will ensure that accurate work steps are included and described. With any flow diagram, outlining the process should include the use of symbols to represent steps; for example, a circle indicates the process start, squares represent action steps, and diamonds represent questions that are asked (decision points). It is helpful to have each step in the process sequentially numbered. If a process is complicated, sub-processes can be further described and numbered. For example, if a process step has three possible decision points, each of those decisions could be numbered as sub-processes 1A, 1B, and 1C. The MSO can use this tool to define current practice or the current state of affairs. The workgroup, or a subset of it, can be charged with making the flowchart, and then the larger group can provide input. Ideally, the team can together observe the actual process to best reflect the actual work happening. This may not be possible in all health care settings or with bigger work teams, but it is beneficial because others who are outside of the

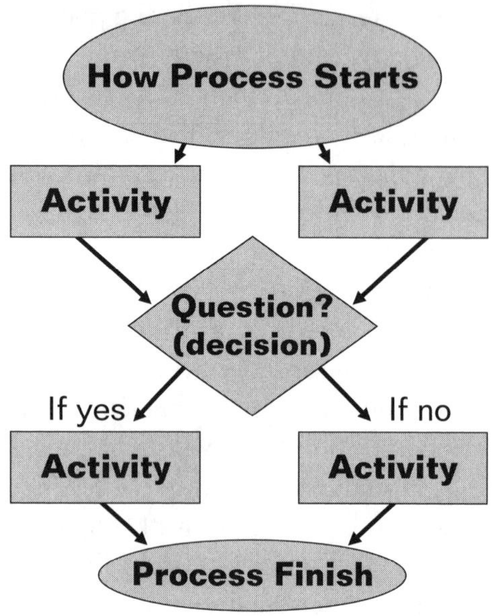

Figure 6-7. Sample flowchart.
Source: Adapted with permission from H. Hagel, *Managing the Patient-Centered Pharmacy*, American Pharmacists Association, 2002.

normal work and may not know the intricacies can objectively observe the workflow and note observations. According to the Veterans Affairs National Center for Patient Safety (VANCPS), it is better to focus on fewer actions that can be accomplished than to create a list of actions that cannot be completed.[31] Additionally, breaking the process into defined steps will help the team sort out ownership of the different steps, and as noted earlier, focus on the steps where there is the most risk and those that are within the team's scope of action. The team can also determine the customers for the CQI effort and their expectations. This is an important step to ensure that you have the right team members involved in development and planning.

The team should review the literature for published practice guidelines, primary literature, other institution approaches to the problem, and national safety or quality guidelines to guide the team's improvement actions. If there are no data to guide your actions, as in the case of many workflow process improvements, it can be helpful to benchmark or survey surrounding similar hospitals or facilities to see how they have approached the same problem. Knowing national standards, such as TJC's NPSG and medication management standards, as well as national core quality and value-based purchasing measures, is very important to help focus team efforts. Once this information is gathered, the team can critically evaluate the available references to help to focus the next steps for improvement.

The last action needed in the "C" step of FOCUS-PDCA is for the work team to define the quality indicator measures that will be used to assess the impact of the intervention. The indicators need to be measurable and specific, with defined data sources and frequency of data collection and reporting. Data sources can include audit information, archived data, patient records, or billing records. If an internal audit is performed, an audit tool should be designed so each person uses the same methods when collecting the data or the data collected will be invalid. If patient records are to be used, the data collection process and goals may need approval from the hospital quality oversight committee or other governing groups, such as the institutional review board. Determining who will collect the data is important as well. These indicators should be represented as rates, for example, *percentage of medications that arrive on the patient unit within 2 hours of order receipt in the pharmacy*, with numerator, denominator, and goal (or target) defined. These targets can be set internally or can come from the literature or national standards. As the indicators are designed, it is important to have a mixture of process and clinical (outcome) indicators if possible. Economic and/or humanistic indicators also can be used, depending on the topic in question.

U (Understand Variation in the Current Process)

In this step, the team gathers the quality indicator data and creates graphs, for example, line charts, bar charts, run charts, or histograms (frequency plots) to analyze data trends. It is recommended to gather indicator data at several different points in time, so the problem's frequency can be determined. In other words, it is helpful to know if there is evidence of a stable problem, sustained over two to three data points, versus a problem detected at one single point in time. Efforts in CQI should be data-driven; knowing baseline performance is essential, and these indicators will be used after the process improvement is implemented to show how actions have been successful. Examples of how to display charts and data are provided in several reference texts.[6,20,32] If many baseline data points are collected, statistical process control charts with defined upper and lower control limits can be used, and this technique will help to define special or actionable causes of variation on which the team can focus. With any process, there is a degree of normal variation to work. Using the statistical process control chart can help the team to identify and focus on time periods when something unique occurred that was outside of normal or expected variance to the process.

Once the baseline data are generated and displayed, the team needs to take part in a brainstorming session to identify all of the problem's potential causes. The key point of group brainstorming sessions is to encourage a free-flow of ideas and allow all ideas to be considered. Brainstorming is used to list as many potential failure mode possibilities as the group is able in the meeting's short time frame. The brainstorming session should be led by a moderator, whose role is to keep the group focused and on track. The MSO can serve as the session moderator, provide objectivity to the session, and ensure equal participation by all members. The moderator should open the brainstorming session by providing an overview of group's charge, the session's goals, and the rules for a productive meeting. *Noted general rules for brainstorming sessions are:*

- Agree on the issue (or in this case, process or sub-process step)
- No suggested idea (failure mode) should be criticized
- Give each participant an equal turn to speak in an identified order, for example, going around the table in a clockwise fashion) with no interruptions between speakers
- Transcribe all ideas on a flipchart or board to capture them
- Set a time limit on the brainstorming session

The brainstorming session can be a bit more unstructured, but in either case, the free-flow of ideas is needed, and a time limit should be set.[4]

S (Select the Process for Change)

The causes of the problem should be prioritized, so the problem's root cause can be selected and targeted for action. It is important to organize the causes into like categories, as this will help to sort out potential actions that can be taken. Focusing the team's effort on what is causing the most problems, or the top several causes that can be successfully impacted by the team, is important, as some of the minor causes may be high effort and low return.

A *cause-and-effect process/diagram* can be used to categorize problems and eventually identify their root causes, which are organized in this diagram. When the brainstorming session is complete, generated ideas listed for each sub-process step can be grouped into major causes and minor causes. These diagrams, known as Ishikawa (after its inventor) or fishbone diagrams (parts of the diagram resemble a rough drawing of a fish), are a visual way to relate varied causes of a particular problem to the resulting effect.[5,33] A sample fishbone diagram is provided in Figure 6-8. The problem, or failure, is put at the far right side of a drawn horizontal backbone line in a text box. Lines extending as a backslash from the horizontal backbone should be drawn to major causes, and these can be typically grouped into three to four major general causes, related to man, materials, methods, or machinery.[4] Another categorization is people, procedures, plant (equipment), and policies.[5] For each general cause header, smaller, much more specific causes are drawn onto the diagram into the "bones" (minor causes) of the fish schematic. The many brainstormed causes will

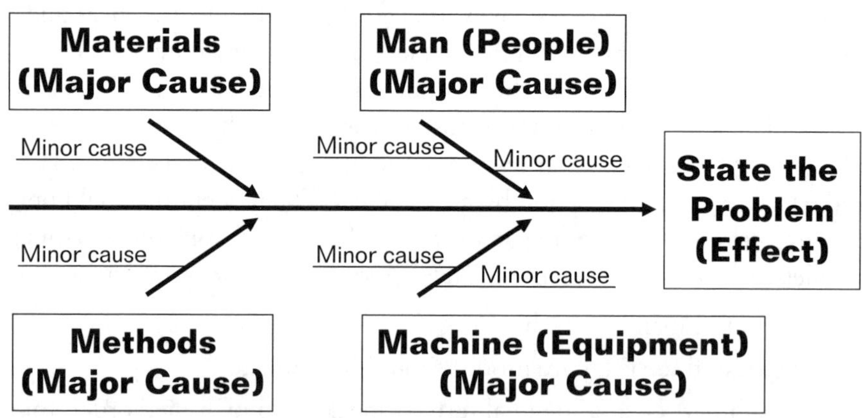

Figure 6-8. Sample fishbone diagram (cause-and-effect).
Source: Adapted with permission from H. Hagel, *Managing the Patient-Centered Pharmacy*, American Pharmacists Association, 2002.

naturally sort into like areas; for example, causes related to technology needs will sort into machinery, or causes related to lack of established standard operating procedures or policies will sort into the methods cause. Once the diagram is complete and all major/minor causes are drawn out, the team can rank the causes in priority to identify the root cause.

The number of like causes is graphed according to frequency, from highest to lowest. The most frequent cause will most likely be the one causing the most problems, so this tool, known as a Pareto chart (named after Vilfredo Pareto, an economist in the 1600s), will help to sort out the "vital few" to focus on versus what can often be the "trivial many" other causes (see Figure 6-9 for a sample Pareto chart).[5,34] The *Pareto chart* is a tool to find an actionable or root cause of a problem or failure. Simply stated, the Pareto principle is that "for many phenomena, 80% of the effects stem from 20% of the causes."[35] The team can also show the increasing frequency of causes as a second Y-axis on the chart, with the first (left) Y-axis being the number of causes and the second one (right) being the cumulative percent of causes. Once identified, the process with the highest frequency will most likely be the one to focus on, as it will result in the most process improvement change; however, as noted above, this cause must be a tangible one, and one that is able to be affected by the group's improvement actions. Any cause that is not high frequency, but may be associated with a tragic outcome, must also be taken into consideration for potential

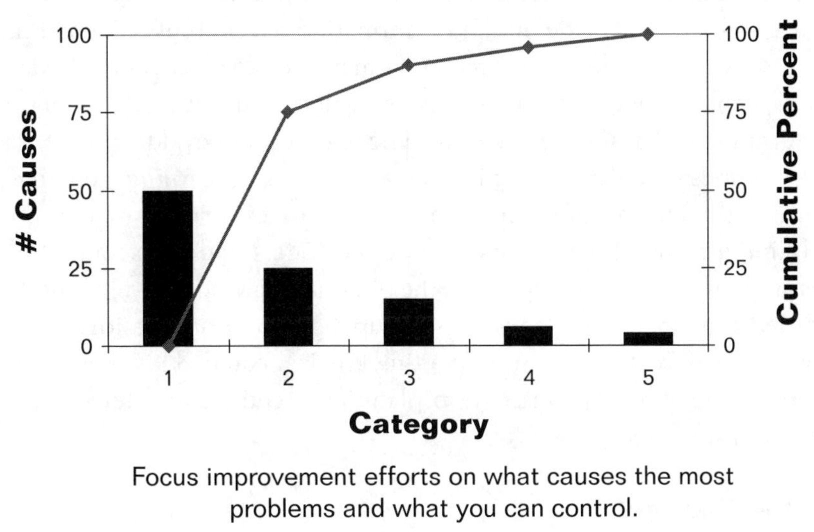

Figure 6-9. Sample Pareto chart.
Source: Adapted with permission from H. Hagel, *Managing the Patient-Centered Pharmacy*, American Pharmacists Association, 2002.

action. The team discussion sessions' work and importance is to identify the causes or failure modes for processes that occur. The Pareto chart is often used as part of CQI processes to quantify how often different causes can occur.

P (Plan the Change)

The team's next step is to plan the change that will occur. So far, the team has identified the problem with baseline data, identified customers and their expectations, reviewed the literature, and prioritized the problem's causes to sort out the root cause. Drawing on the team's expertise, insight, and experience, the action plan for change should be designed. It is important to relate the planned safety initiative to other programs already in place. Figure 6-10 presents a template to assist with developing and presenting a medication safety initiative.

The team should consider the scope of the change and to determine if a test or pilot for the improvement action is needed. A small-scale pilot can be helpful to test out approaches to change, so the efforts of the team are not concentrated on one solution. The pilot's duration, location, and indicator data measurement should be defined to ensure it is conducted for a reasonable amount of time to identify successes and barriers. In case the impact of the change is not what was intended, it is important at the outset to identify stopping points in the pilot.

In addition to determining if the improvement action should be initiated as a pilot test, the team needs to clearly define a critical piece of the plan: the education regarding the change. As the customers and expectations were defined earlier (Clarifying step of FOCUS-PDCA), an educational plan should be designed that is both multidisciplinary and multifaceted, to address different practitioner learning levels, degree of need for detail, and information accessibility. A combination of written and electronic educational materials may need to be developed. Many learners comprehend change and new processes by direct educational sessions, whether group learning or one-on-one teaching. The team should evaluate these traditional learning methods as well as interactive or computer-based learning techniques within the scope of the improvement and available resources. For example, if one aspect of the training plan is for the nurses to better understand the scope of pharmacy services and how often deliveries leave the pharmacy, a video learning module could be recorded and nurses could view this at nursing or unit orientation. As the action steps are planned, it is important that a timeline is created. This timeline can serve as the agenda for the implementation planning meetings and teleconferences to review action steps and progress.

D (Do the Change)

Implementation can be challenging, but it is the most critical piece of the improvement. This step involves taking the actions identified above in the Plan phase, including the different educational approaches and content, and carrying them out. Time must be allowed for implementation, as this includes training, process change (and all supporting documents), and updating or creating materials for education.

Drug Use and Disease State Management Program: Patient Safety Initiative

Initiative Title

Recommendations

- Level of evidence support from clinical trials should appear with each recommendation if pertinent (safety information frequently from ISMP, TJC, and other organizations may be graded as consensus papers)
- Outline specific patients/restriction criteria for appropriate use
- Also include any relationship with existing initiatives (e.g., addition to renal dosing guidelines, inclusion in automatic IV to PO switch program)

Executive Summary

This section serves as a concise summary of the document. Include a clear rationale for the recommendations above.

Background

This section includes information regarding the pharmacology/pharmacokinetics of the focus agent as needed. Include some background on the reason for the need for safe practice recommendations.

Therapeutic Uses

FDA-approved indications should appear exactly as written in the manufacturer package information. Additional off-label uses should be included here particularly if they are the focus of the safe practice recommendations.

Literature Support

Summarize the evidence supporting the recommendations from primary or tertiary literature. Include organization consensus statements pertaining to existing safety guidelines for the agent(s), for example Institute for Safe Medication Practices (ISMP), The Joint Commission (TJC), and Agency for Healthcare Research and Quality (AHRQ). Pertinence to a high-alert medication or National Patient Safety Goal should be discussed here. Case reports and experience papers may also be used to highlight safety.

Toxicity and Cautions

This section typically highlights the reasons for the need for safe practice recommendations for the focus agent with literature support for adverse events seen in practice. Other clinical trials and consensus papers from organizations supporting the safe practice recommendations should be reviewed. Include the black box statement.

Figure 6-10 (continued).

Other Safety Headings

As needed, may include Drug Interactions or Contraindications to support the safe practice recommendations. If included, document drug/drug interactions and contraindications from manufacturer information and clinical studies.

Dose/Administration

The dosing information should include relevant FDA-approved indications and focused review of other dosing for off-label uses derived from the clinical trials.

Adverse Drug-Related Events and/or Medication Errors Experience at This Organization

Highlight and summarize data from the following sources depending on the nature of the safety issue.

- National data and local data
- Adverse drug-related event information (local)

Current Practices

A prospective review of current prescribing practices with the focus agent(s) at this organization, highlighting the opportunity for implementing safe prescribing practices, should be performed. The review should include at least 30 patients. Include information on prescribing patterns, physician services, and indications for use. Include a summary of sample size, time period, outcome measures findings, and appropriateness of use measured against published standard.

Practice at Other Institutions

If appropriate, a national, regional, and/or local benchmarking survey should be done to measure safe practice guidelines and successful implementation strategies at other institutions. A table indicating institution, guideline, and/or implementation strategy is preferred.

References

References should be noted in superscripts throughout the paper with each original thought. The reference list should adhere to the uniform requirements for manuscripts submitted to the biomedical journals.

Written by

The author(s) and reviewer(s) should be included with appropriate degrees and dated with month and year.

Figure 6-10. Drug use and disease state management program: patient safety initiative. *Source:* Courtesy of Drug and Disease Management, Susan Skledar.

Successful implementation depends on the right composition of the team, selecting appropriate communication strategies and appropriate time delineation for learning and testing. In the literature studied, optimal methods for implementation demonstrate computerized reminders and focused education in small groups as generally effective strategies, retrospective feedback as variably effective, and passive education programs (didactic lectures without case application) as least effective.[37] Gross et al. studied optimal implementation strategies and found that physicians reported that the most effective guideline implementation strategies were discussion with colleagues, placement of guideline on front of the patient chart or in progress notes, use of flowcharts or algorithms, and use of preprinted orders.[36]

Education must be done in a thorough fashion, but equally important is redesigning the process to match the improvement. This part of the "do" step can be updating on-line resources, changing technology, or redesigning workflow or daily assignments to support the new work. System changes, when done in conjunction with workflow improvements, can create an environment of success for the new plan, and the front-line work can be done more easily and efficiently. Change that is too complex or not supported by the current technology will result in confusion. For example, if the guideline for a new medication states it can be given only via intravenous (IV) infusion, but the hospital's CPOE system has multiple routes available (e.g., IV push), then the desired practice is not reinforced by the technology.

C (Check the Results of Change)

Post-implementation, the quality indicator data that were collected before the change should be again gathered and compared to the baseline performance. The work team will be busy during implementation with training and reinforcement of new procedures and workflow, but a team member must have responsibility for gathering post-implementation or post-pilot data to determine if the change is positively impacting the work or patient care. Defining the data sources and ownership for data collection during the prior clarifying "C" step is very important, so there is no confusion about this post-implementation. Additional quality measures can be added to the data collection process if needed, especially as the data begin to be generated and problems are identified.

Graphically depicting the indicator data compared to the baseline data is important to compare results, allowing the team to analyze the success of the improvement. Using the same graphs as the baseline data and adding on the post-implementation findings is an easy technique to display change. It is helpful to have the target performance rate (the goal or threshold), which was set during the Clarifying phase of FOCUS-PDCA, on the graph to show if the change achieved the desired impact. At this point, the process flowchart should be redone, with new steps inserted (in different color) as a representation of changed work or care. This will visually show the improvement to other teams or units where the change can be spread if successful. Sharing the results with the team, other stakeholders, and other front-line staff can be an effective way to communicate successes. If barriers such as lack of understanding, differences in findings during different shifts or ineffective communication (e.g., did not reach the intended audience as extensively as planned) are identified, then these barriers can be targeted for next steps, or cycles, of improvement. The team should focus on these barriers and design new action steps to avoid and overcome them. Rapid resolution of problems and accessibility and responsiveness of the work team are very important to create a positive environment for change.

A (Act to Spread or Sustain the Change)

In the final step of FOCUS-PDCA, the team needs to identify lessons learned, evaluate if and how the improvement can be successfully implemented in other areas, and determine the plan for sustained achievement and monitoring. All too often, an improvement effort works very well at the outset, but then processes and behaviors change over time compared to what was happening prior to the change. Continued diligence with monitoring, education, and feedback are important to sustaining, or holding, the gained benefit. Lessons learned can be used to create a better system for design or implementation as the work moves from one pilot area to a larger area or another similar hospital within a health system. Once the improvement is stabilized and is working, assign responsibility for monthly or quarterly ongoing data collection. If the improvements are ongoing, and nearly all of them will be because literature (materials), processes (methods), personnel (man), and technology (machinery) are constantly changing, the next cycles of improvement can be planned. The work team often will stay as a functioning unit, but may meet less regularly or even electronically to review the compliance data, which helps the team to stay focused and identify issues as they arise. Particularly with clinical efforts grounded in the literature, a team member should be assigned responsibility to make sure the guideline recommendations are the most current. As new staff enter the work area and work team, the original team should be open to new ideas and approaches, as CQI action plans must be timely and pertinent to practice.

Failure Modes and Effects Analysis

As noted earlier, the FMEA process can help to identify possible modes of failure in a new, or existing process, and the consequences of those failures. The FMEA is best carried out using a multidisciplinary team of stakeholders, including front-line staff. The MSO can lead the team in working through this process or be a participating member. The MSO should be knowledgeable about the steps in the FMEA process to facilitate the work team's efficiency. A description of the FMEA process is provided below, with an accompanying case example.

Step 1: The Team

The project team should include content experts and front-line staff. Patient safety leaders, risk management, and quality experts also can be involved. The project leader should be identified, as well as the "scribe" and administrative advisors. It may be helpful, especially for clinical staff, to have an alternate member, in case the primary person cannot attend due to a critical patient care issue. Use caution to include the pertinent team members without letting the team become too large that it becomes inefficient for discussion or too difficult to have good attendance at the meeting.

Step 2: Define the Topic

Like the first step explained in the global FOCUS-PDCA process, it is critical to focus your problem or topic. Especially with an FMEA, if the overall process is complex, sub-processes should be defined and analyzed. The topic or problem should be focused, measurable, and timely. For the MSO, using ADE and ME data, TJC alerts, NPSG directives, or high-alert medications, are excellent starting points. Using evidence in the literature to identify best practices, supporting articles, or other institutions' experiences is also beneficial.

Step 3: Process Flow Diagramming

In this step, the team can best understand the problem if a flowchart is used to describe the steps in the process. Process flow diagramming was explained earlier in this chapter.

Step 4: Hazard Analysis

In this FMEA step, the team takes the time to identify the different ways the process can fail or go wrong. Listing the failure modes, or what can go wrong in a process, must be done for each process step. This step can be time-consuming, but it is the crux of the FMEA process. Various tools can be used to identify the failure modes, including focus groups with directed questions and brainstorming sessions with the team.

In the detailed Step 4 Hazard Analysis process of FMEA, the root cause for each failure mode should be listed. The cause-and-effect diagram described above and Pareto chart can help to focus the team on each failure's possible causes. The causes are "why" the failure is occurring. Drilling down to the root of the problem, to focus on the one where you can make the most impact with potential change solutions, is key to project success. Examples of root causes may be knowledge deficits, lack of standardization, distractions in the workplace, or confusing computer order entry screens leading to error. Once this is completed, to compute the criticality index (CI), the potential failure mode's possibility (frequency), severity, and probability of detection must be estimated. Because many failure modes are often identified, the CI is used to determine the exact priority of all root causes in FMEA. Scales are available to assist in this important step in the FMEA process.[30,31] To best display and organize this step, a chart should be constructed to list the failure mode, its cause, its effect, the frequency of failure (likelihood of occurrence), the degree of severity, the chance of failure to detect, and the risk priority.

The frequency of failure is the likelihood of the failure to occur and can be determined from a 1 to 10 score occurrence rating scale from remote (no known occurrence, greater than or equal to 1:10,000 chance) to very high (documented occurrence in literature or practice; 1:10 to 1:20 chance).[30] Next, the failure's severity can be categorized using a 1 to 10 score scale of slight annoyance, to major system problem, to minor injury, to terminal injury or death. Finally, the probability of detection is scored on a 1 to 9 scale from very high (9:10 chance system will detect) to remote (detection cannot occur at any point; 0:10).[30] For each failure mode, these three scores are multiplied to get the CI, which can help prioritize the group's efforts. The team may want to focus on the top three to five highest CI score items for their action plans.

The VANCPS denotes a slightly different approach to calculating the hazard score.[31] The severity rating scale is a 1 to 4 scoring, and each mode is analyzed in severity as catastrophic (4), major (3), moderate (2), or minor (1). Detailed definitions for each step are given in the on-line reference tutorial.[31] A probability rating of frequent (4; likely to occur within a short period) to remote (1; unlikely) is also determined, and the product of these two scores is multiplied for the hazard score. If the team determines the hazard score, for example, is high, and there are no effective control measures for it, then action would need to be taken. Also called the severity-outcome-detection (SOD) rating,[5] this score is helpful to prioritize actions.

Whether the team uses the traditional method with CI or the hazard score method, the next step will be to sort out and prioritize the failure modes that require action. If the CI and hazard score show findings that are slightly different, it remains important to focus the work on a few actionable improvements versus a longer roster of actions that may not be accomplished. Focusing efforts on defined steps that have the most error risk and are within the team's control and influence is most important. Using FMEA to find these risk points is a proactive step in process improvement. Processes of care that are highest risk for the MSO to focus on are those with many and extensive hand-offs, those with interplay of many different disciplines or departments, or those with fragmented care involving many steps.[5]

Step 5: Action

Continuing with the FMEA process, the team must identify which of the identified failure modes and associated CI scores should result in action. The terminology used is that the team must decide whether to eliminate, control, or accept the failure mode cause.[26-31] For example, if there is an effective control measure or safeguard in place already that is working well, the team may decide to keep that control in place and not design new action. If the hazard, however, is not easily known and needs an identification or detection measure, then the team may select it for action. For each failure mode cause that is selected for activity, an improvement action will be described to either eliminate or control that failure mode cause. It is recommended to put the control measure in place at the earliest process step, so it has the best and greatest chance of preventing the failure.

In the industrial improvement models, actions focus on redesign, redundancy, and isolation.[30] Processes and systems can be redesigned for safety and efficiency. Purposeful redundancy (e.g., independent double-check) is important in health care to prevent an error from reaching the patient. Isolating the step with the most risk—for example, preparation of the chemotherapeutic agent in a separate pharmacy area with a built-in pharmacist double-check—is also effective. Automating processes can help with minimizing the chance of human error or mix-up, and continual monitoring of progress and impact is important.

Part of identifying the actions that will occur as a result of Step 4 is to identify the person who will have major responsibility for implementing the action and seeing that it is accomplished and continually monitored. As noted earlier, it is important for higher level administration to be in agreement and support the recommended actions.

Implementation of actions should be carefully done, including process changes, testing of those processes, and rapid evaluation of their impact. With rapid cycle change, a challenge is that change will occur too quickly and front-line staff will not be informed. The identified responsible person must be accountable for informing the work team of changes via written, verbal, and/or electronic means to keep channels of communication open. The team may decide to use planning tools such as timelines and flowcharts to show process steps in the action design, and have frequent meetings to track actions. Steps in the improvement plan should be clearly delineated with target time frames. If there is a process change, logical and measurable steps should be implemented. For clinical (or outcome) improvements, using evidence in the literature for best practices is critical. This will also provide rigor and a scientific basis for the need for the improvement and will help to convince practitioners that the change should be implemented. Literature can also be helpful with identifying other institution practices for approaches to process improvement or care design.

As with FOCUS-PDCA, a pilot, or test, of the action may be warranted and helpful, as it allows for the improvement's implementation on a smaller scale, to test its feasibility and identify process barriers. To make sure all changes are happening in an organized approach, it is suggested that weekly or bi-weekly sessions occur to keep the project on-time. The actions developed should be agreed on by the team, and the action plan itself should be results-oriented and the improvement measures (see next step) usable. Although already in place, front-line staff, if not part of the problem analysis process to this point, should be involved in the action plan development and implementation process.

It should be noted that actions can be complex or simple, and also can be stronger or weaker, depending on the improvement. The VANCPS notes five different criteria for actions that can help to guide the team; an adaptation of those is listed below:[31]

1. Does the action address the root cause of the failure or problem?
2. Is the action specific and concrete?
3. Is the action easy to understand?
4. Should a pilot occur before full implementation?
5. Were those with first-hand knowledge of the process involved in action design?

The ISMP provides additional guidance for the MSO regarding effective strategies for safety/reducing error.[38] Further, ISMP notes that education and providing information, without combining that with other "hard-coded" actions, such as forcing functions and constraints, may not be effective in reducing error. Fixing the system is more effective than "fixing" people and relying on their memory and vigilance to prevent errors and mishaps.[38] The team should consider these guidance factors as improvement actions are designed and implemented.

Actions designed involving equipment or technology change can be effective if the front-line workers understand how to use the new equipment or technology. Actions including double-checks, reminders, auxiliary labels, and repeated education, can be helpful, but are not always fail-safe, as they still include the chance of human error. As noted earlier, the health care industry acknowledges that honest accidents are going to occur. Systems and processes should be implemented to support health care workers to have the tools they need to do their jobs efficiently and effectively.

Step 6: Follow-Up

In the last step of FMEA, process and/or outcome indicator measures need to be designed that can be used to monitor the impact of process changes and improvements. These indicators should be measurable, and data sources need to be identified. Quality indicators can be economic if there is a cost-savings or cost-avoidance element to the work; clinical outcome-oriented (e.g., adverse event reduction); or process-oriented, measuring compliance with specific steps of the change. Humanistic outcome measures, for example, customer satisfaction, also can be determined. These may be more difficult to collect, but are viewed as highly desirable for patient-centered care improvements. Data collection should be done frequently at the improvement's start, and then once the process is stabilized, the data can be collected, weekly, then monthly, then quarterly. It is advisable to assign responsibility for the data collection and reporting, and convene monthly (or quarterly) meetings of the team to make sure the improvements are sustained and identify corrections. The team should revisit the original FMEA to recalculate the CI based on new literature, changing ADE/ME patterns, or even changing health care staff. Key characteristics of the quality indicators include that they be measurable; have defined data sources, numerators, and denominators; be reported as percentages or rates; and have defined measurement periods. Also important is a threshold for improvement that is both achievable and realistic. Incremental thresholds can be utilized that change with time. When a target threshold is achieved, it is time to evaluate what should be done to hit the next goal's threshold. The threshold can be set within internal institution goals and targets or from data found in the literature.

FMEA CASE STUDY: MEDICATION DELIVERY TIMELINESS (MDT)

Step 1: The Team

The team includes the Pharmacy Director and Nursing Administrator as advisors, pharmacists, nurses, pharmacy technicians, information systems specialists, a pharmacy manager, a physician, and a nursing director.

Step 2: Define (and Focus) the Topic

The focus of the FMEA is on improving the timeliness of the pharmacy medication dispensing process. The team's focus, as determined by the process flow diagrams in the next step, will be on accurate and efficient order review by the pharmacist.

Step 3: Process Flow Diagramming

See Figures 6-11 and 6-12 for flowcharts of the MDT process. Time observations also were done on each step in the process, and each step in the chart is numbered in sequence. As depicted in Figure 6-11, process Step 4 is complex, so a sub-process graphic is drawn to define each step in that process as well (Figure 6-12).

Step 4: Hazard Analysis

Figure 6-13 provides the failure modes for each process step. The team will be focusing on Step 4A, which is the step where the pharmacist enters the order into the computer.

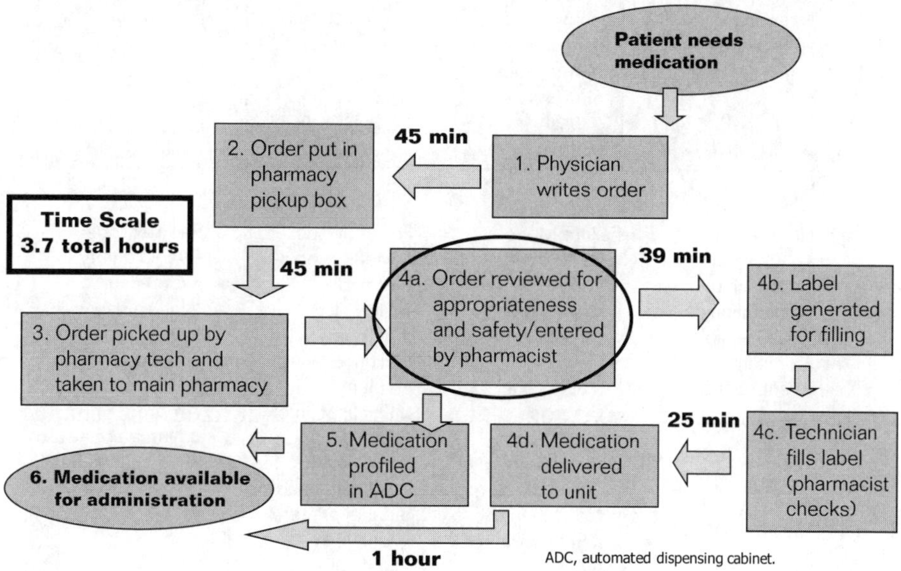

Figure 6-11. Process flow.
Source: Adapted with permission from T. Warholak and D. Nau, *Quality and Safety in Pharmacy Practice*, McGraw-Hill Medical, 2010.

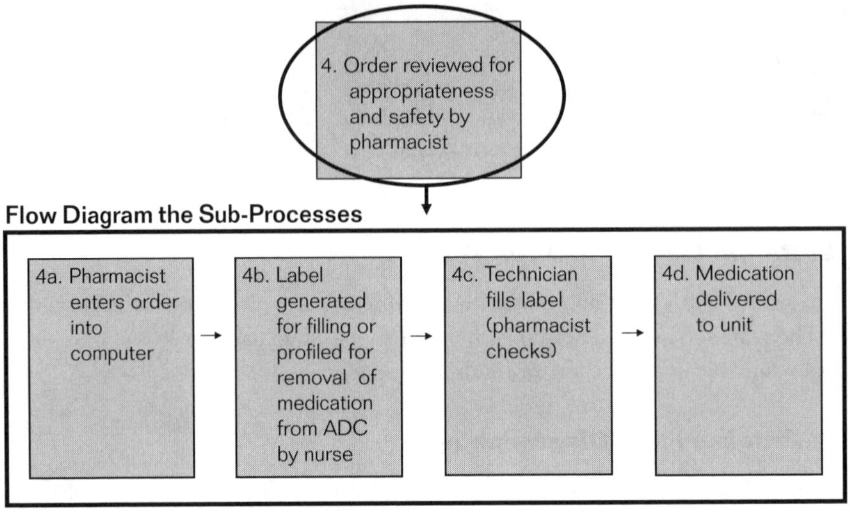

ADC, automated dispensing cabinet.

Figure 6-12. Sub-process graphic.

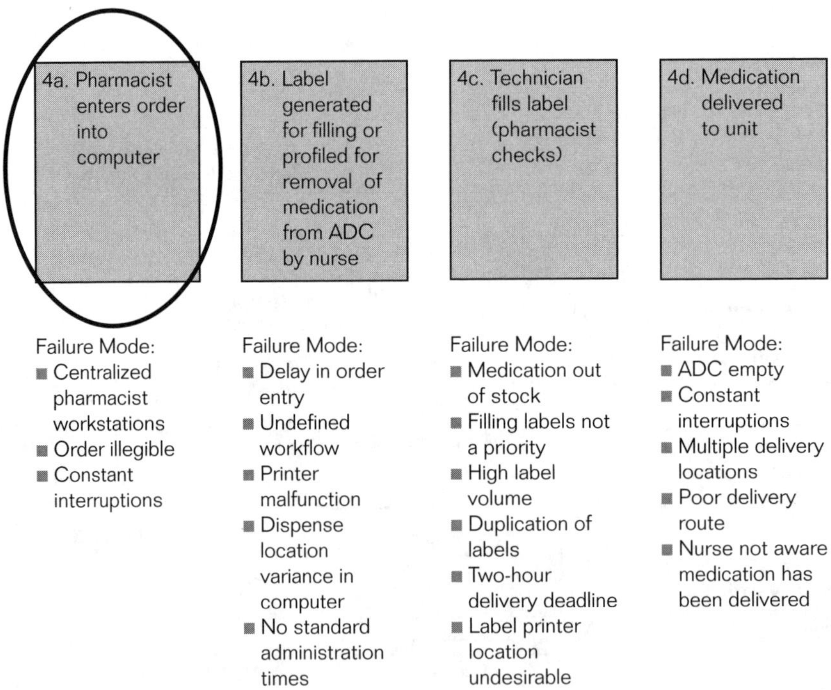

ADC, automated dispensing cabinet.

Figure 6-13. Failure modes for each process step.

Figure 6-14 shows the results of the hazard analysis scoring, using the traditional 1 to 10 scoring methods. For example, the highest-scored failure mode was the illegible orders, with the cause being faxed orders (note: this hospital is not a CPOE hospital), with a score of 8 for frequency and severity, and 10 for chance of failure to detect, resulting in a 640 score. Other high-scoring modes include centralized order entry (geographic challenge) and constant workflow interruptions. All of these identified high CI processes will be the focus of the improvement efforts.

Step 5: Action

Figure 6-14 (column 8) lists the four steps where the actions have been designed. Figure 6-15 displays actions and outcomes, along with data sources for outcome measures (see next step). The actions include concrete steps of eliminating faxing and implementing cell phones and pagers for the pharmacists, and also a bigger overall improvement plan includes implementing a unit-based pharmacy services plan. The FMEA process and plan results were published elsewhere.[39]

Step 6: Follow-Up

Figures 6-15 and 6-16 list the specific actions and outcome measures. Four quality indicator measures were identified, with data sources, rating scales, definitions, and measurement frequency defined. Measurement will be done post-implementation via audit (snapshot) method, as well as monthly data collection. If the data collected show that missing dose calls have increased since the improvement was made, this would be an unexpected finding, so another indicator can be developed to categorize the content of the calls and when they were received. It may be that missing dose calls decrease during the hours when the decentralized services model is active, but increase when the pharmacist is not present on the nursing unit.

Pharmacist enters order into computer

1 **Mode of Failure**	2 **Cause of Failure**	3 **Effect of Failure**	4 **Frequency of Failure (1–10)**	5 **Degree of Severity (1–10)**	6 **Chance of Failure to Detect (1–10)**	7 **Risk Priority (4 × 5 × 6 = 7)**	8 **Design Action**	9 **Describe Design Validation**
Undesirable service geographics (centralized coverage)	Centralized order entry pool	Delay in medication delivery	9	8	8	**576**	☑	Decentralize pharmacists to patient units
Order illegible	Faxing	Delay in medication delivery	8	8	10	**640**	☑	Eliminate faxing during decentralized service hours
	Handwriting (MD or RN)	Delay in medication delivery	8	8	2	128		
Constant interruptions	Multiple phones and faxes	Delay in medication delivery	8	8	5	**320**	☑	Implement cell phones and pagers
	No phone call triage process	Delay in medication delivery	5	8	9	**360**	☑	Implement cell phones and pagers

Figure 6-14. Hazard analysis grid.

Failure Mode	Action	Outcome
Undesirable service geographics (centralized coverage)	▪ Implement decentralized pharmaceutical care model	▪ Nursing satisfaction with pharmacy services (specific questions related to medication delivery)
Order illegible (fax-related)	▪ Eliminate faxing during decentralized service hours	▪ Medication turn-around time ▪ Missing dose calls
Constant interruptions	▪ Implement cell phones and pagers ▪ Technician triage of calls	▪ Missing dose calls ▪ Pharmacy satisfaction: pharmacy vacancy and turnover rates

Figure 6-15. Actions and outcomes.

	Data Source	Measurement Scale	Measurement Frequency
Nursing Satisfaction	Survey of nurses on service line units (all shifts)	Likert Scale (1 to 5) Median comparison	Pre- and post-implementation
Medication Turn-Around Time (TAT) (hr)	Observations on time study log using observations	TAT = Time from when order is written to time medication is available for the patient on the unit	Pre- and post-implementation snapshots
Missing Dose Calls	Phone call tracking log completed daily by pharmacy technicians	% total calls recorded that are for missing doses	Pre- and post-implementation monthly comparison
Vacancy/ Turnover Rate	Human Resources	% positions vacant at site and across health system	Six months pre- and post-implementation

Figure 6-16. Key outcome measures.

Summary

An overview of continuous quality improvement principles, including the FOCUS-PDCA methodology, the FMEA process, and several tools to assist with root cause analysis are presented. Sources of problem identification include external safety and regulatory groups, review of ADE and ME data, and published literature recommendations. Continuing to evaluate practices, particularly focusing on medication and patient safety, is critical for clinicians and patient safety leaders. The MSO has a leadership role in identifying variant processes, mobilizing work teams to solve problems, and a sound understanding of process implementation tools that can be used to facilitate analysis and change. Proactive tools such as FMEA can be used before processes are changed to identify potential failure modes in a process before it is implemented. Pilot programs can be run to test hypotheses of change for best results. Methodologies such as FOCUS-PDCA can be used systematically to solve problems that are identified. Process improvements can be implemented based on internal data and performance, and the MSO should know their internal and external data sources as well as regulatory requirements for reporting. An understanding of these methods and tools is important to engage teams and staff for contribution of ideas and approaches to solving problems that result in sustained improvements and a safer care environment for patients and staff.

PRACTICE TIPS

1. Piloting a change is very much worth the extra effort. A pilot can be quick, and if it is designed with specific indicators of measure can accurately reflect process gaps and points of vulnerability.
2. Quality indicator measures must be data-driven; just as importantly, data sources must be accessible and easy to obtain. Designing a process that relies heavily on manual tracking of findings creates a potential workload burden.
3. Select indicator metrics during the process redesign—do not wait until after the process change is implemented. This focuses the team on what will be measured and should also be the guidance for baseline data gathering.
4. Process redesign should be, as much as possible, hard-coded into the work versus an extra step or series of steps.

References

1. Shewart WA. *The Economic Control of Quality of Manufactured Product.* New York: D. Van Nostrand Company; 1931. Reprinted by the American Society of Quality Control Quality Press, Milwaukee, WI; 1980.
2. Committee on Quality Health Care in America, Institute of Medicine. *Crossing the Quality Chasm: A New Health System for the 21st Century.* Washington, DC: National Academy Press; 2001.
3. Varkey P, Reller K, Resar RK. Basics of quality improvement in health care. *Mayo Clin Proc.* 2007;82(6):735-739.
4. Brassard M, Ritter D. *The Memory Jogger II: A Pocket Guide of Tools for Continuous Quality Improvement and Effective Planning.* Salem, NH: GOAL/QPC; 1994.
5. McLaughlin CP, Kaluzny AD. Defining Quality Improvement. In: McLaughlin CP, Kaluzny AD eds. *Continuous Quality Improvement in Health Care: Theory, Implementations, and Applications.* Sudbury, MA: Jones and Bartlett Publishers; 2006:3-40.
6. Skledar SJ. Continuous Quality Improvement. In: Hagel HP, Rovers JP eds. *Managing the Patient-Centered Pharmacy.* Washington, DC: American Pharmaceutical Association; 2002:217-238.
7. Lynn ML, Osborn DP. Deming's quality principles: a health care application. *Hosp Hlth Serv Admin.* 1991;6(1):111-120.
8. Vogus TJ, Sutcliffe KM. The impact of safety organizing, trusted leadership, and care pathways on reported medication errors in hospital nursing units. *Med Care.* 2007;45:997-1002.
9. Wilson KA, Burke CS, Priest HA et al. Promoting health care safety through training high reliability teams. *Qual Saf Health Care.* 2005;14:303-309.
10. Vogus TJ, Sutcliffe KM. The safety organizing scale: development and validation of a behavioral measure of safety culture in hospital nursing units. *Med Care.* 2007;45:45-54.
11. Edmondson AC. Learning from mistakes is easier said than done: group and organizational influences on the detection and correction of human error. *J Appl Behav Sci.* 1996;32:5-28.
12. Thomas EJ, Sexton JB, Neilands TB et al. The effect of executive walk rounds on nurse safety climate attitudes: a randomized trial of clinical units. *BMC Health Serv Res.* 2005;5(1)28-36.
13. Young D. National medication safety managers see the big picture. *Am J Health-Syst Pharm.* 2004;61:1424-1425.
14. Deming EW. *Out of Crisis.* Cambridge, MA: MIT Center for Advanced Engineering Study Publishing; 1982.
15. Donabedian A. A founder of quality assessment encounters a troubled system firsthand. Interview by Fitzhugh Mullan. *Health Aff* (Millwood). 2001;20:137-141.
16. Donabedian A. The seven pillars of quality. *Arch Pathol Lab Med.* 1990;11:115-118.
17. Young D. Pittsburgh hospitals band together to reduce medication errors. *Am J Health Syst Pharm.* 2002;59:1014,1016,1026.
18. Endsley S, Magil MK, Godfrey MM. Creating a lean practice. *Fam Pract Manag.* 2006;13: 34-38.
19. Statistical Six Sigma Definition. Available at http://www.isixsigma.com/new-to-six-sigma/statistical-six-sigma-definition/. Accessed October 19, 2012.
20. Skledar S. Continuous quality improvement. In: Peterson AM, ed. *Managing Pharmacy Practice: Principles, Strategies, and Systems.* Boca Raton, FL: CRC Press; 2004:205-231.
21. ISMP's List of High-Alert Medications. Institute for Safe Medication Practices. Available at: http://www.ismp.org/Tools/highalertmedications.pdf. Accessed March 10, 2011.

22. *How-to Guide: Prevent Harm from High-Alert Medications*. Cambridge, MA: Institute for Healthcare Improvement; 2012. Available at: http://www.ihi.org/knowledge/Pages/Tools/HowtoGuidePreventHarmfromHighAlertMedications.aspx Accessed October 19, 2012.
23. Sentinel Event Alert, Issue 11. High Alert Medications and Patient Safety. The Joint Commission. Available at: http://www.jointcommission.org/sentinel_event_alert_issue_11_high-alert_medications_and_patient_safety/ . Accessed September 12, 2012.
24. Committee on Identifying and Preventing Medication Errors. Aspden P, Wolcott J, Bootman JL, Cronenwett LR, Editors. *Preventing Medication Errors: Quality Chasm Series*. Washington, DC: National Academies Press; 2006.
25. National Patient Safety Goals. The Joint Commission. Available at: http://www.jointcommission.org/standards_information/npsgs.aspx. Accessed Mar 8, 2011.
26. Cohen MR, Senders, J, Davis NM. Failure mode and effects analysis: a novel approach to avoiding dangerous medication errors and accidents. *Hosp Pharm*. 1994;29:319-324,326-328, 330.
27. Feldman SE, Roblin DW. Medical accidents in hospital care: applications of failure analysis to hospital quality appraisal. *J Comm J Qual Improv*. 1997;Nov23(11):567-580.
28. Senders JW. Theory and analysis of typical errors in a medical setting. *Hosp Pharm*. 1993; 28:506-508.
29. Fletcher CE. Failure mode and effects analysis: an interdisciplinary way to analyze and reduce medication errors. *JONA*. 1997 Dec;27(12):19-26.
30. Williams E, Tally R. The use of failure mode effect and criticality analysis in a medication error subcommittee. *Hosp Pharm*. 1994;9:331-332,334-337.
31. Healthcare Failure Mode Effect Analysis Process. Veterans Affairs National Center for Patient Safety. Available at: http://www.patientsafety.gov/SafetyTopics/HFMEA/HFMEA_JQI.html. Accessed July 19, 2011.
32. Kelly DL, Johnson SP. Measurement and statistical analysis in CQI. In: McLaughlin CP, Kaluzny AD, eds. *Continuous Quality Improvement in Health Care: Theory, Implementations, and Applications*. Sudbury, MA: Jones and Bartlett Publishers; 2006:95-130.
33. Ishikawa K. *Guide to Quality Control*. Trans. Asian Productivity Organization. White Plains, NY: Kraus International Publications. 1987.
34. Juran JM, Godfrey AB. *Juran's Quality Handbook*. 5th ed. New York: McGraw, Hill; 1999.
35. Pareto principle. Available at: http://dictionary.reference.com/browse/Pareto+principle. Accessed September 12, 2012.
36. Gross PA, Greenfield S, Cretin S, et al. Optimal methods for guideline implementation: conclusions from the Leeds Castle Meeting. *Med Care*. 2001;9:1185-1192.
37. Stone TT, Schwiekhart SB, Mantese A, et al. Guideline attribute and implementation preferences among physicians in multiple health systems. *Q Manage Health Care*. 2005;14(3):177-187.
38. Medication Error Prevention "Toolbox." Available at: http://www.ismp.org/newsletters/acutecare/articles/19990602.asp. Accessed September 12, 2012.
39. Weber RJ, Skledar SJ, Sirianni CR, et al. Impact of hospital pharmacist and technician decentralized pharmaceutical care teams. *Hosp Pharm*. 2004;39(12):1169-1176.
40. Spear, S, Bowen HK. Decoding the DNA of the Toyota production system, *Harv Bus Rev*. 1999;77(5):97-106.

Safety in the Medication-Use System

Connie M. Larson

CHAPTER 7

Key Terms

High-Alert or High-Risk Medications—High-alert or high-risk medications have a greater capacity to cause significant patient harm if used incorrectly.

Look-Alike/Sound-Alike Medications—Similar medication names, either written or spoken, which may lead to potentially harmful medication errors when they are confused with each other.[1]

Medication—According to The Joint Commission, any prescription medications, sample medications, herbal remedies, vitamins, nutraceuticals, vaccines, or over-the-counter drugs; diagnostic and contrast agents used on or administered to persons to diagnose, treat, or prevent disease or other abnormal conditions; radioactive medications, respiratory therapy treatments, parenteral nutrition, blood derivatives, and intravenous solutions (plain, with electrolytes and/or drugs); and any product designated by the Food and Drug Administration (FDA) as a drug. This definition of medication does not include enteral nutrition solutions (which are considered food products), oxygen, and other medical gases.[1]

Override—A function related to patient-profiled automated dispensing cabinets (ADC) that allows the user (e.g., nurse) to have access to a medication prior to verification by a pharmacist.

Safety—The degree to which the risk of an intervention (for example, use of a drug, or a procedure) and risk in the care environment are reduced for a patient and other persons, including health care practitioners. Safety risks may arise from the performance of tasks, from the structure of the physical environment, or from situations beyond the organization's control (such as weather).[1]

Unit Dose—Medication to be given to a particular patient at a specific time packaged in the exact dosage required for that time.

Introduction

Just say YES to drugs...for all the right reasons! **Medication therapy** is an essential element of the health care system. Medications are invaluable in the fight to prevent, treat, and cure diseases, although we must be mindful and diligent regarding their use to prevent patient harm and death. Drug therapy can be risky and has been reported to account for up to 19.4% of medical injury in hospitalized patients.[2] In 2008, drug-related adverse outcomes were noted in nearly 1.9 million inpatient hospital stays (4.7% of all stays) and 838,000 treat-and-release emergency department (ED) visits (0.8% of all visits).[3] Identifying and incorporating medication **safety** strategies into the medication-use process are crucial to prevent misuse or errors. We need to make our systems safer to protect our patients and staff.

I believe we have plenty of motivation to want to do better for our patients and for ourselves. We want to help patients—that's why we went in to health care in the first place. As individual practitioners we can encourage mindful and careful practice and performance in our everyday duties. But who is looking at the big picture? Who is tying everything together to make sure we actually are providing safe care—safe medication practices?

Do we need help from regulatory agencies? To motivate us—I hope not. To provide direction based on scientific evidence and identified best practices—definitely. The Centers for Medicare & Medicaid Services (CMS) and The Joint Commission (TJC) are examples of organizations that provide some of the standards and requirements for the medication-use system; their roles are described in more detail in Chapter 4, Accreditation and Regulatory Compliance. Generally, TJC standards describe the elements of a process that need to be in place to achieve compliance with their standards and National Patient Safety Goals, but they do not dictate the process the organization must follow to achieve compliance. However, achieving compliance cannot be the sole goal as it is not necessarily synonymous with safety. Therein lies the challenge—achieving compliance utilizing safe processes specific to the unique needs of the organization, thus improving safety of the medication system overall.

A review of key literature related to system analysis of adverse drug events (ADEs) is essential reading prior to evaluating the organization's medication-use system. Key articles provide a solid foundation on understanding the complexity of the medication-use system and the potential for adverse drug events.[2,4-6] Safeguarding your medication system and reducing ADEs is the medication safety officer's (MSO) primary focus.

TJC and regulatory agencies provide direction for handling **high-alert medications**. High-alert or high-risk medications have greater capacity to cause patient harm if used incorrectly. Organizations should have a list of medications designated as high-alert medications that are present in the facility. Each identified high-alert medication should be evaluated at every component of the medication-use system to identify potential problems and intervention strategies. An example of a high-alert medication list and potential strategies to prevent errors is included in Table 7-1. Other tools (e.g., checklists, flowcharts, and worksheets) are included in this chapter to aid in process review and improvement activities.

A careful review of your medication-use system is essential to the role of the MSO.

Medication Safety Assessment

It is important to understand the organization's risk points in the medication-use system. An assessment of key functions is essential in determining where there are opportunities for improvement that lower the risk for a given process. Equally important is identifying risk points that cannot be eliminated that may require special consideration for development of a safe process.

The medication-use system is a complex process comprised of the following components:

- Procurement
- Outdates/recall management
- Storage/control
- Ordering/prescribing
- Order review for appropriateness
- Preparation
- Distribution
- Administration/documentation
- Monitoring

An assessment of each component to identify risk areas will allow the organization to target and prioritize medication safety improvement initiatives that address critical high-risk medication processes.

Procurement

Formulary Decisions

Obtaining medications from suppliers or wholesalers for use in the organization is a very important function of the medication-use system. Decisions made regarding formulary products to stock and have available for ordering and dispensing requires oversight from a safety perspective. The Pharmacy and Therapeutics (P&T) Committee decision-making process must also include a review of any potential safety issues associated with a new medication product.[7] Formulary decisions affect every aspect of the medication-use system. See Tables 7-2 and 7-3 for medication use safety considerations for a formulary medication review. The ideal situation is to proactively identify and address safety issues before the medication is available for use in the organization. The Medication Safety Committee (MSC) is a good venue for a pre-P&T safety review for medications under formulary consideration.

Table 7-1. High-Alert Medication Safety Strategies

Medication-Use Node	Strategies
Access/storage	■ Apply warning labels and/or distinguish drug names clearly (e.g., tall-man lettering) ■ Use different size containers/manufacturer (look-alike drugs) ■ Sequester and lock drugs if floor stock on units ■ Eliminate or reduce floor stock; stock only in areas of critical need ■ Separate like products when using or storing products ■ Use smallest size package, concentration and dose for floor stock ■ Implement formulary drug restrictions or criteria for use
Ordering	■ Discourage verbal orders for high-alert medications ■ Eliminate the use of non-approved abbreviations ■ Use standardized drug/dose expressions ■ Use ordering protocols ■ Use appropriate dose expression (e.g., mg, mEq), not volume or amp ■ Include dose formula with calculated dose ■ Utilize standard concentration for IV infusion medications
Computer alerts, clinical decision support	■ Rules ■ Pop-ups ■ Interaction checking (allergies, food-drug interactions, drug-drug interactions, duplicate therapy)
Performing independent double-checks	■ Recalculate the dose ■ Use peer review process for unusual drug, dose, regimen ■ Involve patient/family through education ■ Attending physician verifies computer order prior to administration of first dose
Preparation and dispensing	■ Use commercially available premixed IV solutions ■ Establish dose limits and screen orders ■ Use drug preparation guidelines ■ Verify drug preparation ■ Dispense the drug from pharmacy only or emergency stock (drug box or crash cart)
Administration	■ Use drug administration protocols ■ Use dosing charts for IV administration or calculation function on infusion control devices ■ Use infusion control devices for continuous IV infusions ■ Use "smart pump" libraries when this technology is available ■ Use oral syringes for administration of oral products ■ Use bar-code verification when this technology is available
Monitoring	■ Obtain and communicate laboratory values via guidelines ■ Require cardiac monitoring and/or pulse oximetry ■ Require close observation/vital sign monitoring ■ Have antidotes and/or resuscitation equipment close at hand

Table 7-2. Procurement Decisions and Formulary Safety Considerations

Factors	Node	Potential Strategies
Look-alike/ sound-alike	Procurement/ storage	■ Purchasing products from different manufacturers ■ Separating products (pharmacy storage and automated medication cabinets on patient care areas) ■ Tall-man lettering ■ Cautionary sticker on storage bins ■ Cautionary labeling on shelves
	Ordering/ prescribing	■ Pop-up alerts ■ Minimizing/eliminating verbal orders
	Preparation/ dispensing	■ Cytotoxic drug handling procedures (e.g., double-checks) ■ Hazardous medication worksheets (e.g., double-checks) ■ Technician procedure set-up and pharmacist check (e.g., hazardous medication procedure)
	Administration	■ Nurse-independent double-checks
Medications impacted by organ function	Ordering/ prescribing	■ Clinical decision support (rules, pop-ups, alerts) ■ Dosing alerts, dose range checking
Drug-drug, drug-food, drug-lab, drug-POCT interactions	Ordering/ prescribing, dispensing, monitoring	■ Clinical decision support (rules, pop-ups, alerts)
Packaging and labeling	Preparation/ dispensing, administration	■ Investigating other products with better packaging and labeling
Physical/environmental attributes	Storage	■ Appropriate placement in storage devices (e.g., inventory management system, ADC) to minimize errors and ensure appropriate access
	Preparation/ dispensing	■ Packaging needs for non-unit-dose products ■ Special labeling information noted such as caution information for special handling for teratogenic or cytotoxic products, and whether refrigeration is required ■ Special preparation and dispensing needs (e.g., short expiration, complex preparation procedures)
	Administration	■ Special administration information noted (e.g., rate)
Other identified safety issues as part of formulary monograph preparation, (see Table 7-3)	All	■ Medication-use guidelines for complex ordering, dosing, administration, and monitoring ■ Add to drug library for smart pumps (e.g., dose limits) ■ Standardizing concentrations ■ Limiting access (e.g., high-alert medications)

POCT, point-of-care testing.

Table 7-3. Medication-Use Safety Formulary Assessment

Assess for	Finding	Recommendation/Action Plan*
Black box warning(s)		
REMS		
Hazardous substance ▪ Internal list ▪ NIOSH ▪ Waste management		
External safety alerts ▪ ISMP ▪ FDA MedWatch ▪ TJC Sentinel Event Alert		
High-alert medication		
Look-alike/sound-alike		
IV infusion administration		Add/revise smart pump library
Ped/NICU IV administration		Add/revise syringe pump library

FDA, U.S. Food and Drug Administration; ISMP, Institute for Safe Medication Practices; IV, intravenous; NIOSH, National Institute for Occupational Safety and Health; Ped/NICU, Pediatrics/Newborn Intensive Care Unit; REMS, risk evaluation and mitigation strategies; TJC, The Joint Commission.
*Consider each step of the medication-use process.
Source: Courtesy D. Saine, Winchester Medical Center.

Another important aspect related to procurement of medications is identifying if other departments may be purchasing a medication, as defined by TJC, without the knowledge of the pharmacy department. It would not be unusual to find that the Materials Management department could potentially be carrying supplies that would be considered a medication. Some of the products used for wound care are medications rather than a skin care product (e.g., emollients). While one could argue this is probably more of a regulatory than a safety issue, consider the complexities of remotely managing safety-related processes such as drug product bar codes for bar-code medication administration, formulary duplications, recalls, expiration dates, and secure storage. Procurement, storage, and distribution of medications outside the pharmacy requires careful planning between leaders of the pharmacy and that department to ensure practices are in place to support medication-use technologies and comply with regulations and accreditation standards. Another area where purchasing some of their own products/devices could lead to problems is in the operating room (OR). Often the intent is to use devices filled with medications only during the surgery, but then the patient ends up on the inpatient care unit and the nurse does not know how to use the device delivering an anesthetic medication. Education for the staff is often overlooked when new, interesting devices come in to the organization outside of the normal approval channels.

All medications used in your institution should be identified and listed on the formulary approved by P&T. Likewise, all medication infusion devices and other devices need to go through a review and approval process (e.g., New Products Committee) prior to their use. A pharmacist, often the MSO, should be included in the review process if the device is used to administer medications, or if the device uses medications (for example, heparin) during its operation. Of note, these goals can be very challenging to achieve! The MSO should assess the current state and collaborate with leadership to initiate changes as needed. Often, the MSO can provide helpful education on medication safety and medication management standards to help jump-start the process.

Drug Product Shortages

Unfortunately in recent years it has become commonplace to have to deal with drug supply shortages. Drug product shortages can adversely affect drug therapy and medical procedures and lead to medication errors.[8] Many shortages are for high-alert medications, making them even more potentially dangerous. Alternate product choices involving product dose size and concentration can be particularly problematic. For example, hydromorphone may be available as 1-, 2-, and 4-mg syringes. If the 1- and 2-mg syringes are unavailable due to a shortage, utilizing a 4-mg product in situations where the dose may be small is a potentially dangerous substitution. Shortages can wreak havoc on your medication-use system if not handled effectively. A thorough review by the appropriate practitioners is necessary to make sure any alternate products fit well into the various systems and technology already in place. If not, modifications need to be made to address potential safety issues. For the hydromorphone example, consideration of all the options is necessary before a final decision can be made. Considerations may include identifying the areas that have a critical need for the product that may be on shortage. Managing the stock that you do have or any allocations you may obtain, can allow you to minimize the risk by implementing the higher risk product into a more appropriate subset of patients. Figure 7-1, Drug Product Change Evaluation Form, is an example of a tool that can be utilized to manage shortages and product replacements for other reasons, such as cost savings. The MSO, along with the Medication-Use Policy Coordinator, Pharmacy Operations Manager, and purchasing staff are essential to look at alternate products and identify potential problems. Additionally, the multidisciplinary MSC can provide valuable input in the decision-making process if time allows. When a quick turnaround for a product replacement is necessary, key practitioners should be identified (e.g., physicians and nurses) and consulted if needed. Once a revised process is agreed on, education and implementation need to happen in a timely manner based on product supply of old and new product. Just when the updated processes are in place to accommodate the alternate product, the product will again be available and everything will have to be systematically undone for the regular or preferred product. Ideally, all the changes will be effectively taken care of outside of the regular workflow for the frontline staff. Staff need to focus on providing safe patient care and not making telephone calls looking for drugs or trying to implement workarounds to deal with a bad process or poor communication on important changes.

Outdates/Recall Management

Managing outdates such as sequestering expired medications and processing returns is generally handled by the purchasing/stores staff in a larger organization. A process to regularly review the pharmacy drug inventory to identify and remove expired medications must be in place. Unit inspections should be conducted monthly to assess expiration checks for drug supplies in non-pharmacy areas. All health care staff must be on the lookout for expired medications and sequester them when identified.

Recalls are safety notices, either by the manufacturer or the Food and Drug Administration (FDA), to facilitate removal of an unsafe product from the market. *The FDA has three recall classifications based on the level of hazard involved:*

- *Class I:* Dangerous or defective products that predictably could cause serious health problems or death. Examples include a superpotent drug: oversized tablets resulting in a superpotent assay of the drug.
- *Class II:* Products that might cause a temporary health problem or pose only a slight threat of a serious nature. An example is a drug that is under-strength but that is not used to treat life-threatening situations.
- *Class III:* Products that are unlikely to cause any adverse health reaction, but that violate FDA labeling or manufacturing laws. Examples include a minor container defect and lack of English labeling in a retail food.

Written procedures should be established to facilitate removing unsafe medication products from your organization. A key aspect of an effective program is to know all of the medication storage locations in the non-pharmacy areas. It is pharmacy's responsibility to maintain control over drug storage locations and the approved medications for each area. Knowing where recalled medications are stocked can facilitate timely retrieval of recalled medications. It is also important to address ambulatory care areas and prescription supplies, including prescriptions waiting for patient pick-up. A well-defined procedure, implemented quickly, can readily identify medications posing a safety hazard. Figure 7-2 is an example of a document to facilitate retrieving recalled medications.

The MSO needs to be aware of recalls to assess any potential safety issues in the organization. Some recall situations necessitate communication (e.g., e-mail) to the organization. The MSO can facilitate this information and provide specific details related to the organization. Depending on the seriousness of the recall, the MSO should facilitate identifying if any patients received or may have received a recalled medication. In these situations, the medical team should be advised of the recall information and determine the need to communicate to the patient. Additional follow-up for FDA MedWatch reporting can also be done by the MSO if ADEs are identified as a result of a patient receiving medications under recall status.

Drug Product Change Evaluation

Date initiated: ______________ Product approved for future use: ______________

Request for product change due to:

_____ Product not available _____ Temporary–expected date of return: ______________ Return to stock on: ______________

_____ Pricing _____ Permanent

_____ LA/SA

_____ Packaging

_____ Other (*describe*): ______________________________

_____ Current qty on hand

_____ # days supply

Request generated by:

__ Purchasing _____ Medication-use policy Bulk: _____ Unit dose: _____

__ Operations _____ Medication Safety Officer Safety pak product: _____

Generic name: ______________________________ Trade name: ______________________________

New manufacturer: ______________ Dosage strength: ______________ Dosage form: ______________________

Old manufacturer: ______________

Medication-use policy

Formulary revision necessary? _____Yes _____ No Generic rating: ______________

Figure 7-1 (continued).

Medication safety Potential for problems with new/substitute product (*check all that apply*): __Label/packaging __Product (e.g., concentration) _____Clinical information __Storage __Other __No _____ Specify issue(s) if anything checked: ***Interventions*** **(check and describe appropriate strategies):** __CPOE _____ ADC _____ Bulk packager _____Carousel __Education (e.g., FYI vs. medication-use guideline) __Dispensing	Action:

CPOE /pharmacy verification system Orderable changes needed in Gemini: _____No _____Yes Special instructions for orderables: _____No _____Yes Product changes needed in PharmNet: _____No _____Yes Pop-ups, rules: _____No _____Yes	Action:

Automated Dispensing Cabinet Orderable changes in database: _____No _____ Yes _____ ADC _____Carousel Addition to ADC: _____No _____ Yes Deletion from ADC: _____No _____ Yes Change in par level due to size change: _____No _____ Yes Change in location in ADC: _____No _____ Yes Time for change to occur: _____ **immediately** _____**within** _____ **days**	Action:

Figure 7-1 (continued).

Bulk packager Canister bulk no longer available: _____ Temporary _____ Permanent _____ Order new canister if permanent replacement: Canister ordered on: ________________ (date)	Action:
Special considerations TPN compounder Database modification: _____ No _____ Yes Anesthesia trays Other:	Action:
Staff education needed: _____ No _____ Yes If yes, check all that apply: Pharmacy (all) _____ Clinical staff pharmacists _____ Clinical pharmacists/residents _____ Techs/externs _____ Nursing _____ Physicians _____ If all hospital staff, check Pharmacy Medication Alert listserve Responsible party for education:	Action:

Figure 7-1. Drug product change evaluation.
CPOE, computerized provider order entry; ADC, automated dispensing cabinets; LA/SA, look like/sound alike; TPN, total parenteral nutrition
Source: Courtesy C. Larson, University of Illinois Hospital and Health Sciences System.

Product Recall Notice

Recall #

M E M O R A N D U M

TO: All pharmacy medication storage units

FROM: Purchasing/stores

DATE:

SUBJECT: Product recall

DRUG:

RECALL CLASS/REASON:

The lot #s affected are:

(Please see attached letter for specific information regarding the recall.)

Please complete and return to Purchasing/stores (Mailbox in C-300) **By** ____________

( ) No recalled drug found in our area

( ) Yes, we are returning all recalled drugs found (Lot #: ________ Qty: ______)

______________	______________	______________
Area	Signature of person checking	Date

Received From:

___ Satellite

___ Cleanroom

___ Central

___ Automated Dispensing Cabinets (ADCs)

___ Prepack

___ Narcs

___ OR Sat

___ Stores

___ Carousel

FYI: Managers

Figure 7-2. Product recall notice.
Source: Courtesy C. Larson, University of Illinois Hospital and Health Sciences System.

Storage/Control

Control of medications is essential to prevent access by unauthorized individuals and also to have appropriate safeguards in place to prevent diversion of controlled substance medications. Control also implies that the integrity of the medication supplies are maintained and not expired or damaged or recalled. Storage requirements can not only enforce control, but also improve patient safety by limiting access and putting safety strategies in place to highlight important medication information (e.g., look-alike/sound-alike identification).

Over the years, storage of medications has played an increasing role in improving medication safety. The days of readily accessible medications on the patient care units have slowly transitioned into a focus on safety and security. Open bins on patient care units containing dangerous medications (potassium chloride concentrate injection is the classic example) is a thing of the past in organizations that focus on safety and quality. For those of us who recognized the importance of limited access and appropriate medication storage, it has been a long road to travel. The goal was to set up a safer process to provide access to emergently needed medications in a way that would avoid or reduce the potential for medication errors and patient harm.

The simple act of removing potassium chloride concentrate injection from patient care areas was instrumental in reducing harmful patient errors. In retrospect, however, it was not simple at all. I am sure many of us have had to go to battle to justify "inconveniencing" other practitioners and upsetting the status quo when attempting to remove concentrated potassium chloride injection. I can remember working toward this goal many years ago. We worked hard to be as efficient as possible in getting a safer potassium chloride product in a diluted form to the intensive care unit patient care areas in a timely manner to facilitate removal of their concentrated stock. I also remember almost a year later finding out concentrated potassium chloride injection was still available in some areas, and that in some cases the pharmacy would send out the vial if the nurse requested it! Thankfully that was long ago and since then there have been accreditation standards implemented for select medications to limit access and prevent inadvertent use of these high-alert medications (e.g., concentrated potassium chloride, high concentrations of sodium chloride). The Institute of Safe Medication Practices (ISMP) has a long history of identifying problems with concentrated electrolytes and was an early proponent of limiting access to increase safety.

Pharmacy Storage Areas

There are plenty of opportunities to identify potential safety strategies for medication storage in the pharmacy. A wall of alphabetically arranged medications in cardboard boxes or plastic bins presents quite a challenge to prevent dispensing errors. There is too much opportunity to return the wrong drug or strength to the wrong bin, select the wrong medication due to medication in wrong place, or wrong placement of bins for look-alike/sound-alike medications. When bins are utilized, they must clearly indicate the drug product inside so labeling is very important. Different bin colors can be utilized to differentiate different types of medications. High-alert medications are examples that could be stored in a different color bin to indicate the high-alert designation. Ideally, pediatric-specific medications would be stored in a separate section and/or a specific color of bin could be used for these medications. Hazardous medications should also be stored in a separate location and clearly identified. Gloves should be used to handle even unopened hazardous medication products.

Technology has come a long way to assist the pharmacy in more efficient and safe storage of medications. Look-alike/sound-alike medications present a unique problem for medication storage. Separating these medications seems like a good idea but how do you find the product you need and prevent people from moving products back to their original alphabetical location? Placing stickers on bins and using tall-man lettering (e.g., CISplatin) for the drug names are examples of things that can be done to bring attention to the similarities of products, but their effectiveness at preventing dispensing errors is limited. Technology-based solutions offer more benefit when you can physically locate the medications away from each other and the system directs you to the correct product/location (e.g., automated medication cabinets, carousels, and inventory management systems). Bar coding technology can be employed to enhance safety during procurement, storage, preparation, administration, and monitoring phases of the medication-use process.

Patient Care Area Medication Supplies

Review *all* medication storage areas in *all* patient care areas including inpatient nursing units, procedural areas (e.g., cardiac catheterization laboratory, radiology, etc.), ED, OR, post anesthesia care unit (PACU), outpatient clinics, and other areas where medications are kept. All medications should be kept in a controlled area that limits access to appropriate staff. Medications stored outside of approved storage locations, including unapproved medications should be removed and returned to the pharmacy with appropriate follow-up to the area. Floor stock medications are considered readily accessible since they are not dispensed pending a pharmacist review or necessarily require an order (e.g., where the licensed independent practitioner controls ordering, preparation, and administration). Select medications may be made available utilizing the **override** function in the ADC and generally these medications do not undergo a proactive pharmacist review at the time the medication is obtained and administered and, therefore, may be considered as a floor stock medication. All medications obtained via override require an order to be placed as soon as possible to allow pharmacist review in as close to real time as possible so that any detected problems can be acted on in a timely manner.

The preferred process for ADC dispensing is for the medication to be released only after the pharmacist verifies or approves the patient-specific orders due to the safety checks afforded by the pharmacist's review (e.g., allergy screening). A list of floor stock medications for each area should be approved by the MSC and reviewed periodically. Any requests for additions should go through this committee. Limiting ready access to medications is an important safeguard but must be balanced with providing emergently needed medications.

Special attention should be paid to the medication supply restock mechanism for procedural areas or any area where the pharmacist is not reviewing a patient-specific order. If the area has an ADC, make sure they are not stocking other medications or additional supplies elsewhere in the department (e.g., drawers/cabinets). If the area does not have an ADC, then medication stock must be located in a secure area approved by pharmacy. Each medication should be clearly listed and par levels established for acceptable quantities. The mechanism to reorder stock for these areas needs to be defined. Consider a list noting each approved medication and par level and needed restock quantity. The area should not have the ability to order medications that were not approved as stock for a specific area.

Figure 7-3 is an example of a tool that can be used to review medication storage areas for safety and security compliance issues.

Ordering/Prescribing

There has been much published about strategies that could be employed to prevent medication errors related to ordering/prescribing. One main strategy for preventing prescribing errors is the elimination of handwritten medication orders. Illegible handwriting is a major contributor to medication errors.[9,10] Poorly written orders can lead to transcription errors. The pharmacy generally will input the prescriber's written orders into an electronic system that will generate patient medication labels and a medication administration record (MAR) for the nurse. This can result in the wrong drug, dose, schedule, etc. In addition, prior to receiving a new updated MAR for new orders, the nurse may update the current MAR with incorrect information.

Incomplete orders can also result in errors. Components of an ideal medication order are described in Figure 7-4. For example, often medication orders do not contain an indication for use that would be helpful in assessing correct dose, frequency, etc. In addition, having an indication helps identify medication errors when the indication does not match the prescribed medication.

Dosing errors can result in significant patient harm and can be fatal. Dosing errors related to the prescribing mode are multifactorial, as described by Leape et al.[2] Several proximal causes or apparent reasons why the error occurred are described as well as the lack of knowledge of the drug or information about the patient. During the ordering phase, dosing errors may occur when the physician does not know that a particular medication needs to be renally adjusted or have immediate knowledge that the patient's renal function is deteriorating. The prescriber may have forgotten this important information due to distractions or other unexplained reasons. Lack of knowledge of the drug can contribute to each component of the medication order: wrong drug, wrong dose, wrong dosage form, wrong route, wrong time, wrong schedule, and wrong duration.

The use of standardized order forms, pre-printed or electronic, offers several advantages. In addition to eliminating illegible handwriting, they can reinforce an

Medication Storage and Control Rounds

Area inspected:

Date of inspection:________________**Time:**____________________

Name of auditor:________________________________

This area was inspected for compliance with requirements for medication control and storage. The following was identified:

___**Unsecured medications—unlocked medications.**
Example: Medications not locked in the medication room or the ADC.

___**Medications not properly stored but in a locked location.**
Examples: Patient-specific bulk medications not returned to appropriate location; stock bulk medications found in patient-specific drawer; do-not-refrigerate medications found in refrigerator.

___**Medications in unapproved storage area (stashes).**
Example: Patient-specific medications found in locked drawer or room instead of returned to ADC.

___**Bin level does not match amount present.**

___**Keys to medication area not secured.**

___**Punctured multi-dose vial; no date and/or initials.**

___**Single dose vial used as multi-dose.**

___**Opened nitroglycerin SL tabs; no date and/or initials.**

___**Opened bulk bottle; no date and/or initials.**

___**Refrigerator temperature log not properly documented.**

___**Refrigerator not within approved temperature range and "Action" not noted.**

___**Food and/or specimens found in medication refrigerator.**

___**Food/drink in medication area.**

___**Expired medication(s). Please list:**
Automated dispensing cabinet stock________.

___**Expired medication(s). Please list:**
Current patient-specific medication or IVs:_________.

___**Unlabeled medications (medications out of package) but present in a secure location.**
Example: Medications in cup for a patient but left in patient-specific medication drawer. (NOTE: If unsecured, check "unsecured medications" box.)

___**Neuromuscular blocking agents stored without appropriate safety labeling.**

___**Prescription blanks not secured.**

___**Saline bag being used as multi-dose bag for flush.**

___**Unlabeled syringes (oral or injectable).**

___**Medication storage area disorganized and/or dirty.**

___**Unlocked drug box or crash cart.**

___**Crash cart with unapproved items on top or sides.**

___**Controlled drugs found unlocked.**

___**Medication present for patients no longer on the unit.**

___**Respiratory inhalers stored without bag.**

Comments:

Review with Charge Nurse

Nursing signature____

Forward completed form to Pharmacy QA area

Figure 7-3. Medication storage and control rounds.
Source: Courtesy C. Larson, University of Illinois Hospital and Health Sciences System.

Components of an Ideal Complete Medication Order

- Patient name
- Patient-specific information/demographics, particularly age and weight
- Name of the medication; generic only or generic and brand name (particularly for confusing generic names, i.e., combination products, two different formulations)
- Appropriate dose strength units using metric system
- Dosage form
- Route of administration
- Frequency of dosing
- Additional specific instruction, if needed
- Purpose/indication for the medication

Figure 7-4. Components of an ideal complete medication order.

evidence-based protocol or guideline. The order form could be used to facilitate antidote use by including rescue medication orders (e.g., naloxone) along with an intravenous (IV) opioid order. Development and maintenance of standardized forms requires interdisciplinary collaboration.

Goals for order set development include:

- **Safety**—Adhere to organizational policies, legal regulations, standards of care (e.g., professional and accrediting organizations), and medication safety recommendations (e.g., ISMP, National Patient Safety Foundation).
- **Clarity**—Strive for consistent interpretation of orders by all caregivers; eliminate ambiguity in ordering (e.g., medication decisions must be made by the prescriber); state simply and clearly.
- **Optimizing care**—Ensure orders are evidence-based; consider published guidelines/protocols.
- **Reducing cost**—Strive for cost-effective options; reduce redundancy in orders (e.g., multiple as-needed medication choices); encourage use of oral versus injections when appropriate; consider safety, effectiveness, then cost.
- **Preparing for computerized provider order entry (CPOE)**—Create standardized order sets which form the basis for CPOE libraries and decision support.
- **Addressing potential safety concerns**—Address potential safety concerns you perceive with ANY order during the review—do not limit your scope to your professional role! (For example, nurses should question medication doses; pharmacists should question nursing monitoring.) The P&T focus is on medication management, and the purpose of this process is to enhance patient safety.

A sample guideline and checklist for pharmacist review of standard orders is presented in Appendix 7-A. ISMP provides formal guidance on the development of standard order sets.[11]

CPOE systems and electronic medical records (EMR) are bringing many improvements to medication safety along with many challenges. Legibility issues are not an issue with CPOE and, depending on the system, can prevent the need for transcription. CPOE and clinical decision support are discussed in Chapter 8, Medication-Use Technology and Safety.

Order Review for Appropriateness

TJC standards state that a pharmacist reviews all medication orders for medications dispensed in the hospital. Furthermore, there is a responsibility to make sure medication orders are clear and accurate. This is not just the pharmacist's job but includes other health care practitioners (e.g., nurses, respiratory therapists) related to their scope of practice. Any questions related to the accuracy of a medication order must be clarified with the prescriber prior to dispensing or administering.

The clarification process should be considered a special process by the MSO. Extra efforts should be spent with the pharmacy staff to make sure they understand the goals of clarifying medication orders. If the clarification is related to missing patient information the pharmacist requires and those issues are cleared up to the pharmacist's satisfaction, then the order can proceed. If a pharmacist has all the pertinent patient/medication information and identifies a problem (e.g., not renally dosed) with a medication order and feels that the order should be changed then that should be the expected result of a clarification to the physician. If the pharmacist knows the order is incorrect, it is not enough for the physician to respond that this is what is wanted and the order as it is written is OK. The same goes for nurses—they must have their questions addressed. Encourage independent thinking for the nurses and discourage reliance on the fact that a pharmacist approved a medication order. Every practitioner should be empowered to question/clarify medication orders and use the chain of command if the practitioner feels pressured to do things he or she feels might potentially result in patient harm such as dispense or administer an inappropriate drug or dose.

It is important to make sure systems are in place to provide a review for medication orders and that appropriate resources and detailed processes are in place for key medications such as high-alert medications. Hazardous medication order review is a good example of high-alert medications that require a well-defined process to detect/prevent errors. The process should establish a flow from determining the appropriate hazardous medication regimen for the patient, leading to the generation of appropriate hazardous medication orders/adjuvant therapies that include correct dosing/dose, route, timing/duration, and timing relationship to other pertinent medications. A checklist for the ordering process is illustrated in Figure 7-5. Subsequently for the verification and preparation/dispensing process, multiple independent checks should also be incorporated. See sample checklist for order verification process in Figure 7-6.

Hazardous Medication Clinical Checklist and Protocol

Patient Name: **MRN:**

Check all applicable:

☐ Non-weight-based dosing

☐ Weight-based dosing; **dosing weight** = ____kg (actual, ideal, or adjusted)

☐ Dosing based on BSA; calculated BSA:

$$\sqrt{\frac{(\text{Ht }(\_\text{cm}) \times \text{Wt }(\_\text{kg})}{3600}} = \_\_\_\_\_\_\_ \text{ m}^2$$

New order ☐ Change in existing order ☐

Call before making: Yes ☐ No ☐

***** Attach protocol/attending note/other source of reference *****

Comments (if applicable):

Checklist

(Check the following for each hazardous medication and premed)

Clinical Pharmacist initials:

1. Verify orders against study protocol/standard chemotherapy regimen/attending note/other source ______
2. Verify height and weight (within 7 days); calculate BSA ______
3. Check labs (within 7 days); verify any dose modifications or omissions as per protocol for age/organ dysfunction ______
4. Review prior patient chemo profile for previous doses and tolerances ______
5. Correct drug ______
6. Correct dose ______
7. Correct route of administration ______
8. Correct frequency and number of doses ______
9. Correct administration times ______
10. Correct fluid, volume, and infusion rate ______
11. Confirm central line placement ______
12. Correct anti-emetics/premeds, doses, and schedule ______

Date completed ______

Figure 7-5. Hazardous medication clinical checklist and protocol.
Source: Courtesy C. Larson, University of Illinois Hospital and Health Sciences System.

Hazardous Medication Verification Checklist and Profile Form

Patient Name: **MRN:**

Check all applicable:

☐ Non-weight-based dosing

☐ Weight-based dosing; **dosing weight** = ____kg (actual, ideal, or adjusted)

☐ Dosing based on BSA; calculated BSA:

$$\sqrt{\frac{\text{Ht (\_\_cm)} \times \text{Wt (\_\_kg)}}{3600}} = \_\_\_\_\_\_\_\ \text{m}^2$$

New order ☐ Change in existing order ☐

Check applicable:

☐ Clinical Checklist and Protocol Form received

☐ Verbal double-check received from Clinical Pharmacist ____________

(ONLY ACCEPT FOR SCHEDULE CHANGES)

Checklist

(Check the following for each hazardous medication and premed)

	Satellite Pharmacist initials:
Calculate BSA	______
Correct drug	______
Correct dose	______
Correct route of administration	______
Correct frequency and number of doses	______
Correct administration times	______
Correct fluid, volume, and infusion rate	______
Correct anti-emetics/premeds, doses, and schedule	______
Verification of Powerchart orders against written protocol	______
Date completed	______

Profile: *If any changes are made to the original order, create a new updated profile. Staple updated profile to original.*

DOSING SCHEDULE		FINAL RPH INITIALS:	DRUG NAME & ADDITIVES	DOSE	FLUID & VOLUME	ROUTE & RATE
DATE:	TIME:					

Figure 7-6. Hazardous medication verification checklist and profile form.
BSA, body surface area.
Source: Courtesy C. Larson, University of Illinois Hospital and Health Sciences System.

Preparation

Medication preparation is a major pharmacy-controlled activity that deserves a considerable amount of attention to make sure that the basics are in place and good processes have been established that prevent errors. U.S. Pharmacopeia's (USP) <797> *Pharmaceutical Compounding—Sterile Preparations* and <795> *Pharmaceutical Compounding—Nonsterile Preparations*, set practice standards to ensure high-quality compounded sterile and nonsterile preparations. Personnel must be trained and capable of performing defined procedures and ensure the final product has been accurately prepared. Particularly with sterile products, there can be complex procedures involved with many sub-processes and checks and balances to ensure each intermediary step is accurate. IV medication compounding equipment requires special training and procedures to ensure accurate preparations and prevent medication errors.

In general, whenever possible, pharmacy should do all medication compounding. There are exceptions of course, but each exception should be identified and go through a review process before determining that the best course of action is to compound a medication outside of the pharmacy. A common reason for compounding outside of the pharmacy (e.g., procedural area) is that the need for a medication is identified during a procedure and the patient's condition does not allow time to contact the pharmacy and wait for the medication to be prepared and delivered. Ideally, medications necessitating preparation outside of the pharmacy should involve a protocol that outlines the supplies and steps that are needed to properly compound the needed medication. Strategies should be implemented that facilitate accurate preparation outside of the pharmacy. The pharmacy could provide the medication as a kit that includes preparation instructions, the medication, appropriate diluent (e.g., D5W 100-mL bag), and a preprinted label for the final product. These types of protocols should be approved by the Medication Safety and P&T committees.

Medication preparation in the pharmacy has many opportunities for the development of a defined process for ensuring safety due to high-alert medications (e.g., hazardous medications) and problem-prone patient populations (e.g., pediatrics). Pediatric services require attention to detail related to appropriate medication products. Frequently, commercially available products cannot be used or are not available that meet the dosing needs for pediatric patients. Preparation procedures commonly involve dilution of oral and injectable formulations to provide an accurately measured dose that can be administered to very small patients (e.g., premature neonates). It is essential to have appropriate procedures in place to prevent accidental overdoses related to decimal point errors or drug product preparation miscalculations.

Independent double-checks are an important safety feature for high-alert medications for any component of the medication-use process. An independent double-check is a procedure in which two individuals separately check (alone and apart from each other) each component of a process then compare results. Properly done independent double-checks are time consuming and should be reserved for high-risk processes. It is important that each person does not know the results (e.g., drug, dose) of the other.

Again, using the hazardous medication example from above, after determining that the orders are appropriate and verified on the checklist (Figure 7-6), the preparation/verification process must also involve independent double-checks to ensure the accuracy of the preparation process to achieve an accurate final product. Each part of the preparation process must be reviewed carefully to make sure each function has a mechanism to identify potential errors so that the information reflected on the label is exactly what is in the bag. It is unlikely that a preparation error will be caught once the product leaves the pharmacy unless there is a noticeable volume difference or an incompatibility resulting in color change or precipitation. Figure 7-7 is an example of a hazardous medication worksheet that is used to facilitate correct preparation and a comprehensive check of the preparation process.

Flowcharts or flow diagrams are excellent tools to use to orient new staff to an overall process or to staff in general for a revised process. See Appendix 7-B for a sample flowchart of the pharmacy order processing and preparation for hazardous medications.

Parenteral medication safety strategies are extremely important. Most compounded products are clear, colorless solutions. For example, assuming the label is correct based on the patient order, after the bag is dispensed, how will anyone know that the medication infusion was compounded with sodium chloride 23.4% instead of 0.9% as a bag run on the IV compounder?

A summit on preventing harm and death from IV medication errors was conducted by several organizations including ISMP and the American Society of Health-System Pharmacists (ASHP).[12] Best practices were identified and barriers to implementation and suggestions for overcoming barriers were noted. Review of this document will be helpful during the MSO's assessment of the pharmacy IV preparation services in determining work that needs to be done as a priority process improvement project.

Distribution Services

There are many ways to provide medication distribution services and many factors that impact on achievement of a "best practice" for your organization. Some aspects of the distribution service are governed by standards and regulations. The end result may be clearly defined (i.e., all medications are locked); however, implementing a process that ensures safety but does not interfere with timely and appropriate access can be difficult to achieve. Difficulty factors include physical location or layout of a unit or pharmacy, staff resources, and physical properties of the medication (e.g., refrigeration, stability, etc.). One process generally does not work for all units/work areas. It is important to try to minimize deviation from a defined best process to avoid confusion. Different organizations are set up to meet the unique needs of their services, but this can hamper providing patient safety if standardization is bypassed without regard to potential consequences. An analysis of pharmacy distribution operations is a critical knowledge base component for the MSO. An important factor for a safe distribution system involves dispensing medications as **unit-dose**

Hazardous Medication Preparation Worksheet

Patient's Name: ______________________________

Drug: CARMUSTINE (BICNU, BCNU) **Label:** CAR

Product Info: **Route of Administration:**

100 mg/VIAL IV ONLY

RECONSTITUTION INSTRUCTIONS:

Add 3 mL sterile diluent provided and further dilute with 27 mL SWFI

Final concentration: **(Conc: 3.3 mg/mL)**

STABILITY INFO:

Vial stability at room temp: 8 hr

Bag stability at room temp: 8 hr in D5W or NS

PREPARATION INSTRUCTIONS (GLASS ONLY):

DOSE REQUIRED: __________ mg /__________ mL

QA: Check Worksheet/Labels/Profile/Order and Sign Below:

Technician/Student (PRINT NAME): ______________________

First Pharmacist (PRINT NAME): ______________________

Second Pharmacist (PRINT NAME): ______________________

LABELING (additional instructions): **N/A**

DATE						
MFG						
LOT #						
MFG EXP:						
RPH SETUP						
TECH						
RPH CHECK						

NOTES and EXTRA INFORMATION ON DRUG:

- **USE GLASS BOTTLES ONLY!**
- For IV solutions, dilute dose to 250 mL with D5W or NS. If fluid restricted, can use 100 mL, but must be in GLASS.
- WITHDRAW DRUG VOLUME FIRST.
- PROTECT FROM LIGHT.
- Refrigerate until used.
- Precaution: Accidental contact of reconstituted drug with skin has caused transient hyperpigmentation.
- Exposure of drug in vial to temps >31°C will cause drug to liquify and appear as an oil film in vial; discard these vials.
- Infusion rate: IV over 1–2 hours (100 mL/hr).

Figure 7-7. Hazardous medication preparation worksheet.
Source: Courtesy of C. Larson, University of Illinois Hospital and Health Sciences System.

instead of as bulk medications. Bulk medications can be problematic because the nurse must sometimes perform calculations to determine the volume of a liquid. Totally eliminating bulk medications may not be practical but certainly should be a minimal component of any drug distribution system and strongly discouraged for high-alert medications.

Understanding distribution services is critical to establishing a safe foundation for any medication safety program. A poorly designed distribution system could have a negative impact on the entire medication-use system. The bottom line is that the patient at the receiving end of a medication administration receives the correct medication, dose, dose form, route, etc., for the indication in a timely manner.

Automated Dispensing Cabinets

Automated dispensing cabinets (ADCs) are commonly used to control medications that are stored outside of the pharmacy.[13] ADCs can decrease the amount of time before a medication is available on patient care units for administration and ensure greater security of medications, particularly narcotics. Profiled ADCs are the safest because the availability of medications to the nursing staff occurs after the medication orders are appropriately reviewed and verified by a pharmacist. Override medications are available to the nurse without an order or prior to order verification. The availability of medications via the override function should be limited and must go through the approval process of the MSC as previously described.

Medications approved for override and the data associated with their use should be monitored. A process should be in place for the nursing managers to review data for their unit(s). An area for concern is that there must be an order as soon as possible after the override for that medication and subsequent documentation of the administration to the patient to keep the patient's medical record accurate. Also, the review should address inappropriate use (e.g., non-emergency) and appropriate use due to other systemic problems that if properly addressed may eliminate the need for an override. The Nursing-Pharmacy Committee or any structure where both disciplines regularly meet to discuss medications issues should identify systemic problems and bring them to the attention of the MSC.

A potential problem with ADC occurs when the dose of a medication requires multiple dose units (e.g., two tablets) and the nurse must be diligent to remove the correct number of tablets. The nurse is prompted to take the correct number of tablets for the dose, but this can be overlooked. This problem is evident for controlled substances in the ADC because discrepancies can be traced back to identify when the nurse took out the dose incorrectly (e.g., removed one tab for a two-tab dose) and now the inventory count is +1. This problem is hard to identify for non-controlled medications where the inventory is frequently less accurate and the timeline for accessing the medication to identify problems may be hard to effectively evaluate. The end result is the patient is unknowingly underdosed.

Nursing workflow for obtaining medications for patients should be carefully reviewed. Best practices should be defined (e.g., obtain medication for one patient at a time). The ISMP has helpful tools to evaluate your organization for appropriate processes to address medication safety issues. The ISMP Medication Safety Self-Assessment® for Automated Dispensing Cabinets is an excellent tool to thoroughly evaluate your own system.

Administration/Documentation

Certainly every component of the medication-use process is important, but the administration node is the last point to identify and avert a medication error. The organization must ensure that systems in place support safe medication administration. A working knowledge of nursing practices and the identification of key nursing contacts are very beneficial to the MSO.

A general review of nursing policies and procedures related to medication administration is a good place to start; but knowledge of actual practice provides the most beneficial information. Consider shadowing nurses in different environments (e.g., med/surg unit, pediatrics, outpatient, procedural area) and/or surveying nurses to find out if they have any medication administration concerns. The MSC should have at least one frontline staff nurse that should be able to identify current practice variations from policy and procedures, risk points, and opportunities for improvement.

The MAR is a key nursing document that drives the medication administration process. How the MAR is generated can vary. In CPOE systems, the MAR may be generated by the input of the prescriber orders. The printed document may be called a care plan if it details all the orders (e.g., medications, laboratory tests) for a patient. In automated systems, nurses then document on-line medication administration. The MAR then tracks and notes which medications have not been given. Other systems may utilize barcode technology where the medication and the patient are scanned prior to administration. The benefit of this process is that the system should detect if the wrong drug or dose is about to be administered. Besides errors, the alerts may be a result of a recent order change that may have occurred since the time the nurse obtained the medication. Sometimes the pharmacy generates the MAR for nursing after the orders are transcribed into the pharmacy system. The nurse then hand writes the administration time on the paper document. Paper documentation can be difficult to read due to poor handwriting and may lead to interpretation errors.

Nursing practice often varies by unit. Medication administration in an intensive care unit (ICU) setting involves the use of more high-alert medications, since the patient is more thoroughly and frequently monitored and recommended monitoring equipment is available. It is necessary to differentiate acceptable medication administration practices in an ICU versus a general care floor or an intermediate area, where there is a minimum level of monitoring equipment (e.g., telemetry) helping the nurse safely and properly care for/monitor the patient.

Medication safety strategies that impact administration can target identified problems. Other examples of medication administration strategies include independent double-checks, labeling/packaging interventions that highlight key safety information, ADC dispensing alerts, bar-coded medication verification, MAR automated medication comments that convey special administration precautions, and smart pump infusion technology.

As noted previously, hazardous medications require special attention. The administration step, particularly for these highly toxic medications, is the last chance to identify an error so, generally, additional checks are required prior to administration. Nurse-independent double-checks to ensure that the medication dose matches the order and the protocol are common. Infusion pump settings are another part of the process that could benefit from an independent double-check.

Accurate documentation of medication administration is very important when assessing if the patient's medication therapy has been effective and is another important factor in the prevention of medication errors. If a dose is not properly documented as administered or not administered, the confusion may result in the patient receiving an extra dose that could result in an adverse drug event. Correct interpretation of drug levels relies on accurate documentation of the timing of medication administration and the timing of the sample.

Monitoring

Patient medication therapy monitoring is an important aspect of patient care. Medications are fraught with potential problems if not used correctly or if problems are not identified in a timely manner. By their nature, high-alert medications generally require special considerations for monitoring to ensure that the intended outcomes have been achieved and any adverse effects are appropriately addressed.

Institutional clinical care guidelines or treatment protocols that identify best practices must include information related to appropriate monitoring. Identification of medications that have special precautions related to administration is closely tied with special monitoring requirements that define the appropriate type of patient care area where a drug may be administered. It is helpful to identify these medications that may require more frequent monitoring (e.g., vital signs), specific monitoring equipment (e.g., telemetry), or specific laboratory tests. Table 7-4 is a sample of a document that clarifies which medications can be given IV push and the appropriate practice setting based on the level of nursing care/monitoring available.

Medication Management

The 2011 ISMP Medication Safety Self-Assessment® for Hospitals is a tool provided by ISMP to help you assess the overall safety of medication practices in your facility and identify opportunities for improvement. These assessment tools were used in 2000 and 2004, and participants were able to compare improvements they made over time and compare their experience with the aggregate experiences of demographically similar hospitals. Even though the survey is closed, the tool is still very relevant to current medication safety concerns. In any type of system evaluation it is important to have all the key stakeholders present to ensure that your assessment is accurate. Multidisciplinary staff directly involved in the process need to provide input because having a policy and procedure for a process is no guarantee that something is being done.

Other ISMP self-assessment tools include the 2005 ISMP Medication Safety Self-Assessment® for Antithrombotic Therapy in Hospitals and the 2012 International Medication Safety Self-Assessment® for Oncology. Once your assessments are complete, you should be able to determine your strengths and weaknesses. TJC has singled out anticoagulation therapy through a National Patient Safety Goal for a higher level of oversight to improve patient safety. The rationale as noted by TJC: Anticoagulation therapy poses risks to patients and often leads to adverse drug events due to complex dosing, requisite follow-up monitoring, and inconsistent patient compliance. The use of standardized practices for anticoagulation therapy that include patient involvement can reduce the risk of adverse drug events associated with the use of heparin (unfractionated), low molecular weight heparin, and warfarin. The goal goes on to define specific criteria that must be addressed and programs implemented. The MSO should be involved in making sure that any action plans developed involve sound, workable processes so the programs will be successful. Appropriate monitoring of the components of programs should be periodically evaluated.

Following completion of a self-assessment, the development of a medication safety plan is essential to address identified problems in a systematic manner using appropriate continuous quality improvement tools. It can be a daunting project if it appears as if there is too much to tackle in a reasonable time frame with limited resources. Prioritization of the needs will facilitate placing the focus on the highest risk processes requiring attention and should drive the organization to make sure resources are made available.

Completion of these tools and the overall assessment should help to identify areas where clinical pharmacy services would be the most valuable. Practice models vary by institution depending on a multitude of variables including patient population served, organizational mission philosophy, medical services provided, and available resources. Clinical pharmacy services may be provided by a number of different mechanisms that range from no direct patient interaction to a high level of direct patient care involvement. To effectively utilize clinical pharmacy services, evaluate your particular system to determine what the biggest needs are in the organization, how critical processes are currently handled, and what gaps may exist that prevent achievement of a best practice model for that process.

A valuable component to a medication safety plan is to incorporate the use of clinical pharmacists on the patient care units. Literature supports the use of clinical pharmacists as part of the team doing patient rounds.[14-17] The presence of a pharmacist during the discussion and decision-making process for a patient's overall treatment helps to address eliminating potential problems early on in the medication-use process facilitating use of the correct medication, dosing, etc.

Table 7-4. Sample Medications Given by IV Push Administration in Adults

Drug	Intensive Care	Stepdown with Telemetry	Stepdown	General Care	Monitoring When Given IV Push	Usual Adult Dose	Administration Rate	Usual Concentration	Adverse Effect from Administering Too Rapidly	Comments
Flumazenil	X	X	X	X	Vital signs, ECG, oxygen saturation rates every 5 min for 30 min	0.2–0.5mg	**Reversal of benzodiazepine sedation:** Give over 15 to 30 seconds **Benzodiazepine overdose:** Give over 30 seconds	0.1 mg/mL	Serious withdrawal symptoms (i.e., seizures, confusion, agitation) in those dependent on benzodiazepines	**Resedation:** Monitor closely. Repeat doses may be given at 20-minute intervals as needed with maximum of 1 mg/dose and 3 mg/hour. **Benzodiazepine overdose:** If patient has not responded 5 minutes after receiving a cumulative dose of 5 mg, the major cause of sedation is not likely due to benzodiazepines.

Table 7-4 (continued).

Drug	Intensive Care	Stepdown with Telemetry	Stepdown	General Care	Monitoring When Given IV Push	Usual Adult Dose	Administration Rate	Usual Concentration	Adverse Effect from Administering Too Rapidly	Comments
Furosemide	X	X	X	X		20–40 mg	Give over 1 to 2 minutes **Maximum rate:** 40 mg/minute	10 mg/mL	Ototoxicity occurs as a result of high peak levels	
Haloperidol	X				Monitor ECG	Delirium in ICU: 2–10 mg every 20–30 minutes until calm then 25% of max dose every 6 hours		5 mg/mL	Torsades de Pointes and QT prolongation observed particularly when administered by the IV Push route	Contraindications: Parkinson's disease, severe CNS depression, bone marrow suppression, severe cardiac or hepatic disease.

Definitions:

IV Push is the direct injection of a medication over a period of 5 minutes or less; the term is also synonymous with IV bolus and rapid administration.

Appropriate care setting is one in which a particular medication may be administered by the IV Push route.

Please consult other references for clarifications and/or additional information.

Source: Courtesy C. Larson, University of Illinois Hospital and Health Sciences System.

If resources do not allow pharmacist participation in patient rounds, consider drug-specific pharmacist services for key high-alert medications. Oncology and anticoagulation medication use are good examples where a higher level of pharmacist services can improve safety. Pharmacokinetic monitoring for therapeutic drug-monitored medications such as aminoglycoside and vancomycin therapy is another area where pharmacist expertise can help decrease costs and improve outcomes related to inappropriate use, dosing, dosing intervals, and laboratory costs.[18]

Another effective medication safety program to consider is pharmacist participation in the medication reconciliation process.[19,20] Pharmacist participation in taking the patient's medication history can be an effective method and provides an accurate list of home medications. The most accurate list possible helps improve care when the patient must be hospitalized and then transitioned back to the home.

ASHP and the ASHP Research and Education Foundation provide guidance on utilizing pharmacist leadership, including all levels of pharmacy personnel to facilitate the safe and effective use of medications through their Pharmacy Practice Model Initiative. There are several readings that can help pharmacy departments evaluate their systems and develop a pharmacy practice model for their organization[21-23] as well and tools and resources on the ASHP website.[24]

Risk Evaluation and Mitigation Strategies

The Food and Drug Administration Amendments Act (FDAAA) of 2007 gave the FDA the authority to require a Risk Evaluation and Mitigation Strategy (REMS) from manufacturers to ensure that the benefits of a drug or biological product outweigh its risk. A REMS is a required risk management plan that uses tools, as specified in FDAAA, beyond routine professional labeling (the package insert). A REMS is an enforceable document that describes the elements that an applicant is required to implement. At the Center for Drug Evaluation and Research, the Office of New Drugs and the Office of Surveillance and Epidemiology both have responsibilities for the review of proposed REMS and the evaluation and modification of existing REMS. The REMS components can include the following:

- *Medication Guides*—paper handouts that come with many prescription medicines. The guides address issues specific to particular drugs and drug classes and contain FDA-approved information to help patients avoid serious adverse events. The FDA maintains a list of medications or biologics that have a medication guide. However, with recent changes, not all medication guides are a part of each REMS.
- *A Communication Plan*—requirement targeted to health care providers, e.g., letters to professional societies. It includes information about serious safety risks and processes to ensure safe use.
- *Elements to Ensure Safe Use (ETASU)*—components include special training, experience, or certification for prescribers and special certification for

pharmacy to dispense. ETASU may involve dispensing limits (e.g., hospital setting), patient monitoring, or patients enrolled in a registry.

- *Implementation Systems*—often linked to an ETASU. They may involve audits related to restricted distribution system or a pharmacy/health care setting to ensure compliance with the ETASU.

The FDA website has information regarding currently approved REMS.[25] ASHP has a REMS resource center on its website.[26] The P&T Committee should be the group to assess the requirements of any REMS and the impact to the medication-use process.

Summary

Achieving safety with medication-use processes is very complex. The target(s) may move or change when you least expect it. So much of what is put in place can be very fragile, so it is important to identify and monitor the biggest risk areas for your organization. There may be new standards or regulations to address or new equipment to operationalize—all these things can add new challenges/problems, so it is important to constantly assess your medication-use system. Pharmacists are the medication experts, and it is imperative that their expertise is fully utilized as an integral member of the health care team. Given the opportunity, pharmacists make invaluable contributions that enhance medication and patient safety when involved in direct patient care activities working with physicians, nurses, and other health care personnel. As the MSO, you are in a unique position to champion the medication-use expertise that the pharmacy can offer to advance medication and patient safety.

PRACTICE TIPS

1. Take the time to review actions considered to address drug shortages. A critical eye for potential safety problems will help to reduce errors when identified and addressed proactively.
2. When implementing a new form or tools to standardize a process, review the forms after implementation and ask staff for their feedback on likes/dislikes. Do not assume everything is going well!
3. When considering using forms and other tools developed outside your organization, remember it will probably need to be tweaked to fit your particular system.
4. Identify and establish your go-to people for the various aspects of the medication-use system.

References

1. The Joint Commission. Available at: https://e-dition.jcrinc.com/MainContent.aspx. Accessed July 18, 2012.
2. Leape LL, Bates DW, Cullen DJ et al. Systems analysis of adverse drug events. *JAMA.* 1995;274:35-43.
3. HCUP Statistical Brief #109. April 2011. Agency for Healthcare Research and Quality, Rockville, MD. http://www.hcup-us.ahrq.gov/reports/statbriefs/sb109.pdf.
4. Kohn LT, Corrigan JM, Donaldson MS, eds. *To Err Is Human: Building a Safer Health System.* Washington, DC: National Academy Press; 1999.
5. Bates DW, Cullen DJ, Laird N et al. Incidence of adverse drug events and potential adverse drug events: implications for prevention. *JAMA.* 1995;274:29-34.
6. Lesar TS, Briceland L, Stein DS. Factors related to errors in medication prescribing. *JAMA.* 1997;277:312-317.
7. Murri NA, Somani S. Implementation of safety-focused pharmacy and therapeutics monographs: a new university health-system consortium template designed to minimize medication misadventures. *Hosp Pharm.* 2004;39:653-660.
8. Fox ER. Birt A, James KB, et al. ASHP Guidelines on managing drug product shortages in hospitals and health systems. *Am J Health-Syst Pharm.* 2009;66(15):1399-1406.
9. Vitillo JA, Lesar TS. Preventing medication prescribing errors. *Ann Pharmacother.* 1991;25:1388-1394.
10. Brodell RT, Helms SE, KrishnaRao I, et al. Prescription errors: legibility and drug name confusion. *Arch Fam Med.* 1997;6:296-298.
11. The Institute for Safe Medication Practices. ISMP'S Guidelines for Standard Order Sets. Available at: http://www.ismp.org/tools/guidelines/StandardOrderSets.asp. Accessed July 16, 2012.
12. Proceedings of a summit on preventing patient harm and death from i.v. medication errors. *Am J Health-Syst Pharm.* 2008;65:2367-2379.
13. Pedersen CA, Schneider PJ, Scheckelhoff DJ. ASHP national survey of pharmacy practice in hospital settings: dispensing and administration. *Am J Health Syst Pharm.* 2006;63:327-345.
14. Kane SL, Weber RJ, Dasta JF. The impact of critical care pharmacists on enhancing patient outcomes. *Intensive Care Med.* 2003;29:691-698.
15. Leape LL, Cullen DJ, Clapp MD, et al. Pharmacist participation on physician rounds and adverse drug events in the intensive care unit. *JAMA.* 1999;282:267-270.
16. Kucukarsian SN, Peters M, Mlynarek M, Nafziger DA. Pharmacists on rounding teams reduce preventable adverse drug events in hospital general medicine units. *Arch Intern Med.* 2003;163:2014-2018.
17. Kaushal R, Bates DW, Abramson EL, et al. Unit-based clinical pharmacists' prevention of serious medication errors in pediatric inpatients. *Am J Health-Syst Pharm.* 2008;65:1254-1260.
18. Bon CA, Raehl, CL. Clinical and economic outcomes of pharmacist-managed aminoglycoside or vancomycin therapy. *Am J Health-Syst Pharm.* 2005;62:1596-1605.
19. Gleason KM, Groszek JM, Sullivan C, et al. Reconciliation of discrepancies in medication histories and admission orders of newly hospitalized patients. *Am J Health-Syst Pharm.* 2004;61:1689-1695.
20. Nester TM, Hale LH. Effectiveness of a pharmacist-acquired medication history in promoting patient safety. *Am J Health-Syst Pharm.* 2002;59:2221-2225.
21. Shane R. Critical requirements for health-system pharmacy practice models that achieve optimal use of medicines. *Am J Health-Syst Pharm.* 2011;68:1101-1111.

22. Siska MH, Tribble DA. Opportunities and challenges related to technology in supporting optimal pharmacy practice models in hospitals and health system. *Am J Health-Syst Pharm.* 2011;68:1116-1126.
23. Myers CE. Opportunities and challenges related to pharmacy technicians in supporting optimal pharmacy pract models in health system. *Am J Health-Syst Pharm.* 2011;68:1128-1136.
24. American Society of Health-System Pharmacists. Pharmacy Practice Model Initiative. Available at: http://www.ashpmedia.org/ppmi/. Accessed July 16, 2012.
25. U.S. Department of Health & Human Services, Food and Drug Administration. Available at: http://www.fda.gov/Drugs/DrugSafety/PostmarketDrugSafetyInformationforPatientsandProviders/ucm111350.htm. Accessed July 16, 2012.
26. American Society of Health-System Pharmacists. REMS Resource Center. Available at: http://www.ashp.org/REMS. Accessed July 16, 2012.

Appendix 7-A: Guidelines and Checklist for Pharmacist Review of Standardized Order Sets

Key Questions:

☐ Does the title reflect (adequately describe) the order set intent?

- If it applies to a limited population, state in title (e.g., adults; critical care).

☐ Are all the required statements present?

- Beginning of order set: "Any order preceded by a box must be checked to activate the order."
- Approval dates, any unique numbers.

☐ Is there a designated prompt and space for patient allergies/ADRs?

☐ Is the "order flow" logical and easy-to-follow?

- Try to group similar types of care/orders together, e.g., medications and IV fluids; laboratory tests.
- Think about error reduction and human factors; reduce opportunities for omissions.

☐ Are there ways to reduce "hand-offs" within patient care? "Hand-offs" contribute to error.

☐ Does the order set appropriately reference unit standards of care or specify standard concentrations where helpful, especially helpful for high-alert medications or those infrequently used?

☐ Are all units consistent throughout the order set?

- **Use mL or ml.** Do NOT use "cc" (easily mistaken for "units" or "u" or the number "4" or zero, especially when handwritten).

☐ Have all acronyms or non-medication abbreviations been defined? When acronyms or non-medication abbreviations are used, make sure they are defined the first time they are used in the order set. Example: BG (blood glucose).

☐ Does shading or use of underlines have the potential to obscure clean order copies? If so, re-design to eliminate this contribution to error.

☐ Have you screened for errors in detail?

- Make sure spelling is correct.
- Make sure punctuation doesn't interfere with clear interpretation of order.
- Eliminate use of symbols such as <or>.

Appendix 7-A (continued).

Medication Orders:

☐ Are orders written in manner consistent with organizational policies?

- No abbreviation of medication names.
- No use of prohibited abbreviations (e.g., QD, U, etc.).
- PRNs must include an indication and frequency for dosing.
- Always use generic names. Include brand name(s) AND indication to decrease error with sound-alike/look-alike (SALA) drugs. Include indication for all SALA drugs.
- Generic names are generally written in lower case, unless at beginning of a sentence or using tall-man lettering. Brand names generally begin with a capital letter.
- Pediatric orders: see additional requirements (e.g., weight-based prescribing).

☐ Consult High-Alert Medication Policy

- If a high-alert drug, follow all safety strategies listed.
- Use tall-man lettering per organizational list.
- If a restriction in prescribing is desired or required, incorporate the approval documentation INTO the order set; do not rely on memory!
- If administration is restricted, make sure order set is consistent with policy.

☐ IV infusion orders should contain the following elements:

- Initial bolus, or IV push dose, if any.
- Initial dosage per unit of time (e.g., 1 mg/hr, or 1 mg/kg/hr).
- Titratable drips should specify dosage range (minimum and maximum), the specific outcome goal for titration, and instructions for how to titrate.
- Example: "titrate for comfort" is not acceptable. "Titrate to pain score of less than 3" is OK.
- Increase/decrease by 1 mg/kg/hr every 10 minutes until goal achieved.

☐ When a dose is written as "dose amount per patient weight," the prescriber MUST calculate the actual dose to be administered. This is a principle for safe medication ordering; it allows independent verification by the RN and RPh. It also contributes to accurate documentation of actual dose given. Example: 2 mg/kg × _____kg = _________mg IV × 1 dose. (Note: this standard may be modified for automated systems with functionality to display both the weight-based dose and final dose.)

☐ All medications must be on the formulary.

Appendix 7-A (continued).

- ☐ "Blanket" orders, such as "resume pre-op meds" or "meds as at home," are not acceptable.
- ☐ When it is possible to designate a specific dose, do so, rather than "fill in the blank."
- ☐ Do not use frequency ranges (e.g., 4–6 hr not OK; use q4h instead). Minimize use of dose ranges; consistency in carrying out orders with dose ranges is difficult to achieve. If dose ranges must be used, tie them to a specific outcome (e.g., a specific pain score).
- ☐ Include administration instructions, especially for unusual or complex therapies. Always consider possible errors and ways to avoid them!
- ☐ **Independently verify all calculations.**
- ☐ Make sure the dosage unit for a particular medication is the safest used for ordering and that the units are consistent throughout the order (e.g., don't mix mg and mcg). If usually ordered in mcg, then use those units on the order sheet. Minimize need for mathematical conversions.
- ☐ **Make sure the dosage units, concentrations, and dosing parameters used for all IV medication infusions are consistent with the Smart Pump Library.**
- ☐ If laboratory testing or other monitoring is needed for a particular medication therapy, make sure these are included in the order set (appropriate laboratory tests, at appropriate intervals/timing, etc.).
- ☐ Minimize duplication of treatments.
    - Do you need all the choices (e.g., is there a need for four choices of laxatives)?
    - If choices needed, be specific as to when to use one medication rather than another. This is now an accreditation standard.
- ☐ Make sure significant drug interactions are not present. If treatments require use of medications with potential interaction; include tests/monitoring to mitigate patient harm or to enhance the early recognition of interaction.
- ☐ Look for opportunities to build in discontinue dates for medications, if appropriate. For example, ketorolac ×24 hours; prophylactic antibiotics ×2 doses post op.
- ☐ Unless there is a P&T approved protocol (such as heparin protocol), the order must be a directive by the prescriber. The prescriber cannot "delegate" the choice of medications to be made by a non-prescriber.
    - Example: "Give clindamycin if allergic to penicillin." The prescriber must make the assessment and drug choice. This statement cannot stand alone as an order.

Appendix 7-A (continued).

- Instead, use a check box system for the prescriber to choose:
  - Clindamycin 900 mg IV ×1 (patient allergic to penicillin).

☐ Do the detail work.

- Make sure medications are spelled correctly.
- If symbols must be used, make sure they are correct.
- Avoid use of acronyms, such as "SSI"; spell it out.

Source: Courtesy D. Saine, Winchester Medical Center.

Appendix 7-B: Inpatient Hazardous Medication (HM) Process Flowchart, Pharmacy Satellite/Cleanroom

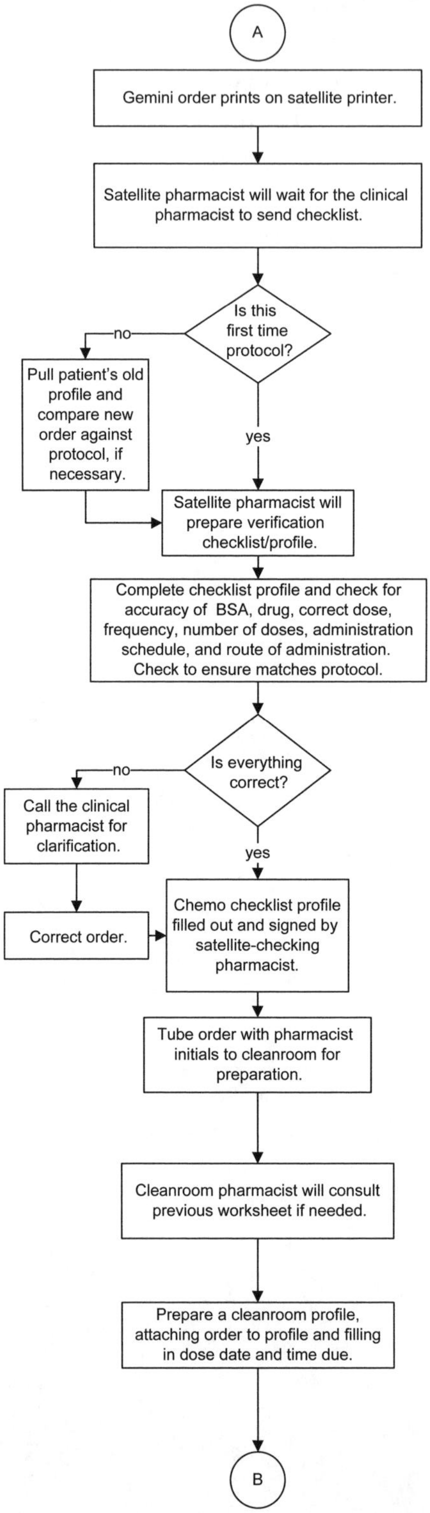

Appendix 7-B (continued).

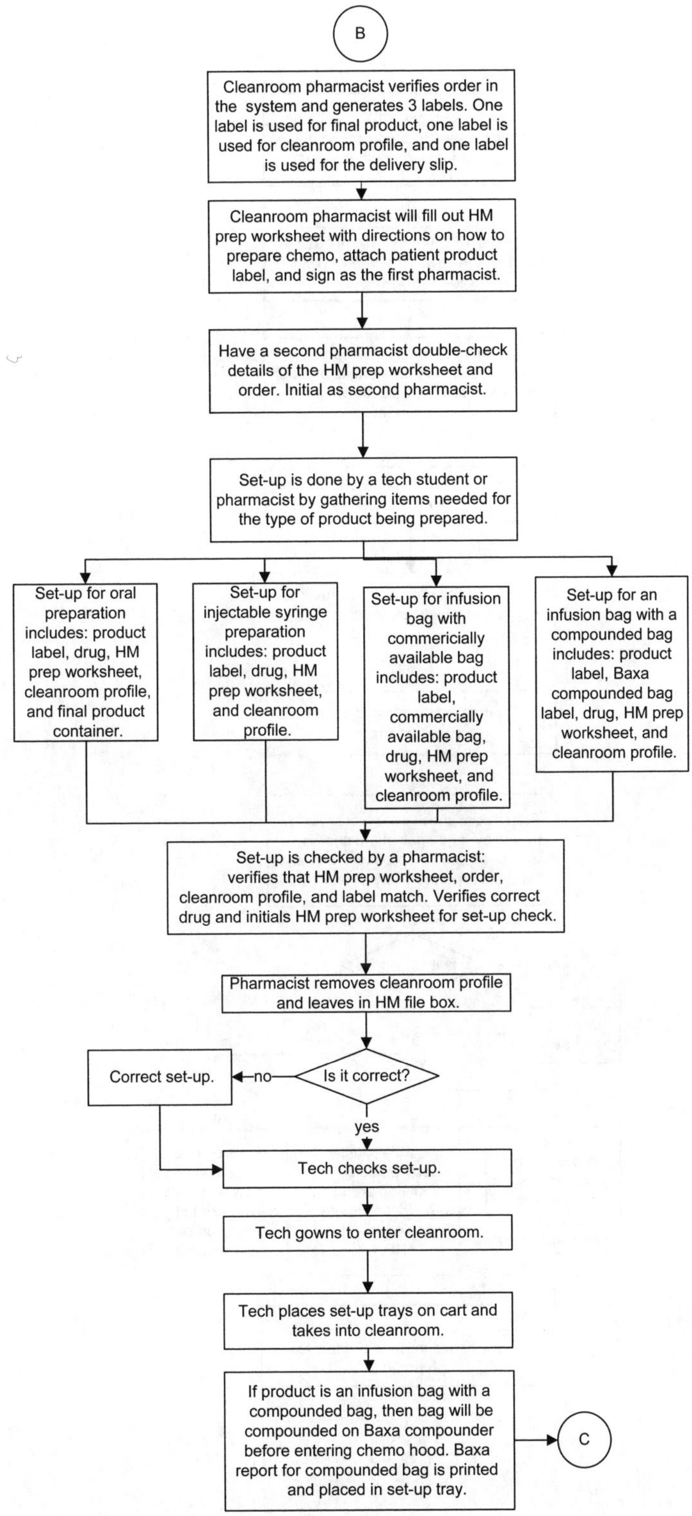

Appendix 7-B (continued).

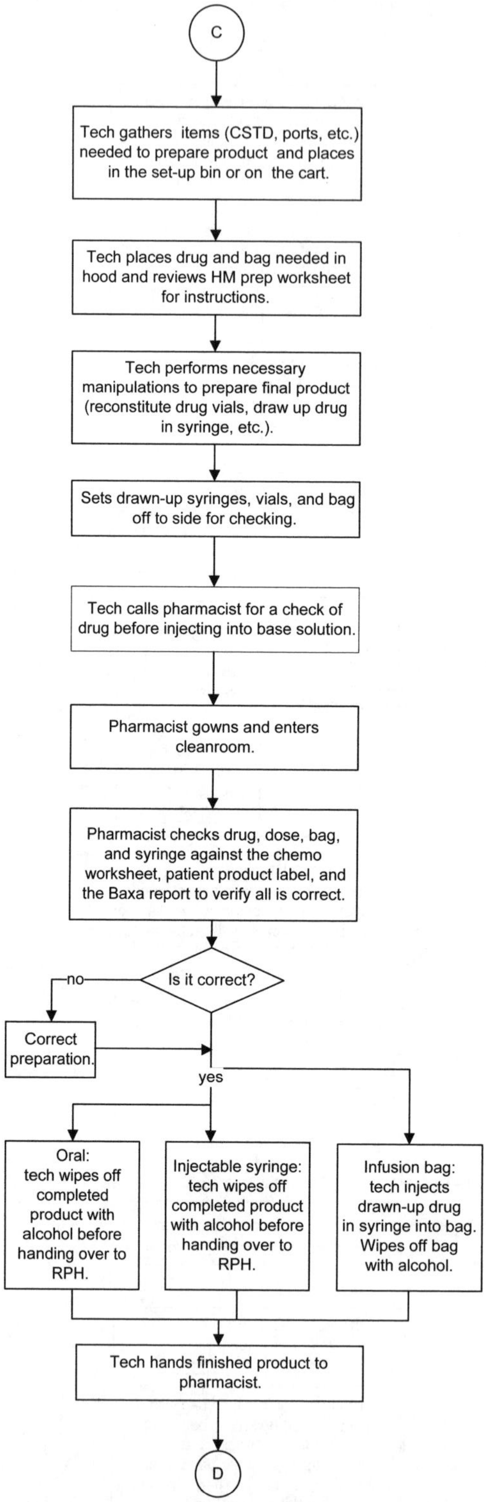

Appendix 7-B (continued).

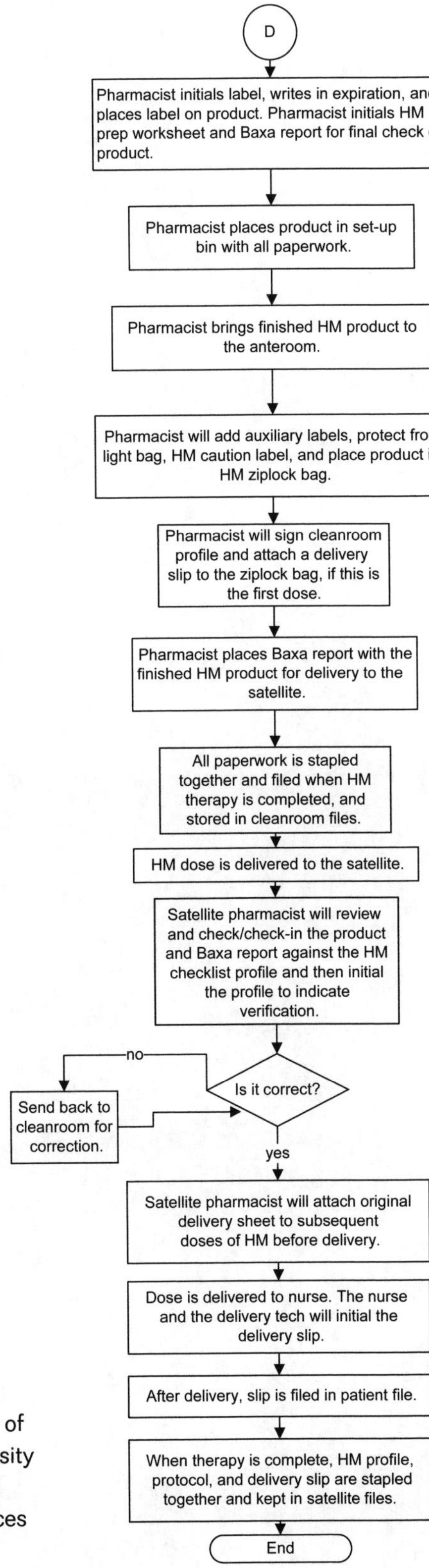

Source: Courtesy of C. Larson, University of Illinois Hospital and Health Sciences System.

Medication-Use Technology and Safety

Lisa M. Hanlon Wilhelm

CHAPTER 8

Key Terms

Alert Fatigue—Tendency to disregard or not thoroughly review pop-up alerts/warnings in an information system due to high-volume, low-significance, or nuisance alerts.

Computerized Provider Order Entry (CPOE)—Direct entry of medical orders into a health care system's electronic health records by licensed independent practitioners or other staff with specific ordering privileges and not by clinical or administrative support staff; may or may not include direct integration with other information systems such as pharmacy, laboratory, or radiology.

End-User—Primary user of a technology product, often frontline staff involved in direct patient care.

Gap Analysis—A process tool to evaluate and compare differences between two items; often used to compare actual performance with desired performance and to identify action steps needed to achieve the desired state.

Meaningful Use—Term used to describe a component of the 2009 American Recovery and Reinvestment Act that provides governmental monetary incentives for health care organizations that implement specific levels and elements of an electronic health record and various health care technologies.

Super-User—An individual, often an end-user, who has received additional training in use of a particular technology and functions as a resource for purposes of training or problem-solving/ trouble-shooting.

Workaround—A method for achieving a task by not following proper procedures; a shortcut; often a creative solution to circumvent a problem without eliminating it.

Introduction

Should we regard technology as friend or foe? The use of technology has had an incalculable impact on the evolution of human work. Considered among the greatest engineering achievements of the twentieth century, computers, electronics, the Internet, imaging, and health technologies enhance our daily lives and the delivery of health care.[1] The term *technology* comes from the Greek word *technología* which means systematic treatment.[2] As modern patient safety science is evolving, a systems-approach to preventing medical errors has become fundamental.[3-5] The use of technology is a major tool in strategies to improve efficiency, patient care, processes, and safety. Technological interventions can result in significant medication safety improvements such as better adherence to clinical practice guidelines, reduction of medication turnaround time, and decreased medication errors.[6-9] In fact, several professional organizations, regulatory and accrediting bodies, and payers have established recommendations on the use of technology to reduce errors, in particular, medication errors.[6-9]

Gap Analysis

Technology in broad terms has two forms: enhanced and replacement. *Enhanced technology* is something that improves an existing invention, making it better, faster, or producing more of it. By contrast, *replacement technology* is when one technology literally replaces another, using entirely different principles, and renders the first one obsolete.[10]

Both forms are prevalent in health care. However, "the effects of technology are unpredictable. They are among the best examples of the law of unintended consequences."[10] In health care, there is an ever increasing number of studies describing such unintended consequences.[11-15] In fact, in December 2008, The Joint Commission (TJC) released a Sentinel Event Alert (SEA), *Safely Implementing Health Information and Converging Technologies*, in response to the increased incidence of adverse events reportedly caused by health information technology. The alert discusses that "unintended consequences typically stem from human-machine interfaces or organization/system design." Thirteen suggested actions to prevent patient harm related to technology are included in the alert (see Figure 8-1). The medication safety officer (MSO) should evaluate these recommendations through a **gap analysis** to determine any opportunities for medication safety improvement. A *gap analysis* is basically a comparison between the current state (what is) and the future or ideal state (what should be). Identifying the gaps will aid the MSO in establishing priorities, action plans, and next steps. Many gap analysis tools are readily available on the Internet ranging from simple to sophisticated. A simple gap analysis can be created using a spreadsheet or table. An example is shown in Table 8-1.

Joint Commission Suggested Actions to Prevent Patient Harm Related to the Implementation and Use of Health Information Technologies

1. Examine workflow processes and procedures for risks and inefficiencies and resolve these issues prior to any technology implementation. Involving representatives of all disciplines—whether they are clinical, clerical, or technical—will help in the examination and resolution of these issues.
2. Actively involve clinicians and staff who will ultimately use or be affected by the technology, along with IT staff with strong clinical experience in the planning, selection, design, reassessment, and ongoing quality improvement of technology solutions, including the system selection process. Involve a pharmacist in the planning and implementation of any technology that involves medication.
3. Assess your organization's technology needs beforehand (e.g., supporting infrastructure, communication of admissions, discharges, transfers, etc.). Investigate how best to meet those needs by requiring IT staff to interact with users outside their own facility to learn about real world capabilities of potential systems, including those of various vendors. Conduct field trips to look at integrated systems (to minimize reliance on interfaces between various vendor systems).
4. During the introduction of new technology, continuously monitor for problems and address any issues as quickly as possible, particularly problems obscured by workarounds or incomplete error reporting. During the early post-live phase, consider implementing an emergent issues desk staffed with project experts and champions to help rapidly resolve critical problems. Use interdisciplinary brainstorming methods for improving system quality and giving feedback to vendors.
5. Establish a training program for all types of clinicians and operations staff who will be using the technology and provide frequent refresher courses. Training should be appropriately designed for the local staff. Focus training on how the technology will benefit patients and staff, i.e., less inefficiency, fewer delays, and less repeated work. Do not allow long delays between orientation and system implementation.
6. Develop and communicate policies delineating staff authorized and responsible for technology implementation, use, oversight, and safety review.
7. Prior to taking a technology live, ensure that all standardized order sets and guidelines are developed, tested on paper, and approved

Figure 8-1 (continued).

by the Pharmacy and Therapeutics Committee (or institutional equivalent).

8. Develop a graduated system of safety alerts in the new technology that helps clinicians determine urgency and relevancy. Carefully review skipped or rejected alerts as important insight into clinical practice. Decide which alerts need to be hard stops when using the technology and provide appropriate supporting documentation.
9. Develop a system that mitigates potential harmful CPOE drug orders by requiring departmental or pharmacy review and sign off on orders that are created outside the usual parameters. Use the Pharmacy and Therapeutics Committee (or institutional equivalent) for oversight and approval of all electronic order sets and clinical decision support alerts. Assure proper nomenclature and printed label design, eliminate dangerous abbreviations and dose designations, and ensure MAR acceptance by nurses.
10. To improve safety, provide an environment that protects staff involved in data entry from undue distractions when using the technology.
11. After implementation, continually reassess and enhance safety effectiveness and error-detection capability, including the use of error tracking tools and the evaluation of near-miss events. Maximize the potential of the technology in order to maximize the safety benefits.
12. After implementation, continually monitor and report errors and near misses or close calls caused by technology through manual or automated surveillance techniques. Pursue system errors and multiple causations through the root cause analysis process or other forms of failure-mode analysis. Consider reporting significant issues to well recognized external reporting systems.
13. Re-evaluate the applicability of security and confidentiality protocols as more medical devices interface with the IT network. Reassess HIPAA compliance on a periodic basis to ensure that the addition of medical devices to your IT network and the growing responsibilities of the IT department haven't introduced new security and compliance risks.

Figure 8-1. The Joint Commission suggested actions to prevent patient harm related to the implementation and use of health information technologies (HIT) and converging technologies.[16]

Source: © The Joint Commission, 2011. Reprinted with permission. The entire Alert can be viewed at: http://www.jointcommission.org/sentinel_event_alert_issue_42_safely_implementing_health_information_and_converging_technologies/

Table 8-1. Sample Gap Analysis: Excerpt from a Smart IV Pump Implementation

Issue	Current State	Ideal State	Discrepancy (Gap)	Next Steps	Responsible Party
Standard concentrations for all continuous infusions for adult populations.	Most continuous infusions are standard concentrations except for norepinephrine, milrinone, and vasopressin, which differ throughout the ICUs.	Standard concentrations for all infusions.	Norepinephrine, milrinone, and vasopressin are utilized differently between different critical care units	Meet with all adult ICU committees, (surgical, neuro, medical, and cardiac) to determine standard.	MSO and Critical Care Committee(s). Final approval through Pharmacy and Therapeutics Committee.
Standard infusion times for intermittently infused medications, i.e., antibiotics.	Few standard infusion times established, only vancomycin and aminoglycosides have standard infusion times per policy.	Standard infusion times for all intermittent medications.	Intermittent medications that do not have a standard infusion time.	Review formulary, determine standard infusion times.	Nursing representatives, clinical pharmacists.

The implementation and maintenance of technologies intended to improve medication safety need careful consideration and comparison of how the technology functions with the actual work it is intended to replace or enhance. Proactive planning and preparation can minimize unintended consequences. Pharmacists should always be involved in the implementation of any medication-related technology. The MSO, in particular, has a special role in the implementation of new medication-related technologies to ensure that medication safety is preserved and achieved. This includes reviewing the literature and case reports, site visits to see how other institutions are using the technology, team selection and participation, participating in hands-on demonstrations, and project leadership. The MSO should partner with pharmacy informatics colleagues within the organization to ensure consistent pharmacy representation in the planning and implementation of medication-related technologies.

Project Management and Process Redesign

Implementing any new technology requires planning, organizing, and managing complex multidisciplinary processes. A solid project management plan is a critical first step. Organizations may provide formal in-house project management support or utilize outside consultants. If not, project management resources and tools are readily available in bookstores and via the Internet. A high-level outline identifying the basic components of a project management plan is shown in Figure 8-2.

Ideally, project leadership should come from an individual with project management experience and training in performance improvement methodologies. *Project management* is the application of knowledge, skills, tools, and techniques to identify activities to meet project requirements. It focuses on planning, organizing, leading, and controlling an organization's resources to accomplish a specific objective. Conventional management focuses more on organizational activities such as human resources, finance, marketing, and operations.[17] Many information technology (IT) departments utilize project management methodology. It is vital that the MSO have a good working relationship with the IT department. Collaboration with IT and pharmacy informatics staff is fundamental when implementing any new medication safety technology.

Understanding project management techniques, such as identifying scope and constraints, creating a work breakdown structure, and planning and scheduling tools, can be very helpful in the implementation of a new medication safety technology on time and on budget. MSOs should become familiar with project management basics and, if planning to lead a project, should consider training and or certification in project management. The MSO may hold a variety of roles within the implementation of a new technology ranging from project manager, project lead, subject matter expert, or team member. The role depends upon many variables including existing project management support, organizational size and resources, and experience level of the MSO.

Setting clear expectations of what the new technology "is" and "is not" is vital. Adequate resources should be allocated for planning, implementation, and maintenance. Many technologies do not reduce the need for resources, especially staff. In many situations any time savings resulting from the new technology must be reassigned to other functions supporting the technology or the technology creates additional work that must be accommodated. Where medication safety is a concern, the MSO may need to advocate for these resources.

Managing expectations helps with social and cultural acceptance, which can be more challenging than acceptance of the technology itself, especially for major workflow changes such as **computerized provider order entry (CPOE)**, and electronic health records (EHR). Executive leadership and clinical champions are essential roles in facilitating the social and cultural acceptance of new technologies. MSOs can function in these capacities as appropriate to the organization. These individuals should be highly respected, visible, and accessible to the **end-users**

Sample Project Management Plan Outline

- Specific project goal(s)
  - Project charter
- Scope of the project
  - Work breakdown structure
- Executive/leadership sponsor(s)
- Clinical champion(s)
- Team of key stakeholders
- Timelines
  - Overall project
  - Each individual objective/activity
    - Defining sequence
    - Identifying resources needed
- Project/action plan with assigned responsibilities
  - Plan for downtime
    - Written policies and procedures
- Ongoing list of issues
- Communication plan
- Training plan
- Resource assessment and allocation
  - Project budget
  - Human resources
- IT infrastructure/support
  - Planning
  - Go-live
  - Post implementation
- Pre/post data collection
  - Identify risks
  - Plan for quality assurance
- After-action review
  - What worked well
    - Celebrate successes!
  - What could we have done better
    - Lessons learned
- Planning for ongoing maintenance/support

There are many project management templates available online for free and for purchase.

Figure 8-2. Sample project management plan outline.

throughout the planning, implementation, and maintenance phases of the project. Key stakeholders should include representatives from all clinical disciplines impacted by the technology including pharmacists, nurses, physicians, physician extenders, (e.g., physician assistants, nurse practitioners, etc.), and respiratory therapists.[18-20]

Process/workflow redesign should begin with creating a flowchart of the current state process and then creating a flowchart of the future state/ideal process. Although these processes can be quite time-consuming, they are worth the investment in the end. Do not assume that the technology will fix current process issues. Problematic process issues in the current state will need to be addressed and corrected prior to implementing the technology. Otherwise, the technology can exacerbate the underlying initial problem. These are often referred to as latent errors. When creating a flowchart of current processes, remaining focused on the current rather than the ideal process can be very challenging for some individuals. The project manager/facilitator should be sure to record ideas generated for the ideal process in a separate document. Areas that are problematic should be further evaluated through a gap analysis.[21]

It is important to consider the entire medication-use system when implementing a new technology. Because working within the medication-use system is the specialty of MSOs, they are best suited to facilitate this process. Other stakeholders and end-users may be solely focused on the segment of the system that they represent.

Remember to look beyond the obvious steps involved and consider impact further up or down the process. Conducting a proactive risk assessment on the new technology such as a failure mode and affects analysis (FMEA) (see Chapter 6 for further discussion of FMEA) can identify vulnerabilities that must be addressed in advance of the roll-out.[22] The MSO should ensure planning for scheduled and unexpected downtimes of the technology including the development of written policies and procedures.

Clinical workflow should be the primary driver of all processes. If the technology requires the clinician to step out of their current workflow, it could result in resistance, **workarounds**, or noncompliance, and may result in patient harm. Often workflow must be changed to accommodate the technology. Obtaining key clinician buy-in and conducting thorough training will aid in the adoption of the new process. This is where the clinical champions can be very helpful. The MSO is essential in communicating with and establishing consensus among the clinical champions and end-users.

When redesigning processes and workflows, it is imperative to include end-users such as staff nurses, staff pharmacists, physician extenders, staff and resident physicians, and unit clerks or secretaries in the decision-making process. Involving frontline clinical staff will provide an accurate picture of the current workflow as well as identify barriers early on that could result in dangerous workarounds. These are also key people to involve as **super-users** or trainers during roll-out.

Depending on the type of technology being implemented, it may also be beneficial to complete risk or readiness assessments.[21] Professional organizations such as the American Society of Health-System Pharmacists (ASHP) and the Institute for Safe Medication Practices (ISMP) have several tools and resources available on their websites. Electronic list serves are also a very good way to share experiences and solicit feedback from other organizations. Be careful not to rely solely on information from vendors.

Example Technologies

CPOE and Clinical Decision Support

CPOE has been identified as an important technological intervention to improve medication safety. The number of published articles on CPOE has been steadily increasing.[23] Wolfstadt et al. concluded in a review that only 5 out of 543 studies looking at CPOE with clinical decision support (CDS) found significant reductions in adverse drug events (ADEs).[24] A review by Kaushal et al. evaluated the effects of

CPOE and CDS on medication safety and found a reduction in medication errors. However, the studies were on "home grown" systems not commercial systems.[25] Eslami et al. reviewed computerized physician medication order entry articles and reported "studies on safety showed some positive effects of CPOE but tended to be non-randomized and were focused on medication error rates, not powered to detect a difference in adverse event rates." [23] Overall, CPOE with CDS is considered to positively impact medication safety. However, published reports with mixed results warn of negative effects if not implemented carefully.[11-15,23-25]

Adoption of CPOE in U.S. hospitals has been slow due to the complexity and cost of implementation. CPOE implementation timelines can be at a minimum 2 to 3 years. Implementation delays are a common occurrence and should be expected. One source states that only 14% of all U.S. hospitals have achieved the expected 10% CPOE level required for stage 1 of **meaningful use**.[26] The 2011 ASHP national survey of pharmacy practice in hospital settings reports 34.2% of U.S. hospitals have CPOE with CDS, increased from 18.9% the previous year. The ASHP survey reports that larger hospitals are more likely to have CPOE.[27]

There are many possible types of CPOE functionality. It is generally accepted that direct order entry by the prescriber provides the most safety. If and how the electronic orders integrate with the pharmacy, laboratory, and radiology systems, as well as the medication administration record (MAR) are also important considerations. Integration of the above-mentioned systems should minimize opportunities for error by reducing manual entry of information and providing immediate access to clinical information. Eliminating steps in any process eliminates opportunities for error.[3-5]

CDS "encompasses a variety of tools and interventions such as computerized alerts and reminders, clinical guidelines, order sets, patient data reports and dashboards, documentation templates, diagnostic support, and clinical workflow tools."[28] Basic medication-related CDS functions are allergy checking, dose range checking, formulary compliance, duplicate therapy checking, drug-drug interaction checking, electronic MAR (eMAR), and order sentences built with key medication order components (e.g., strength, schedule, dose form) that facilitate appropriate orders. Advanced medication-related CDS can be implemented after basic CDS is implemented and working well. These functions include advanced dosing guidance for monitoring patient-specific factors such as age, weight, renal functions, hepatic function, fluid status, cumulative doses, as well as medication-associated laboratory values, and patient monitoring.[29]

A major concern with any level of CDS is rule or **alert fatigue**. Just like the annoying "pop-ups" that occur when using the Internet, CDS can manifest as alert boxes that quickly become disregarded as clinicians grow weary of high-volume, non-clinically significant alerts referred to as nuisance alerts. This desensitization to alerts can decrease the effectiveness of this tool intended to enhance medication safety. As with CPOE, CDS should be implemented with extensive planning and testing to minimize unintended consequences.[30-37] One study found higher compliance with alert recommendations by "tiering" alerts according to clinical significance. "Only the most serious drug-drug interactions would require a response by the clinician." A Level 1 alert required one of the orders to be stopped. Level 2 alerts required a reason for override, and Level 3 alerts were for information only and did not require any action. Organizations should consider not using any clinically insignificant informational alerts so as to decrease the "noise" of too many alerts.[38]

One organization studied the incidence and types of alerts in their CPOE/CDS system reporting an average of 1226 alerts per day and 11 alerts per patient. The most frequent alert that fired (57%) was related to duplicate medication class. The value of alerts was found to be inversely related to the quantity because a mere 1.4% of the orders were then abandoned. The study published a list of recommendations to help reduce false-positive alerts that is a useful resource for MSOs (see Figure 8-3).[39]

Non-CDS CPOE improvements include ensuring that medication ordering is specific to each medication. Order sentences ideally incorporate a complete order that directs the prescriber to commercially available dose strengths and appropriate dosing schedules for that medication. This is helpful in situations where medications

Recommendations to Help Reduce False-Positive Alerts

1. Collect and analyze site-specific alert data; identify and evaluate frequent alerts.
2. Evaluate protocols and medication order sets for alert potential as part of the approval process.
3. Do not wait for computerized provider order entry (CPOE) to address potential alert fatigue; address it with the current pharmacy system.
4. Any new alerts should be carefully considered before adding. Is it specific enough, or will it only contribute to alert fatigue?
5. Require the vendor database to enable customization of alerts to the individual user or subspecialty.
6. Require the vendor database to allow suppression of an alert for a specific alert once it has been overridden.
7. Update allergy profiles so previously tolerated medications do not alert in the future.
8. Consider including alternative therapy suggestions in the alert.
9. Analyze medication error reports for missed alerts and consider coding that information into the ADE database.
10. Do not blindly accept drug interaction programming. Many systems have a high number of less clinically significant interactions.

Figure 8-3. Recommendations to help reduce false-positive alerts.
Source: Adapted with permission from Cash, JJ. Informatics exchange: Alert fatigue. *Am J Health-Syst Pharm.* 2009;66:2098-2101.

come in multiple dose forms (e.g., immediate release [IR], sustained release [SR]) where the dose interval is different. Also, to reinforce safe medication administration practices it is helpful if during the ordering process, for example, only the routes appropriate for that medication are accessible to the prescriber.

The MSO, as well as other pharmacists from the organization, should be included in all phases of planning, implementation, and maintenance of CPOE and CDS. The MSO should be fully engaged in the design, review, and evaluation of medication order sets, drug dosing protocols, alert levels, dose-range checking, drug naming conventions, drug and order set mnemonics, and alert prioritizations. There is an ever increasing pool of resources available to aid in the planning and implementation of CPOE and CDS (see Figure 8-4 for a list).

Bar Code Medication Administration

Bar code medication administration (BCMA) is another technological intervention recommended and widely accepted as a means to reduce medication errors.[7-9,40-42] It is estimated that 35% of medication errors occur in the administration phase where there are few to no double-checks in the process before reaching the patient.[40] Studies suggest that BCMA systems can reduce administration medication errors by up to 50%.[40-42] However, one study reports that less than 10% of the errors detected by BCMA were rated as moderate or severe. Over 90% of errors detected had minimal severity potential.[41] BCMA is often the last line of defense against administration errors, and if implemented carefully, can improve medication safety.[43] There are at least 20 different vendors of BCMA systems.

> There is no universal right "technology" solution due to the complexity and variability of institution-specific factors ... BCMA technology is comprised of a number of hardware and software components that may include a bar code printing system for both wristbands and medication packages in the pharmacy; portable bar code scanners interfaced to computers located near the patient; a communications network (usually wireless) tying the portable bedside computers to a centralized computer server; software applications running on the server that process the incoming information and return information to the bedside computers; and interfaces for communication between the server/software and other hospital databases, such as the pharmacy information system, the order entry system, and the admission, discharge, transfer (ADT) system.[40]

According to the 2011 ASHP national survey of pharmacy practice in hospital settings, 50.2% of U.S. hospitals use BCMA, a significant increase from 34.5% reported in the previous year.[27] A multidisciplinary team including frontline clinicians especially

Resources for Computerized Provider Order Entry and Clinical Decision Support Implementation

Preparing for CPOE Implementation

ASHP guidelines on pharmacy planning for implementation of computerized provider-order-entry systems in hospitals and health systems. *Am J Health Syst Pharm.* 2011; 68:e9-e31; doi:10.2146/sp100011e.

Stablein D, Welebob E, Johnson E, et al. Understanding hospital readiness for CPOE. *Jt Comm J Qual Saf.* 2003;29(7):336-344.

Massachusetts Hospital CPOE Initiative CPOE Readiness Roadmap Guide. Massachusetts Technology Collaborative. Available at: (http://masstech.org/ehealth/cpoe.html)

Metzger J, Fortin J. Computerized physician order entry (CPOE) in community hospitals: Lessons from the field. Oakland, CA: California Health Care Foundation; 2003. Available at: http://www.chcf.org/topics/view.cfm?itemID=20729)

The Physician Order Entry Team (POET) in the Department of Biomedical Informatics and Clinical Epidemiology at Oregon Health & Science University. www.cpoe.org has several consensus recommendations:

1. Considerations for a successful CPOE implementation. Available at: http://www.ohsu.edu/academic/dmice/research/cpoe/findings.php#considerations
2. CPOE issues still under debate. Available at: http://www.ohsu.edu/academic/dmice/research/cpoe/findings.php#issues
3. Principles for a successful CPOE implementation. Available at: http://www.ohsu.edu/academic/dmice/research/cpoe/findings.php#principles
4. Types of unintended consequences of CPOE. Available at: http://www.ohsu.edu/academic/dmice/research/cpoe/findings.php#unintended

Clinical Decision Support (CDS)

Osheroff JA, Pfifer EA, Teich JM, et al. Improving outcomes with clinical decision support: An implementer's guide. HIMSS. 2005. Available at: http://marketplace.himss.org

Osheroff JA. Improving medication use and outcomes with clinical decision support: a step-by-step guide. HIMSS. 2009. Available at: http://marketplace.himss.org

Figure 8-4. Resources for computerized provider order entry and clinical decision support implementation.

nursing, pharmacy, and respiratory therapy should be involved in the planning for BCMA implementation. The MSO is again a key member of any BCMA team. Other patient-care areas using bar-coding technology such as laboratory, blood bank, and admissions should be considered. As with CPOE/CDS, there is an expanding body of knowledge around the safe implementation of BCMA.[40,43]

Major medication safety concerns with BCMA are workarounds. *Workarounds* are actions that do not follow standard procedure or protocol and are often referred to as shortcuts. These shortcuts undermine and minimize the potential gains in medication safety from BCMA. Koppel et al. reported 15 types of BCMA-related workarounds and 31 separate causes of the identified workarounds. The workarounds were categorized as omission of process steps, steps performed out of sequence, or unauthorized process steps. Classes of probable causes of BCMA workarounds were classified as technology, task, organizational, patient, or environmental-related.[45] A common workaround with BCMA is scanning a dummy or duplicate label instead of the actual medication or the patient directly. Ways to minimize this type of shortcut are to involve staff nurses when designing workflow, establish safeguards to prevent the printing of dummy or duplicate labels, and educate nurses and others on the dangers of shortcuts. Proactively soliciting feedback from users, through frequent rounding on patient care units or through a standing interdisciplinary committee, followed by action to address problems is another method to reduce workarounds.[46] Conducting an FMEA prior to implementation of BCMA is a good way to identify those potential shortcuts (failure modes) and design your processes to prevent them.

The MSO can assist in developing or enhancing the pharmacy's operations to support BCMA. As with other technologies discussed, creating a flowchart of the entire process, in combination with FMEA or a gap analysis, is a good starting point. To ensure scan readability and accuracy, a sample of every product should be scanned on its arrival in the pharmacy, prior to placing in the pharmacy storage area. For this process, the pharmacy technician should use the same equipment nursing uses for BCMA. The MSO should confirm that redundancies are included in the process for mapping bar codes and adding new products to the system, (e.g., pharmacist verification of a technician's work). When adding bar code labels to products, designate guidelines for safe attachment; for example, be sure the drug name and all critical information remains visible or is placed on a permanent part of the drug device—not on removable caps of inhalers or syringes. A reference guide, such as the example shown in Table 8-2, can be helpful for consistent dispensing and method of bar-code placement. Be sure to collaborate with end-users on a process for notifying the pharmacy when the product bar code is not readable or incorrect, as well as the action required by pharmacy or others. The MSO may select any of these processes as a basis for performance improvement metrics.

Automated Dispensing Cabinets

Automated dispensing cabinets (ADCs) are "computerized drug storage devices or cabinets that allow medications to be stored and dispensed near the point of care, while controlling and tracking drug distribution."[47] ADCs have evolved into the primary method of drug delivery in many hospitals. Their use has positively impacted drug distribution by improving accessibility, security, and billing processes. ADC software capabilities range from simple to complex. More complex systems offer integration with automated refilling systems as well as bar coding for restocking and administration. Most systems offer some type of alerts and/or basic decision support as well. It is generally accepted that "profile" ADCs, those that are interfaced with

Table 8-2. Respiratory Therapy Medications

Generic	Brand	Strength	Form	Size	NDC#	Manufacturer	Barcode Process*	Storage Area	Comments	Dispensing
Albuterol	Proventil	90 mcg	Inh	17 gm	1727072101	Armstrong	2	Area B	Out of box**	Mulitdose
Albuterol	Albuterol	2.5 mg	Neb	3 mL		Dey	1	Area B		ADC/cartfill
Budesonide/ formoterol	Pulmicort respules	0.25 mg	Neb	2 mL	186198804	AstraZeneca	5	Area A	Dispense in repackaged bag. Fill in 2 week exp. date at time of dispensing	Multidose
Flunisolide	Pulmozyme		Neb	2.5 mL	5024210039	Genetech	2	Refrigerator store in foil pouch	Dispense unit dose in blue refrig. zip lock	Cartfill

***Barcode Process:**
1. Use manufacturer barcode,
2. Flag label,
3. Unit dose and liquid cups,
4. Unit dose and oral med,
5. Needs repackaging,
6. Robot packaging.

****Out of Box:**
1. Remove inhaler from box.
2. Flag patient label away from mouthpiece.
3. Dispense in security bag.

Inh, inhalers; Neb, inhalation solutions.

Source: Courtesy of D. Saine, Winchester Medical Center.

the pharmacy computer system and require pharmacist verification of the patient's medication orders prior to withdrawal from the ADCs, provide optimal medication safety. Non-profile machines, where the medication is accessible without, or prior to pharmacist review of orders, are often employed in areas such as the emergency department (ED), operating room, post-anesthesia care unit, and labor and delivery. These areas are then lacking the important safeguards of a prospective pharmacist review of medication orders. Non-profile areas should be minimized as much as feasible. In hospitals with CPOE, the ED is one area where profiled ADCs are starting to gain momentum because of the many medication safety benefits previously described. Many ED patients are ultimately admitted and ED orders and medication administration documentation provides continuity of care. Extra flexibility for overrides may be needed during the transition period and pharmacy turn-around-time reports for verification can be utilized to provide data for wait time for medication access in an area that traditionally had relatively open access.

Medication errors can result from ADCs being restocked incorrectly due to look-alike/sound-alike medications next to each other, access to more than one medication at a time, or pockets overflowing and spilling over to other pockets. Bar code restocking in combination with BCMA can reduce these types of errors. Bar code restocking without BCMA is more problematic. A bar-coded medication bag could be filled with the wrong medication or a combination of the correct and incorrect medication, often a look-alike medication. If each individual bar-coded medication is scanned into stock and out of stock for filling and into patient medication bins on the patient care areas, then the likelihood of an error is much less; but, this is a cumbersome process and generally would not be done.

ADCs possess the ability to have pop-up alerts or warnings as designated medications are being withdrawn from the unit. This functionality, when used judiciously can help to decrease medication errors or provide important drug information at the point of dispensing. Some examples of possible alerts include medications that are: high-alert, look-alike/sound-alike, restricted, require special handling/monitoring, on shortage, concentrated solutions, extended-release formulations, etc. The MSO, in conjunction with nursing or a medication safety team should determine the use of ADC alerts and periodically review/change them as appropriate so as not to contribute to alert fatigue.

Medication errors can also result from medications removed via override. Medications available on override are accessible for withdrawal prior to pharmacist verification of the order. Overrides should be reserved only for medications needed in emergent/urgent situations. When routine medications are available on override, medication errors are more likely to occur.[48] Override lists for each patient care area should be established based on criteria that address potential safety issues with each medication for that area (see Figure 8-5).

Sample Automated Dispensing Cabinet Override Criteria

1. Medications for which the delay in waiting for pharmacist review could compromise the patient's clinical condition.
   a. Emergency or "code" medications to treat:
      i. Hypoglycemia
      ii. Hyper/hypotension
      iii. Arrhythmias
      iv. Hemorrhage
      v. Anaphylaxis/severe allergic reactions
      vi. Acidosis
      vii. Severe electrolyte abnormalities
      viii. Seizures
      ix. Severe agitation
   b. Reversal agents, antidotes, or rescue medications
   c. Medications for intubation
   d. Other urgently needed medications
      i. Albuterol
      ii. Surfactant
      iii. Oxytocin
2. Medications for patient comfort
   a. IV opiates
   b. IV antiemetic

Figure 8-5. Sample automated dispensing cabinet override criteria.

The medication safety committee/team and Pharmacy and Therapeutics (P&T) Committee should approve all override medications. Questions for consideration of potential override medications include:

- How critical is the immediate administration of the medication?
- Does the mechanism and onset of action justify it being on override?
- Does the delay it takes for pharmacist review/verification jeopardize patient safety?

Although there is no formal consensus on an appropriate ADC override rate, professional guidelines recommend minimizing the number of override medications to only those that are emergent/urgent. The MSO should ensure that processes are in place for pharmacist retrospective review of override orders, auditing override rates, and evaluating the potential for medication errors in the ADC override process.

ISMP[47] and ASHP[49] have guidance documents available on their websites to aid in the safe use and implementation of ADCs. In 2007, ISMP released a report listing the 12 core processes associated with safe ADC use[47] (see Table 8-3 for a summary and recommendations). MSOs should critically evaluate their ADC systems, processes, and policies for compliance with the ISMP and ASHP recommendations.

Table 8-3. Safe Automated Dispensing Cabinet (ADC) Use: Core Processes, Risks, and Possible Solutions

Core Process	Safety Risk	Possible Solution
Environment for ADC	Poor lighting or temperature control, distractions, distance to supplies/ patient.	Proactive planning for placement or remodel. Install in area with minimal distractions.
ADC security	Unauthorized access to medications, password protection.	Clearly defined policies and procedures around access, passwords, updates, terminations, etc.
Non-profile machines	Medication withdrawn and administered without a pharmacist review.	Minimize/eliminate non-profile ADCs. Store a limited variety and quantity of medications. Consider independent double-check process for removals from non-profile machines.
Information and display on ADC	Incomplete information or error-prone display.	Ensure complete patient name and medication information are clearly visible—avoid abbreviation and truncation. Use tall man lettering where appropriate. ADC med name should match med label and MAR.
Inventory selection and PAR levels	Unsafe or inadequate inventory.	Establish criteria for inventory selection, customize for usage and patient population. Use P&T or Medication Safety Team oversight. Use unit dose or ready-to-use unit of use products. Limit inventory levels to avoid accidental overdose.
ADC configuration	Look-alike names and packaging. Restock or removal errors.	Use single, lidded compartments; avoid matrix drawers. If must use matrix, avoid controlled substance, high alert, drugs with high potential for diversion. Plan drawer layouts: one drug strength per compartment. Set up mock drawers to visualize look-alike errors. Monitor if drawer inventory changes.
Restocking process	Restock errors: wrong drug available for withdrawal.	Bar-coding verification for pharmacy fill and cabinet fill processes; ensure consistency of drug name across medication-use process. Differentiate look alike/sound alikes.
Medication withdrawal	Wrong medication selection; administration of wrong medication, dose, route, or frequency.	Configure ADCs in pharmacy profile mode; Work with nursing to ensure medication withdrawal for one patient at a time.

Table 8-3 (continued).

Core Process	Safety Risk	Possible Solution
Overrides	Medication withdrawn and administered without a pharmacist review can result in patient harm from unrecognized allergies, contraindications, interactions; incorrect medication, dose, route.	Establish criteria for overrides. Develop process for retrospective review of medication orders obtained via override. Routinely monitor and audit overrides. Limit quantity and drug concentrations available on override.
Transport from ADC to patient bedside	Administration to wrong patient; diversion; medications stored inappropriately.	Transport in original unit-dose packaging to bedside; Ensure adequate number ADCs, placed for safe workflow. Work with nursing to develop process.
Returns	Returning medications to wrong bin can lead to withdrawal and administration errors.	Create process for all returns to go to a one-way return bin.
Staff education/ competency	Unfamiliarity with functionality can lead to unsafe workarounds or delay in care.	Ensure adequate training on orientation, after any upgrades, and periodic competency assessments.

ADCs, automated dispensing cabinets; MAR, medication administration record; P&T, Pharmacy and Therapeutics.
Source: Adapted with permission from Institute for Safe Medication Practices. Guidance on the Interdisciplinary Safe Use of Automated Dispensing Cabinets. Available at: http://www.ismp.org/Tools/guidelines/ADC_Guidelines_Final.pdf.

Smart IV Pumps/Intelligent Infusion Devices

Computerized infusion devices with software programmed to prevent medication errors have become known as *smart pumps* or *intelligent infusion devices* (IIDs). Smart IV pumps contain drug libraries in which drug-specific dosing guidelines, concentration limits, infusion rates, and times can be programmed. The dosing can be standard or weight-based with limits that are hard or soft stops. One way that drug libraries can be separated is by care areas such as adult medical/surgical, adult critical care, and adult oncology to facilitate population-specific dosing guidelines and minimize opportunities for medications to be administered inappropriately. Smart IV pumps are important tools in preventing medication errors, especially with high-alert medications such as heparin and insulin infusions, where pump programming errors can result in significant patient harm, even death.[50-53] Husch et al. report that smart IV pumps could prevent 97% of pump programming errors.[54]

According to the 2011 ASHP National Survey, 67.9% of all U.S. hospitals use smart IV pumps.[27] As with other technological interventions, significant multidisciplinary planning should precede their implementation. Because nursing primarily uses the IV pumps, the datasets, infusion parameters, and dosing limits should have significant nursing input and review to optimize the use of the safety features. Dosing and infusion parameters should be consistent with clinical practice to avoid unnecessary overrides. Standard drug concentrations must be established and followed prior to implementation. Not using the smart functionality on the pumps literally eliminates the safety features and should be strongly discouraged if not prohibited unless under very specific circumstances such as the medication cannot be added to the library. The MSO should be familiar with nursing practice and work closely with nursing leadership to develop policies for use. Alert fatigue can occur with IV pump alerts. Rothschild et al. found that 25% of IV pump alerts were ignored.[55] Ideally, overrides and other data reports should be available from the pumps to evaluate for continuous quality improvement (CQI) purposes. This is best accomplished through the use of a wireless server for the pump software so that CQI data can be downloaded on demand and analyzed without having to physically touch every pump. Modifications based on the quality improvement data can be made to the drug libraries to minimize overrides and non-use of the smart functionality. Conducting a proactive risk assessment such as an FMEA is recommended to minimize workarounds. Such actions are often under the direction of the MSO.

Research suggests that future directions of Smart IV pumps should include integration with CPOE, BCMA, MARs, and pharmacy computer systems to enhance their medication safety capability.[56] One institution has integrated their eMAR, BCMA, and IIDs into a bar code–driven workflow. Known as IV interoperability or auto programming, all three technologies interface and function as an integrated system eliminating the need for manual programming of the pump. Preliminary results from this one institution's experience look quite promising as they demonstrated a 32% reduction in reported errors with heparin infusions.[56] Although more research and experience is needed with medication device interoperability, it will likely be a significant opportunity for the MSO.

Other Dispensing Technologies

Several other medication technologies exist that are used to improve efficiency, accuracy, and safety especially in the dispensing phase of the medication-use system. Some of these technologies include carousel dispensing technology, robotics for unit-dosing, cart fill, IV compounding, and medication delivery, and unit-dose packagers. There are numerous organization case reports on the successful use of these technologies but few if any large-scale studies. As with any new medication safety technology, the MSO is central to its safe implementation. Automation of dispensing processes can result in improved efficiency. A thorough project management plan including evaluation of the literature, site visits, workflow study and redesign are crucial to a successful implementation.

Other Considerations

The MSO will want to ensure downtime, data management/CQI, and systems integration and interoperability are safely and effectively addressed. It is important to note that these processes cannot be designed, tested, or implemented in isolation—the MSO will be a part of a greater collaborative effort.

Downtime

All technology experiences downtime whether it is planned or unexpected. When clinical processes rely on technology to function, it can paralyze workflow and ultimately patient safety if downtime processes are not defined, communicated, workable, and accessible. The MSO should facilitate the creation of downtime procedures for medication-related technologies. This includes the creation of paper back-up forms, plans for back entry of data, automatic backup of systems and snapshot reports that can be run to access patient information and drug information. The MSO should partner with IT and pharmacy informatics on downtime procedures.

Data Management/CQI

Many medication-related technologies have the capacity to produce data. In addition to monitoring medication error reports, MSOs should evaluate data mining capabilities of the technology and develop a plan to monitor the effectiveness of the new technology during implementation, immediately after implementation, and long term. The medication safety or other appropriate committees should regularly review the data evaluating opportunities for improvement. These technologies may provide more data on actual occurrences rather than relying on self-reported incident reports.[4]

Integration and Interoperability

Reducing the number of manual entry steps in a process is a proven method of decreasing medication errors.[4] The next step in the evolution of medication-related technologies is integrating multiple technologies into one seamless system.[57] A 2007 ASHP survey showed that 86% of all U.S. hospitals had their pharmacy computer system either integrated within a suite of products by one vendor or interfaced with technology from other vendors. However, the same survey showed that only 19.6% of U.S. hospitals had all three: eMAR, BCMA, and electronic nursing documentation.[58] As more technologies have the ability to integrate, interface, and/or interoperate, new opportunities open up for the MSO. When integrating multiple technologies, for example, the pharmacy system, eMAR, and IIDs, the systems may not support the same type of dosing for infusions. This may occur if the IIDs have weight-based dosing but the pharmacy system and eMAR display in volume/time (e.g., mL/hr) so the nurse does not have the appropriate information to program the pump for weight-based dosing. When this occurs, the MSO should work with others to develop and implement safeguards in the medication-use process to prevent error and patient harm.

Summary

Technology is generally accepted as a means to improve medication safety. However, unintended consequences and new causes of error should be expected when implementing a medication-related technology. Project management planning, proactive risk assessments, and multidisciplinary teams are critical components of a successful roll-out. There is a rapidly evolving body of literature and resources surrounding the use of technology in health care. Two common themes are the importance of adequate resources and careful planning to ensure optimal results. Table 8-4 summarizes opportunities for the MSO to enhance safety with selected technologies. The MSO has a key role in the implementation and use of medication-related technologies: to ensure that medication safety is preserved and achieved.

PRACTICE TIPS

1. The MSO should be involved in planning for *all* new medication-related technologies. Identify potential safety "go-live" issues during planning and help team members understand the interrelationships, implications, and possibilities of current and proposed medication-use technologies and the impact on medication safety.
2. Always include representation from end-users when implementing new technologies. Clinical workflow should be the primary driver of processes and tools.
3. The MSO should partner with clinical informatics colleagues within the institution/health-system for medication safety. Build strong working relationships with pharmacy informatics and other groups or departments involved in medication-use process technologies such as clinical transformation, CPOE, and nursing informatics.
4. Remember to plan for monitoring of the new technology, downtime, and long-term support after implementation. The MSO will want to ensure safety is not compromised after technology implementation through monitoring and data analysis, and his or her expertise is helpful in identifying critical safeguards for downtime and ongoing support.

Table 8-4. MSO Opportunities to Improve Medication Safety with Selected Technologies

Common Medication Safety Issues with Selected Technologies	Opportunities for the MSO
Computerized Physician/Provider Order Entry/Clinical Decision Support	
■ Drug naming conventions/mnemonics within the system—are they clear and consistent? ■ Non-evidenced—based or approved standard protocols/order sets. ■ Look-alike drug names ■ Alert fatigue ■ Interaction checking ■ Duplicate checking ■ Other custom alerts developed internally ■ Inconsistency in dosage units (mg versus Gm, elemental versus salt form for electrolytes)	■ Work closely with pharmacy informatics on development of drug name mnemonics and be sure they are consistent with other related systems, e.g., ADC, billing, etc. ■ Participate in the development and review of CPOE order sets and protocols. ■ Include prevention of look-alike/sound-alike error prevention strategies in the development of CPOE order sets. ■ Monitor rules and alerts (CDS) that fire to end-users within CPOE. Take steps to reduce nuisance or those that are nonclinically significant. ■ Partner with pharmacy informatics to develop more specific and sophisticated CDS. ■ Aid in the development of testing scenarios that evaluate potential medication errors. ■ Educate end-users on any error-prone processes within the CPOE system. ■ Plan for downtimes, expected and unexpected, as well as software upgrades. ■ Look for opportunities to integrate and/or interoperate with other medication technologies.
Bar Code Medication Administration	
■ What type of bar code does the system use and what information does it contain? ■ Does the wireless system have the capacity to adequately support BCMA? ■ Patient ID band must have barcode ■ Hardware (computer) and scanners not in every patient room ■ Products for which the unit of use does not contain a barcode ■ Potential for workarounds, e.g., scanning of "dummy labels" instead of the actual product or patient ■ Overrides	■ Participate in the evaluation and selection of the BCMA system. ■ Review formulary and ensure all medications are mapped to drug codes. ■ Develop a process for adding barcodes to products that do not contain the unit of use or the packaging limits its readability. ■ How does the BCMA handle partial, multiple, and range doses? ■ Work closely with nursing to flowchart medication administration, documentation, and monitoring. ■ Conduct a FMEA prior to BCMA implementation. ■ Develop policies, procedures, and training. ■ Plan for downtimes and software upgrades. ■ Routinely monitor noncompliance or exception reports.

Table 8-4 (continued).

Common Medication Safety Issues with Selected Technologies	Opportunities for the MSO
Intelligent Infusion Devices	
■ Non-standard concentrations ■ Non-standard infusion times ■ Alert fatigue ■ Non-use of drug library ■ Overrides	■ Participate in evaluation and selection of IIDs. ■ Facilitate dataset/drug library development with other clinical staff. ■ Develop policies, procedures, and training. ■ Manage updates to drug library and software or hardware upgrades. ■ Review overrides and update drug library as appropriate. ■ Champion the use of wireless technology to update and monitor IIDs. ■ Work closely with nursing to assess incidence of not using the smart pump drug libraries.
Dispensing Technologies	
■ Inefficient workflows ■ Routine maintenance ■ Downtime ■ Training ■ Double-check/verification	■ Flowchart workflows, conduct time-motion studies, and assess error reports pre- and postimplementation. ■ Ensure equipment is properly maintained: watch for peak-use times. ■ Develop downtime and upgrade procedures. ■ Ensure adequate training and orientation. ■ Establish processes to ensure the use of the technologies is optimized. ■ Develop policies, procedures, and training.

ADC, automated dispensing cabinets; BCMA, bar code medication administration; CDS, clinical decision support; CPOE, computerized provider order entry; IIDs, intelligent infusion devices; FMEA, Failure Modes and Effects Analysis.

References

1. National Academy of Engineering. Greatest Engineering achievements of the 20th century. Available at: http://www.greatachievements.org/ Accessed July 10, 2008.
2. Technology. Dictionary.com. *Dictionary.com Unabridged (v 1.1)*. Random House, Inc. Available at: http://dictionary.reference.com/browse/technology Accessed: July 14, 2008.
3. Leape LL. Error in medicine. *JAMA.* 1994;272:1851-1857.
4. Leape L, Kabcenell A, Berwick D. *Institute for Healthcare Improvement's Breakthrough Series Guide Reducing Adverse Drug Events.* Boston, MA: Institute for Healthcare Improvement; 1998.
5. Leape LL, Bates DW, Cullen DJ, et al. Systems analysis of adverse drug events. ADE Prevention Study Group. *JAMA.* 1995; 274:35-43.
6. The Institute of Medicine. *To Err Is Human: Building a Safer Health System*. Washington, DC: National Academy Press; 1999.
7. The Institute of Medicine. *Crossing the Quality of Chasm: A New Health System for the 21st Century.* Washington, DC: National Academy Press; 2001.
8. The Leapfrog Group. Available at: www.leapfroggroup.org. Accessed March 9, 2009.
9. National Quality Forum. (2003). Safe practices for better health care. Washington, DC. Available at: http://www.qualityforum.org/News_And_Resources/Press_Kits/Safe_Practices_for_Better_Healthcare.aspx Accessed June 1, 2011.
10. Klein M. The technological revolution. *Footnotes. The Newsletter of FPRIs Wachman Center.* 2008;13(18). Accessed September 9, 2012.
11. Ash, J, Sittig D, Poon E, et. al. The extent and importance of unintended consequences related to computerized provider order entry. *J Am Med Inform Assoc.* 2007;14(4):415-423.
12. Ash J, Berg M, Coiera E. Some unintended consequences of information technology in health care: The nature of patient care information system-related errors. *J Am Med Inform Assoc.* 2004:11:104-112.
13. Nebeker J, Hoffman J, Weir C, et al. High rates of adverse drug events in a highly computerized hospital. *Arch Intern Med.* 2005;165:1111-1116.
14. Koppel R, Metlay J, Cohen A, et al. Role of computerized physician order entry systems in facilitating medication errors. *JAMA.* 2005;293:1197-1203.
15. Teich JM, Merchia PR, Schmiz JL, et al. Effects of computerized physician order entry on prescribing practices. *Arch Intern Med.* 2000;160:2741-2747.
16. The Joint Commission. *Sentinel Event Alert Safely implementing health information and converging technologies.* Issue 42. December 11, 2008. Available at: http://www.jointcommission.org/sentinel_event_alert_issue_42_safely_implementing_health_information_and_converging_technologies/ Accessed September 4, 2011.
17. Project Management Institute. *A Guide to the Project Management Body of Knowledge: PMBOK Guide.* Newtown Square, PA: PMI; 2008.
18. Bruce A, Langdon K. *Essential Managers Project Management*. New York: DK Publishing Inc; 2000.
19. Healthcare Information and Management Systems Society. Klinedinst JW. The project management discipline: An introduction. Available at: http://www.himss.org/content/files/PM_Discipline_Intro031307.pdf?whhdl. Accessed July 10, 2008.
20. Healthcare Information and Management Systems Society. Why have a project methodology in health care and how to deliver successful projects. HIMSS Project Management Task Force. January 7, 2008. Available at: http://www.himss.org/content/files/WhyHaveProjectManagementMethodology.pdf?src=enews20080109 Accessed July 11, 2008.
21. Mitchell J. Root-Cause Analysis and Healthcare Failure Mode and Effects Analysis: Two Proactive Harm-Prevention Strategies. In: Manasse H, Thompson K, eds. *Medication Safety: A*

Guide for Health Care Facilities. Bethesda, MD: American Society of Health-System Pharmacists; 2005:237-251.

22. Gordon B. Medication Safety Self-Assessments. In: Manasse H, Thompson K, eds. *Medication Safety: A Guide for Health Care Facilities*. Bethesda, MD: American Society of Health-System Pharmacists; 2005:299-318.
23. Eslami S, de Keizer, N, Abu-Hanna A. The impact of computerized physician medication order entry in hospitalized patients: A systematic review. *J Am Med Inform Assoc.* 2007;14(4):400-406.
24. Wolfstadt JI, Gurwitz JH, Field TS, et al. The effect of computerized physician order entry with clinical decision support on the rates of adverse drug events: A systematic review. *J Gen Intern Med.* 2008;23(4):451-458.
25. Kaushal R, Shojania K, Bates, D. Effects of computerized physician order entry and clinical decision support systems on medication safety: A systematic review. *Arch Intern Med.* 2003;163:1409-1416.
26. KLAS. CPOE adoption milestone still out of reach for most U.S. hospitals. Available at: https://www.klasresearch.com/News/PressRoom/2010/CPOE.aspx. Accessed June 1, 2011.
27. Pedersen C, Schneider P, Scheckelhoff D. ASHP national survey of pharmacy practice: Dispensing and administration—2011. *Am J Health-Syst Pharm.* 2012;69(6):768-785.
28. Osheroff JA, Teich JM, Middleton B, et. al. A roadmap for national action on clinical decision support. *J Am Med Inform Assoc.* 2007;14:141-145.
29. Kuperman GJ, Bobb ,. Payne TH, et al. Medication-related clinical decision support in computerized provider order entry systems: A review. *J Am Med Inform Assoc.*2007;14(1):29-40.
30. Metzger J, Welebob E, Turisco F. Effective use of medication-related decision support in CPOE. *Patient Saf Qual Healthcare.* 2008;Sep/Oct:16-24.
31. Van Der Sus H, Aarts J, Vulto A, et. al. Overriding of drug safety alerts in computerized physician order entry. *J Am Med Inform Assoc.* 2006;13:138-147.
32. Paterno M, Saverio M, Gorman P, et al. Drug-drug interaction alerts by severity increases compliance rates. *J Am Med Inform Assoc.* 2009;16:40-46.
33. Agency for Healthcare Research and Quality. Emerging lessons: computerized provider order entry with clinical decision support. Available at: http://healthit.ahrq.gov/portal/server.pt?open=514&objID=5562&mode=2&holderDisplayURL=http://prodportallb.ahrq.gov:7087/publishedcontent/publish/communities/a_e/ahrq_funded_projects/test_emerging_lessons/health_briefing_12282006111158/computerized_provider_order_entry_with_clinical_decision_support.html. Accessed July 12, 2008.
34. Shamliyan T, Duval S, Du J, et al. Just what the doctor ordered. Review of the evidence of the impact of computerized physician order entry system on medication errors. *Health Svs Res.* 2008;43(1Pt1):32-53.
35. Ammenwerth E, Schnell-Inderst P, Machan C, et al. The effect of electronic prescribing on medication errors and adverse drug events: A systematic review. *J Am Med Inform Assoc.* 2008;15(5):585-600.
36. Gross PA ,Bates DW. A pragmatic approach to implementing best practices for clinical decision support systems in computerized provider order entry systems. *J Am Med Inform Assoc.* 2007;14(1):25-28.
37. Dixon, BE, Zafar, A. *Inpatient Computerized Provider Order Entry (CPOE) Findings from the AHRQ Health IT Portfolio*. Agency for Healthcare Research and Quality. AHRQ Publication No. 09-0031-EF. January 2009 Available at: http://healthit.ahrq.gov/images/jan09cpoereport/cpoe_issue_paper.htm. Accessed September 4, 2011.
38. Sittig D, Ash J, Zhang J. Lessons from "unexpected increased mortality after implementation of a commercially sold computerized physician order entry system" *Pediatrics.* 2006;118:797-801.

39. Cash JJ. Informatics exchange: Alert fatigue. *Am J Health-Syst Pharm.* 2009;66:2098-2101.

40. Cummings J, *UHC Technology Report: Bar-coded Medication Administration.* University HealthSystem Consortium. June 2005.

41. Johnson C, Carlson R, Tucker C, et al. Using BCMA software to improve patient safety in Veterans Administration medical centers. *J Healthc Inf Manag.* 2002;16(1):46-51.

42. Larrabee S, Brown MM. Recognizing the institutional benefits of bar-code point-of-care technology. *Jt Comm J Qual Saf.* 2003;29:345-353.

43. Sakowski J, Newman J, Dozier K. Severity of medication administration errors detected by a bar-code medication administration system. *Am J Health-Syst Pharm.* 2008;65:1661-1665.

44. American Hospital Association, Health Research and Educational Trust, Institute for Safe Medication Practices. *Pathways for Medication Safety: Assessing Bedside Bar-coding Readiness.* Chicago: Heath Research and Educational Trust, 2002.

45. Koppel R, Wetterneck T, Telles J. Workarounds to barcode medication administration systems: Their occurrences, causes, and threats to patient safety. *J Am Med Inform Assoc.* 2008;15:408-423.

46. Patterson ES, Rogers ML, Render ML. Fifteen best practice recommendations for bar-code medication administration in the veterans health administration. *Jt Comm J Qual Saf.* 2004;30(7):355-365.

47. Institute for Safe Medication Practices. Guidance on the interdisciplinary safe use of automated dispensing cabinets. Available at: http://www.ismp.org/Tools/guidelines/ADC_Guidelines_Final.pdf Accessed September 4, 2011.

48. Kester K, Baxter J, Freudenthal K. Errors associated with medications removed from automated dispensing machines using override function. *Hosp Pharm.* 2006;41:535-537.

49. American Society of Health-System Pharmacists. ASHP guidelines on the safe use of automated medication storage and distribution devices. *Am J Health-Syst Pharm.* 1998;55:1403-1407.

50. Eskew J, Jacobi J, Buss W, et.al. Using innovative technologies to set new safety standards for the infusion of intravenous medications. *Hosp Pharm.* 2002;31:1179-1189.

51. Malashock C, Shull S, Gould D. Effect of smart infusion pumps on medication errors related to infusion device programming. *Hosp Pharm.* 2004;39(5):460-469.

52. Williams C, Maddox R. Implementation of an i.v. medication safety system. *Am J Health-Syst Pharm.* 2005;62:530-536.

53. Wilson K, Sullivan M. Preventing medication errors with smart infusion technology. *Am J Health-Syst Pharm.* 2004;61:177-183.

54. Husch M, Sullican C, Rooney C, et.al. Insights from the sharp end of intravenous medication errors: Implications for infusion pump technology. *Qual Saf Health Care.* 2005;14:80-86.

55. Rothschild JM, Keohane CA, Cook EF, et al. A controlled trial of smart infusion pumps to improve medication safety in critically ill patients. *Crit Care Med.* 2005;33:533–540.

56. Prusch AE, Suess TM, Paoletti RD, et al. Integrating technology to improve medication administration. *Am J Health-Syst Pharm.* 2011;68:835-842.

57. Siska MH, Tribble DA, Opportunities and challenges related to technology in supporting optimal pharmacy practice models in hospitals and health systems. *Am J Health-Syst Pharm.* 2011;68:1116-1126.

58. Pedersen CA, Gumpper KF. ASHP national survey on informatics: Assessment of the adoption and use of pharmacy informatics in U.S. hospitals—2007. *Am J Health-Syst Pharm.* 2008;65:2244-2264.

Medication Error Reporting and Analysis

Marjorie Shaw Phillips

CHAPTER 9

Key Terms

Adverse Drug Event—Harm resulting from use of a medication.

Adverse Drug Reaction—An idiosyncratic reaction or other adverse effect of a medication that is not preventable (i.e., not a medication error).

Adverse Event—An undesirable occurrence associated with the use of a medical product in a patient, directly associated with care or services provided within the jurisdiction of a medical facility.

Data Mining—The process of extracting meaningful (useful and potentially actionable) information from large databases such as administrative and clinical health records (sifting through volumes of data to find hidden material of value).

Detection Sensitivity Level—The rate at which errors that occur are actually reported and recognized by the organization. A high detection sensitivity level is demonstrated through a high error reporting rate.

Food and Drug Administration MedWatch—The Food and Drug Administration safety information and adverse event reporting program.

Medication Error—An error occurring in any step of the medication-use process; any preventable event that may result in incorrect medication use or patient harm.

Near Miss—An error process that is stopped or interrupted either by chance or through a check-and-balance in the medication-use process, such as recognition of the problem and intervention by an experienced practitioner. Other similar terms include *close call* and *good catch*.

Non-Punitive—An approach that uses positive feedback to individuals who report errors (including self-reports) rather than punishment when an error is detected and contributes to a culture where open communication about errors is encouraged.

Patient Safety Organizations—Entities registered with and listed with the Agency for Healthcare Research and Quality under the Patient Safety Act and Patient Safety Rule, which provide confidentiality and privilege protections for patient safety work product.

Taxonomy—The practice and science of classification. The National Coordinating Council for Medication Error Reporting and Prevention taxonomy is a classification system to describe and analyze the details around individual medication errors events.

Introduction

It should be a goal of every health care organization to continually improve systems to prevent harm to patients due to **medication errors**. Health care organizations should monitor actual and potential medication errors that occur within their organization and investigate the root cause of errors. The goal is to identify ways to improve the medication-use system to prevent future errors and the potential for patient harm. A consistent organizational framework is needed to monitor and measure medication safety. The role of the medication safety officer (MSO) is central in this medication error assessment and monitoring process, both to pinpoint improvement opportunities and to assess the effectiveness of interventions already underway to improve patient safety. Encouraging reporting, monitoring, and open discussion of medication errors is key in establishing a culture of safety, or a *Just Culture*. See chapter 5 for further discussion of Just Culture.

What Is a Medication Error?

Achieving consensus on what constitutes a medication error is central to understanding the causes of medication errors and taking a comprehensive approach to achieving a safer medication-use system. Early medication error researchers and public policy makers often defined medication errors simply as a deviation from what the physician prescribed. This narrow focus excludes steps in the medication-use process that are frequently associated with harmful events such as prescribing and patient monitoring. When medication errors are looked at more broadly, pharmacy intervention programs to optimize medication use and actions to improve patient understanding and adherence to their medication regimen become significant components of the overall safety effort.

In July 1995, the National Coordinating Council for Medication Error Reporting and Prevention (NCC MERP), an independent body comprised of 27 national health care organizations representing the collaboration of key national health care and consumer organizations, was formed to begin addressing growing concerns related to medication errors (see www.nccmerp.org). As a first step the NCC MERP established this definition:

> A medication error is any preventable event that may cause or lead to inappropriate medication use or patient harm while the medication is in the control of the health care professional, patient, or consumer. Such events may be related to professional practice, health care products, procedures, and systems, including prescribing; order communication; product labeling, packaging, and nomenclature; compounding; dispensing; distribution; administration; education; monitoring; and use.[1]

This definition becomes a powerful tool for improving medication safety across the continuum of medication use because it recognizes the importance of studying errors whether or not they are caught before they reach the patient and even if harm did not occur in that instance. Medication errors overlap with other categories of drug-related incidents, such as **adverse drug events** (ADEs), medication misadventures, or **adverse drug reactions** (ADRs). It is important for the MSO to differentiate among these events to ensure an appropriate and timely response. David Bates and colleagues at Brigham and Women's Hospital have provided a visual framework that is helpful to explain the overlap among these types of events (Figure 9-1). For each medication error detected or reported, there must be an assessment of the patient outcome or potential for harm.

Because ADRs are by definition not preventable or ameliorable (i.e., not medication errors), the focus of the response will be on patient management, reporting (internally and, if applicable, externally through the FDA MedWatch system), and education to increase health care provider awareness. Events that may initially be considered unexpected when the effects of a medication are incompletely known, often can be prevented once increased knowledge is obtained of necessary therapeutic monitoring, or actions to manage potential interactions with other medications, foods, or disease states. Thus, reporting and information sharing on ADRs are important to medication safety.

Detecting Medication Errors

Measuring medication errors is an important tool for identifying and reducing the preventable risks associated with the medication-use process and also for assessing the impact of system improvements. It is critical that practitioners and organizational leaders understand the difference between *reported* medication errors and the actual level of medication safety achieved in a health system. Reported medication error rates are simply a measure of the ability of the organization to recognize and report medication-related problems. Therefore, an organization with a large number of

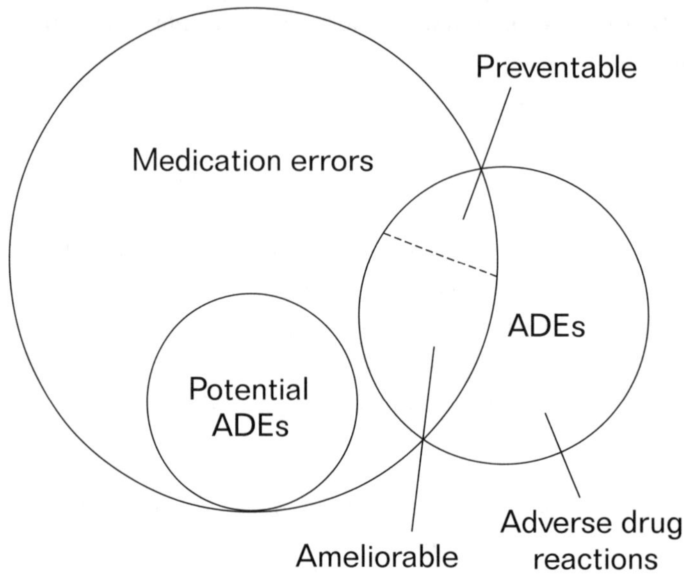

Figure 9-1. Detection and classification of adverse drug events.
Source: Reproduced from Morimoto T, Gandhi TK, Seger AC, et al. Adverse drug events and medication errors: Detection and classification methods. *Qual Saf Health Care.* 2004;13:306-314. Used with permission from BMJ Publishing Group Ltd.

error reports may actually (and in many cases is likely to) have a lower true underlying medication error rate than an organization where few reports are received, analyzed, and acted on.

Heinreich[2] developed the iceberg model of accidents and errors, an analogy that applies to medication errors and error reporting as well as to the automobile accidents he studied. The part of the iceberg above the water (all that is visible to the observer) represents errors that cause major harm; the larger part of the iceberg below the water is no-harm events or events that cause only minor injuries as well as **near misses**. Sometimes the only thing that separates an accident that causes no injury from one with major harm is sheer chance. A near miss is an error process that is stopped or interrupted; either by chance or through a check-and-balance in the medication-use process (such as recognition of the problem and intervention by an experienced practitioner). An example of a near miss is when the pharmacist discovers the errant preparation of a morphine infusion containing 10 times the correct amount of drug, during the sterile product checking process (recognition of the problem). The pharmacist does not dispense the product, discards it, and begins the preparation process again with appropriate coaching and education of the technician involved (interventions). While an error occurred, the incorrect product was prevented from reaching the patient through a check-and-balance in the medication-use process.

Recognition or detection of medication errors is a first step in medication safety management. Within an organization, it is important for the detection or identification rates to be high, because unexpected risks or hazards that are not detected can have disastrous consequences. Kaplan and Battles coined the term **detection sensitivity level** (DSL) to describe the rate at which errors are actually reported and recognized by the organization.[3] A high reporting rate indicates a high DSL, and a low reporting rate indicates a low DSL.[4] To achieve a high DSL, an organization must eliminate barriers to reporting. As the amount of information about errors goes up and the organization implements targeted risk-reduction strategies, risk will eventually go down. As medication errors are investigated and analyzed and safety strategies are implemented, the DSL rate may remain high; however, the severity of events (e.g., number of harmful events) should go down. Therefore, a high DSL is a sign of an effective patient safety culture. Organizations that are not aware of near-miss events and other unsafe conditions (low DSL) will have less opportunity to improve and implement corrective actions before a similar event occurs that results in patient injury.

Self-reporting programs or spontaneous voluntary reports from health professionals, patients, and families, are the most readily recognized means of detecting medication errors. Because so many errors go unrecognized and/or are unreported, it is important to use additional detection methods. These methods include use of observation or physical evidence, such as through chart review, the results of interviews, or the use of computer information systems and other technology (automation). Interventions made by health care professionals, such as pharmacists, are often tracked in a separate database and are near-miss reports that should be analyzed along with other medication error events. Each error-detection approach has both strengths and limitations. Interestingly, these methodologies are complementary because each method is likely to detect events that would go unrecognized using the other approaches (Table 9-1).

Voluntary Reporting

Incident or event reports are the most basic type of voluntary reporting process. Information about a medication variance or unsafe condition is provided by a health care professional or other staff member identifying that an error has occurred. Patient and family complaints that are determined to be subsequent to an error may also serve as a report source. One limitation of voluntary reporting is that many medication errors go undetected and thus will not be reported.

There are also a number of potential barriers to receiving voluntary error reports.[5] There may be a concern about discoverability of data (increased liability if the error becomes public) as well as punishment (disciplinary action or other negative consequences) if the reporter was involved in the event. In addition, there is a natural reluctance to report incidents involving peers, physicians, or others in positions of authority (such as a supervisor). In some organizations, participation in the reporting process is limited to a few individuals, such as nurse managers, or a few key

Table 9-1. Comparison of Medication Error Detection Methods

Approach	Focus	Strengths	Weaknesses	Comments
Observation method	Administration	■ Is consistent ■ Is standardized ■ Has greatest capture of events at single point in time	■ Resource intensive ■ Does not consider prescribing errors ■ Most of the events are not serious (e.g., wrong time)	Useful research methodology to measure the impact of changes (error rate over time)
Chart review	Prescribing Documentation of administration Adverse drug events (ADE) (outcomes)	■ Looks at medication use in the context of individual patient	■ Resource intensive ■ Limited to accuracy and completeness of medical record documentation	Concurrent approach that allows follow-up with staff interviews to gather more information
Computerized methods (see also automation)	Potential ADEs	■ Is low cost ■ Can follow up with chart review for details ■ May catch potential problems before harm to patient	■ High rate of false positives ■ Details on causes may not be captured	
Automation ■ Point of care ■ Infusion device ■ Pharmacy bar coding ■ Pharmacy alerts ■ CPOE alerts ■ Clinical decision support	 Administration Administration Dispensing Dispensing Prescribing Monitoring	■ Can work prospectively to prevent errors from occurring while collecting data	■ May lead to alert fatigue or workaround (bypassing technological support or ignoring alert) ■ May cause false sense of security (system will catch problems)	

Table 9-1 (continued)

Pharmacist interventions	Prescribing Monitoring	▪ Is by-product of current daily clinical responsibilities	▪ Pharmacists may under-report due to time involved	
Voluntary reporting and incident reports	All medication use nodes	▪ Is more likely to be high-yield events (harm or potential for harm)	▪ Dependent on staff recognizing error, numerous barriers to reporting (time, perceived negative consequences)	Can follow up immediately with staff involved to get more information
Executive walk rounds	All medication use nodes	▪ May increase reporting rates, particularly of unsafe conditions; promotes safety culture in organization	▪ Limited by staff recall of events after the fact	Important to building a safety culture

physicians and pharmacists. Lack of time for reporting is often cited as a reason for not reporting errors, particularly if reporting is seen as a low priority for the institution. Lack of awareness of the benefits of reporting (seeing the reports as another form of "bean-counting") also makes it less likely that staff members will participate. Gragg[6] also noted that the effectiveness of voluntary reporting may be limited due to delays in the reporting process (making it difficult to gather additional information needed for analysis), incomplete data (the report may be missing key information such as the drug involved or factors on what contributed to the cause of the error), and an insufficient volume of reports to guide improvement efforts.

Cultivating a "culture of safety" can help motivate reporting of errors and unsafe conditions once they are recognized by staff. All members of the health care team need to be aware of the organization's definition of a medication error and understand that reports will be used to improve medication-use processes and address reported problems rather than to punish the practitioners. A **non-punitive** approach includes positive feedback to individuals who report errors (including self-reports) and the offer of suggestions to prevent future events. Some hospitals go further and provide incentives for individual reporters or rewards and recognition for the nursing units with the highest number of reports. Small tokens, such as an ice cream, pizza, gift cards for individuals, or a unit-based meal or party can bring positive visibility to the error reporting program. Rather than rewarding areas that are error free, health-system leaders and the MSO should be asking what can be done to increase the number of reports. Instead of zero errors, the dual goals should be to maximize the number of reports and to avoid events that result in harm to the patient. It helps increase the perceived value of reporting when the staff is made aware of cases when error reports result in process improvement, the introduction of new technology, or other safety enhancements. To support a non-punitive culture, some organizations use the term *medication-use variance* to describe an unplanned and preventable event that deviates from the intended course of medication use because it may have fewer negative connotations than medication error.[7] An on-line reporting process with immediate notification of reviewers (pharmacy, risk management, quality management, nursing supervisors) when an error occurs can increase the timeliness of analysis and response after an event. Allowing anonymous reports may decrease the fear of reprisal; however, it may be more difficult to gather additional data related to the event (factors that contributed to the error and its eventual detection).

The leadership message must be that most errors are caused by failures of the medication-use system (rather than individuals), and safety can be improved through modifying policies, procedures, processes, and safety nets. Performance evaluation systems (such as those previously common for nurses) that rate the employee based on the number of errors made (and may even trigger termination based on the number of errors) are counterproductive because they only stifle reporting. A non-punitive approach does not remove individual responsibility for a medication error. Individuals whose willful neglect, criminal intent, or failure to follow clear policies and consistently-reinforced safeguards should still be subject to disciplinary action.

Another effective technique called *executive walk rounds* can stimulate additional error reports as well as involve all levels of staff in problem-solving to improve safety. The American Hospital Association (AHA) suggests sending executives on regular visits to patient care areas along with someone from that unit. The executives ask frontline health care professionals specific questions about unsafe conditions or near misses and communicate to staff that it is a high priority to collect information and analyze these events.[8] This approach is effective only when coupled with a process to follow up on identified issues and bring resolution strategies back to the staff. The Institute for Healthcare Improvement (IHI) has several resources on its website, www.ihi.org, to guide senior executives in what they call patient safety executive walk rounds™. Although active involvement of senior executives in walk rounds is important to establishing a culture of safety in the organization, the MSO can play a leadership role in the initiation of this activity, as well as facilitating follow-up actions, communication, and feedback to the staff after each session. The IHI recommends the creation of safety briefings, which share the results of insights and safety tips contributed by staff in previous sessions, in addition to prompting additional information sharing. The MSO may choose to accompany an executive on their rounds, prepare safety briefings for the executive to use, conduct separate medication safety walk rounds (perhaps in conjunction with a pharmacy technician, nurse manager, or other clinician), or use a combination of these approaches. Sample questions for medication safety–focused walk rounds are listed in Figure 9-2.

- Can you think of any medication-related events in the past few days that have resulted in harm to a patient?
- Can you think of any near misses that almost caused a patient harm but did not?
- What aspect of our medication process is likely to lead to the next case of patient harm?
- How are you involved in medication safety?
- What do you think this area could do on a regular basis to improve medication safety?
- What high-risk medications do you use routinely? What special safeguards are in place?
- What medications are on the "Override List"? How and when are overrides used?
- When you make a medication error, do you always report it?
- If you prevent or intercept a medication error, do you always report it?
- If you make or report a medication error, are you concerned about personal consequences?
- Do you know what happens with information that you report?
- Are you aware that we are actively promoting a Just Culture?
- Have you discussed medication safety issues with your patients and their families?
- Can you think of a time when your intervention prevented harm to a patient who would otherwise have been harmed by a system flaw?
- What specific intervention could leadership (or the MSO, or the Medication Safety Committee) direct to make the work you do for your patients safer?

Figure 9-2. Sample questions for medication safety walk rounds.

Interviews of patients and families are another potential means of prompting voluntary reports of medication variances and suggestions for improved medication processes. After their study showed patients experienced many events that were not documented in the medical record, some serious and some preventable, Weissman et al. suggested adding questions about **adverse events** to post-discharge patient interviews.[9]

Observation Method

Observation as a method of detecting and counting errors in drug administration dates back to the early 1960s,[10] and there is evidence that it is valid, efficient, and accurate.[11, 12] This technique involves a trained observer documenting all the details of medication administration on a single medication pass or shift and then comparing the information to the medication orders. A series of studies in the 1960s utilized the observation method to evaluate the unit dose concept, which is now the standard of care in U.S. hospitals. Since 1984, the Centers for Medicare & Medicaid Services (CMS, formerly the Health Care Financing Administration or HCFA) has used observation by surveyors as part of its long-term care site visits; a deficiency is cited for one or more significant errors or greater than or equal to a 5% observed error rate on a medication pass observation with 20 to 25 opportunities for error.[13] CMS-funded research in the early 2000s compared error detection methods in a sample of 36 hospitals and nursing homes in Georgia and Colorado.[14] A research pharmacist confirmed 457 of 2556 comparison doses to be in error for a true occurrence rate of 17.9%. The authors concluded that "the true frequency of [errors of potential clinical significance] was best estimated by direct observation" and suggested the most efficient approach to reducing clinically significant errors may be to "simply focus on reducing the rate of all errors detected by direct observation."[14] The most frequently detected error types were wrong time (greater than 60 minutes before or after dose due) or dose omission. Although a very personnel-intensive approach, the observation method has the advantage of providing the most complete picture of medication errors at a single point in time. Limitations of the observation method when used alone are that it may not recognize prescribing errors (because the medication order is used as the gold standard), and it also assumes that the content of a product matches its label unless there is obvious evidence to the contrary.

Chart Review

Another approach to identification of medication errors is by concurrent or retrospective review of the medical record. The chart review methodology for detecting medication errors used for research conducted at Harvard-affiliated hospitals uses trained data collectors who spend about five minutes per inpatient chart scanning medication orders, progress notes, flow sheets, and laboratory test results and then compare the findings with the medication administration record.[15] The collectors look for specific signals or triggers, such as a sudden change in patient condition, transfer to the intensive care unit, changes or clarifications in physician orders, orders for antidotes, and outdated narcotic orders. By conducting the review concurrently, patient care staff can be asked to complete a report form providing details on the event and describe any consequences for the patient.

Chart review performed at the intensity required for a research study is not sustainable on a daily basis but may be useful for targeted measurement to assess the impact of a process change (a before-and-after sample design). The IHI has developed an easy-to-use ADE measurement kit (available at www.IHI.org with free registration). By reviewing a random sample of charts (e.g., 10 per week), hospitals can obtain monthly estimates of their ADE rates over time.

Information Technology

Computerized search methods to detect ADEs and medication errors include use of International Classification of Disease (ICD) codes, recognizing new drug allergies, computerized event monitoring, and **data mining** (free-text searching for pairs of terms, such as warfarin and bleeding).[16] A complete electronic medical record is not needed to use computers to help identify errors. Simple flags can be built into existing pharmacy and laboratory computer systems and run inexpensively to identify triggers or events that may signal an ADE or impending ADE, such as the use of a rescue medication or an abnormal laboratory result. Rules can be written to generate an alert to the practitioner that would help avert patient harm. When potential ADEs are identified, additional review of the medical record (chart) will be needed in most cases to confirm that an error occurred and to gather additional information about the event for analysis. There are also outside drug information and pharmacy service vendors who offer electronic surveillance and reporting software for detecting and monitoring patients at-risk. These subscription decision-support services guide prospective and concurrent interventions by interfacing with or manage data from pharmacy, laboratory, and other electronic medical records system components.

Information on averted errors can be captured as a by-product of the use of automation, equipment, and information systems that support medication use. Computerized order entry systems, "smart" infusion devices, and point-of-care verification systems such as bedside scanning all can generate information on the number and types of alerts that resulted in the practitioner canceling or modifying their action. In addition to documenting the value of technological safety enhancements, analysis of these errors is important to learn more about the human factors that led to such errors, as well as the latent risks if the safety technology is bypassed.

Combining information from a variety of electronic information sources is also valuable. For example, likely errors can be detected by comparing the product selected and time stamp from an automated dispensing cabinet entry to charting of administration on the electronic medical record (either entered manually or as a by-product of bar code medication administration or other point-of-care technology documentation of the dose).

Practitioner Interventions

Practitioner interventions may be defined as the detection of errors, deficiencies, discrepancies, or opportunities for improvement in patient care and averting those errors as part of systematically performing normal patient care functions within the practitioner's scope of activity.[17] In most cases the intervention averts the errors before they reach the patient or concurrently while some sort of "recovery" is possible, for example, by changing the dose or the drug. Intervention reporting systems measure errors that are produced by the system that is in place as well as the care system's ability to recover from those errors. The ability to detect errors can be improved by providing better decision support, training of staff, adding staff, and by changing the way care is provided (e.g., increasing the availability of information through the use of preprinted order sheets or by requiring weight and allergy status documentation on the order). Professional consensus on what constitutes safe and appropriate medication use, such as through medical staff-approved drug use criteria can increase the likelihood of reporting because practitioners will be more comfortable intervening. Compared to the information in the literature about pharmacist practitioner intervention programs, very little information is available about intervention reporting by patients and families, nurses, physicians, and other health care team members. Intervention documentation systems typically suffer from underreporting due to the resources needed to maintain these records. Participants in the Pharmacy Practice Model Initiative (PPMI) Summit in 2010 recognized the importance of generating pharmacist intervention documentation but stated to be most beneficial it should be captured as a by-product of daily pharmacy care activities and charting in an electronic medical record, rather than through a parallel documentation function.

Analysis of Medication Error Reports

Analysis of medication errors must include categorization of individual reports to identify patterns and trends, as well as detailed review of the narrative (a detailed story of the event) to look for root causes and opportunities for improvement. It is important to verify or validate information in individual reports before beginning analysis because there may be incomplete data or misinformation. The reporter's perspective often addresses only a portion of the story and fails to acknowledge all the active and latent failures that led to the event. One key component of each medication error report should be to ask the reporter and any individuals involved in the analysis, "What can/should be done to prevent this from happening again?" Knowledge of the medications most often involved in harmful events (or events with a high potential for harm, also called *close calls*), the most frequent types and causes of errors, and where and when different errors are most likely to occur, can help set priorities and guide improvement efforts. Close calls are opportunities for learning and afford the chance to develop preventive strategies and actions. Therefore, close calls should receive the same level of scrutiny as adverse events that result in actual injury.

NCC MERP has developed a medication error **taxonomy** tool to help health care practitioners and organizations characterize, track, and analyze medication errors in a standardized, systematic manner.[18] The taxonomy is useful for developing a medication error database and designing an error reporting or data collection form. Health care organizations should develop systems and procedures to collect adequate information needed to analyze and report medication errors at the time the events occur (ideally, all the elements identified in the taxonomy). Since the taxonomy was developed in the late 1990s, detail may be lacking in some areas of focus in the contemporary health care organization, such as technology and informatics. It is also important to balance the need for detail with usability of the data and not make the database unwieldy. The approach taken with a paper form (which then requires data entry) would be different than with web-based or other electronic reporting process that has reporters doing some or all of the data entry. For example, national error reporting vendors provide a comprehensive table of medication generic and trade names; however, this would not be practical to maintain at a local level. Allowing each user to enter drug names as free text will make it very difficult to run summary reports by medication. At a minimum, the ability of the reporting system to utilize the organization's drug formulary would be helpful for ease of submitting and generating reports. Limiting the number of required fields for a reporter will help maximize reporting, whether on a paper or electronic form.

One key component of the taxonomy is the NCC MERP medication index that classifies an error according to the severity of the outcome on a scale from A to I (Figures 9-3 and 9-4). The index considers factors such as whether the error reached the patient and, if the patient was harmed, to what degree. The Council encourages the use of the index in all health care delivery settings and by researchers and vendors of medication error tracking software. The index is being used in the Institute for Safe Medication Practices (ISMP) Medication Error Reporting Program (MERP) database MEDMARX™, an anonymous, Internet-accessible, subscriber-based reporting system developed by the U.S. Pharmacopeia (USP) and transferred to Quantros in December 2008; ISMP-Canada's Analyze-ERR program, the mandatory statewide Pennsylvania Patient Safety Reporting System (PP-PSRS); and commercial patient safety event reporting programs. Categorizing outcomes can present a challenge for the reporter, as the degree of harm may be unknown at the time of the report. One way to handle this is to encourage the reporter to select the best option at the time of the report submission, and as reports undergo further review the classification is updated as appropriate. An alternative design would be for the reviewer, rather than reporter, to classify the severity of the event.

When working to enhance a medication error reporting program, the focus should be on increasing the reporting and analysis of reports that did not result in patient harm (category A through D) with the goal of decreasing harmful events (E through I). Excessive focus on trends and "the numbers" through monthly statistical reports can be counterproductive if it results in a de-emphasis on the analysis of root causes that should lead to corrective actions and process improvement. However, review of summary information on a quarterly, semi-annual, or annual basis is often helpful to refocus safety improvement efforts as well as identify areas of the organi-

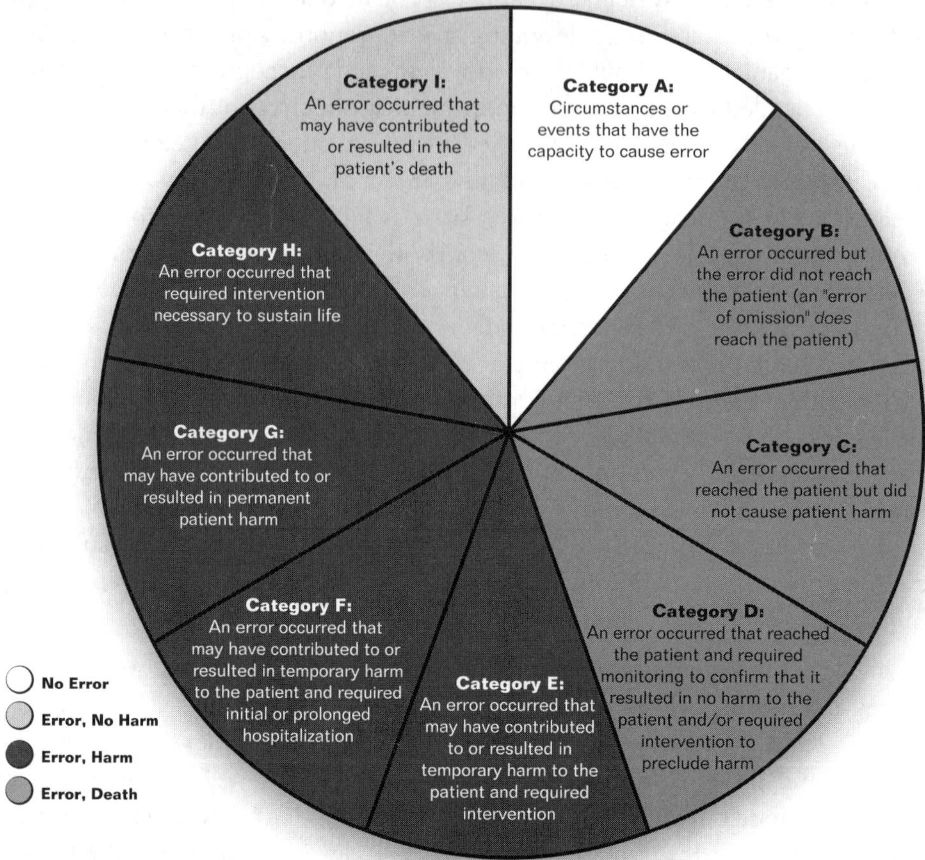

Definitions

Harm—Impairment of the physical, emotional, or psychological function or structure of the body and/or pain resulting therefrom.

Monitoring—To observe or record relevant physiological or psychological signs.

Intervention—May include change in therapy or active medical/surgical treatment.

Intervention Necessary to Sustain Life—Includes cardiovascular and respiratory support (e.g., CPR, defibrillation, intubation, etc.)

Figure 9-3. Sample questions for medication safety walk rounds.
Source: Reprinted with permission.

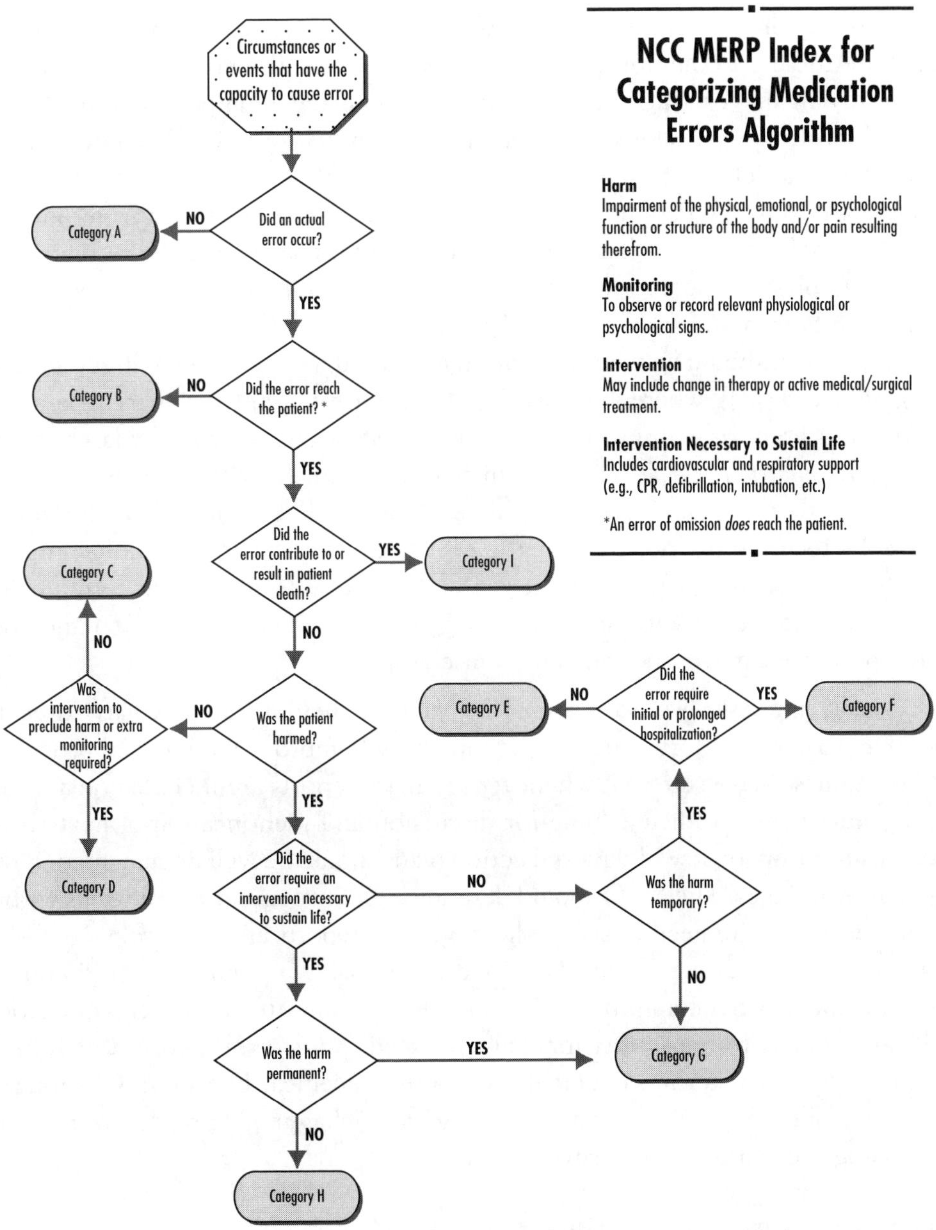

Figure 9-4. NCC MERP index for categorizing medication errors algorithm.
Source: Reprinted with permission.

zation that are underreporting. Graphical information can help a Medication Safety Committee address questions such as "What medications are most problem-prone? What are the most common causes of error? What are the greatest opportunities for improvement?" or "Has the latest intervention made an impact on errors?" It is also helpful to compare local patterns in error reports to national reporting data, by review of articles published by USP's Center for the Advancement of Patient Safety (CAPS) in the Patient Safety CAPSLink™.[19] Unfortunately, this resource is only archival because USP has eliminated its direct involvement in error reporting. Some examples of report formats to consider are listed in Figures 9-5 through 9-9. Pareto charts are a useful way to visually display the most frequent causes and types of errors, which should be where attention is focused. Named after Vilfredo Pareto, this graphical display, where the individual values are represented by bars in descending order, is used to highlight the most important among a (typically large) set of factors. The *Pareto Principle* (also known as the Law of the Vital Few, or the 80-20 Rule) states that for many events roughly 80% of the effects come from 20% of the causes. By focusing on the vital few, the MSO can have a more substantial impact. Reports of errors by location are most useful as a tool to identify underreporting errors and reward units with higher reporting numbers. It is important to remember that reports are a means, not an end themselves.

Visually interesting reports are of no value if they are not regularly used to focus improvement efforts and take action that will improve patient care processes and outcomes. Make sure that whenever summary reports are included on a meeting agenda there is sufficient time for discussion and identification of next steps. Conclusions from review of data and action plans should be well documented in the committee minutes. The MSO should determine all the committees or teams within an organization who need to see medication error reports and their role in reviewing or acting on the data. Typically, a Medication Safety Committee (or Pharmacy and Therapeutics Subcommittee), Patient Safety Committee, or other work group will have primary responsibility for analyzing medication error reports. Other bodies (e.g., Performance Improvement Committee, Medical Executive Committee, and Board of Directors) will want to see higher level aggregate reports or minutes containing the work group's analysis and actions.

Medication Error Tracking Software

Many institutions use a home-grown relational database[20] or a risk management (incident reporting) error tracking software package to support their medication error prevention programs. Alternatively, several vendors offer electronic solutions for capturing, analyzing, and managing medication error reports, including MEDMARX℠, the University Health-System Consortium (UHC) Patient Safety Net (PSN), and the ISMP-Canada Analyze-ERR program.[21] Whether solely internal or both internal and external to the organization, a medication error reporting system should help establish processes to detect and correct errors, identify trends or patterns to guide priority-setting, and encourage changes to the medication-use system

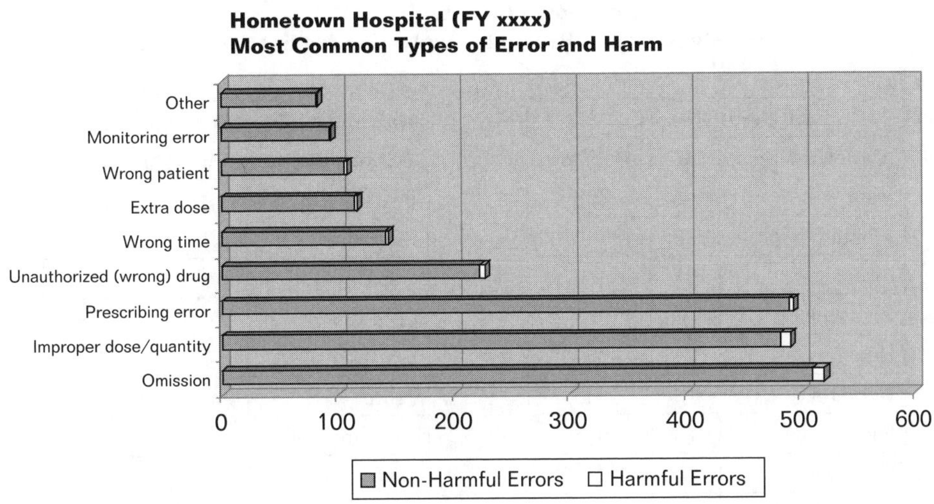

Figure 9-5. Medication errors by type (sample report).

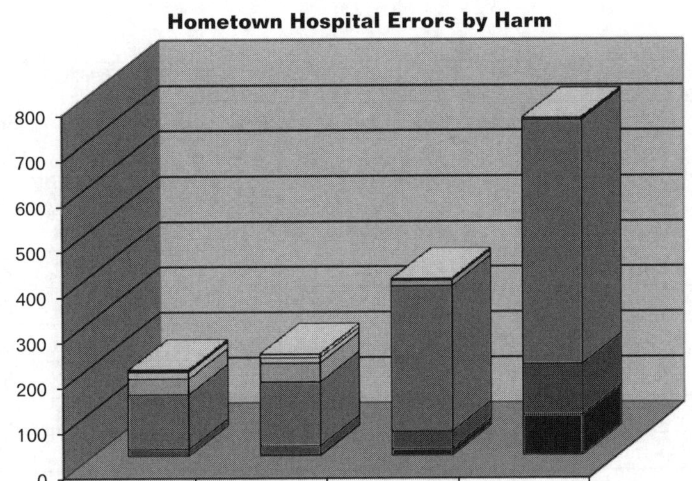

	FY2009	FY2010	FY2011	FY2012
Death (Category I)	4	8	1	0
Serious Harm (Category G-H)	15	12	2	1
Harm (Category E-F)	35	42	13	5
No Harm (Category C-D)	120	140	320	537
Caught (Category B)	15	20	38	112
No Error (Category A)	0	2	15	89

Figure 9-6. Medication errors by severity (sample report).

Hometown Hospital (FY 2013)
Commonly Reported Products Involved in Medication Errors

All Error Records		
Generic Name	**n**	**Percent**
Insulin	44	3.6
Albuterol	32	2.7
Morphine	31	2.6
Potassium Cl	26	2.1
Heparin	24	2.0
Warfarin	18	1.5
Furosemide	18	1.5
Cefazolin	17	1.5
Acetaminophen	16	1.3
Vancomycin	16	1.3

Harmful or Fatal (Categories E–I)		
Generic Name	**n**	**Percent**
Insulin	9	8.7
Morphine	7	6.8
Heparin	5	4.8
Potassium Cl	4	3.9
Warfarin	4	3.9
Fentanyl	3	2.9
Hydromorphone	2	1.9
Vancomycin	1	1.0
Furosemide	1	1.0
Meperidine	1	1.0

Figure 9-7. Medication errors by product (sample report).

	Jan	Feb	Mar	Apr	May	Jun	Jul	Aug	Sep	Oct	Nov	Dec
2 South	23	19	13	15	12	21	25	22	31	28	15	14
3 North	2	5	3	1	2	0	0	0	3	8	12	23
3 West	15	14	11	15	8	12	22	34	39	47	42	49
3 South	12	15	10	11	19	17	23	22	25	37	28	41
4 North	42	58	62	68	59	55	48	44	59	45	47	51
4 West	15	12	14	18	22	56	49	53	61	46	42	48
4 South	27	29	33	48	27	43	39	42	51	57	52	47
ICU	48	15	39	51	47	36	41	47	38	44	51	43
Operating Room	3	5	1	2	5	1	2	6	2	3	10	14
Pharmacy	32	23	41	27	29	31	48	36	41	32	31	10

Shaded area represents low reporting with opportunity for improvement.

Figure 9-8. Medication errors by location (sample report).

Hospital Quality and Safety Report Card—Error Reports by Category (A to I)

	Jan	Feb	Mar	Apr	May	Jun	Jul	Aug	Sep	Oct	Nov	Dec
No Error												
Category A												
Error, No Harm												
Category B												
Category C												
Category D												
Error, Harm												
Category E												
Category F												
Category G												
Category H												
Error, Death												
Category I												

Figure 9-9. Medication errors scorecard for hospital board (sample report).

to reduce the potential for future errors. Because it is important that an electronic reporting system captures all the key data elements needed for analysis (drug name, therapeutic class, type of error, causes of error) and a detailed narrative description of the event and follow-up actions, creating and maintaining a home-grown database that is fully functional for medication safety is a time- and resource-intensive proposition. Each of the commercial error report management software programs has its own strengths and weaknesses. The ability for staff members to report events over the organization's intranet is a high value feature, as is a multi-user interface (for pharmacy, risk management, quality management, and department managers) that provides immediate notification of new reports requiring review, analysis, or follow-up. The availability of canned reports that meet basic reporting needs, as well as ease-of-use in custom reports are other important features.

Limiting the number of required fields for medication error reports is one key to maximize reporting. When designing a local database for medication errors or customizing a commercial product, consider the quality, quantity, and value of the data that will be collecting. Requesting a lot of information from frontline reporters could seriously decrease the number of errors reported. The highest value information you can extract from staff members is a detailed narrative of what occurred, their thoughts on root causes of the event, and actions that should be taken to prevent the error from happening again. Save some data entry for quality and medication safety reviewers (such as determining the category of error and severity or harm codes). This will make the initial reporting process less intimidating and also ensure that fields used for sorting and reporting are coded consistently.

The MSO must be actively engaged in the organization's development, or selection and implementation, of a new or replacement reporting program. Educating risk management and information services staff on required elements and needed reports for medication safety is crucial before decisions are made. The selection of an error report management software program may be dictated by the Risk Management Department or senior administration, guided by the organization's group purchasing organization, or mandated as part of a state patient safety reporting process, such as exists in Pennsylvania. One question to ask when building or purchasing a separate medication error report tracking system is how it will work with the database management program used for other types of medical errors and incident reports. To avoid the need to reenter information, the ability to easily transfer or interface data should be a key decision criterion. Although internal medication error report management is usually the primary reason for selection of error tracking software, the ability to share reports nationally or include them anonymously as part of a state-, national-, or consortium-based reporting program is also key to maximizing learning from local error reports.

Medication Error Reporting Programs

The Patient Safety and Quality Improvement Act of 2005 (Patient Safety Act) authorized the creation of **patient safety organizations** (PSOs) to improve the quality and safety of health care delivery in the United States. PSOs are entities registered with and listed with the Agency for Healthcare Research and Quality (AHRQ) under the Patient Safety Act and Patient Safety Rule, which provide confidentiality and privilege protections for patient safety work products. PSOs create a secure environment where clinicians and health care organizations can collect, aggregate, and analyze data about medical errors, with the goal of identifying and reducing the risks and hazards associated with patient care.

Reporting events to a national reporting program allows health professionals to serve the public health beyond their organization by alerting other health professionals of problems so that injury to other patients can be prevented in the future. All health care organizations are encouraged to submit confidential reports to these reporting agencies so that others can learn from these experiences. In the United States, a national reporting program for medication errors is operated by ISMP, a PSO certified through AHRQ. Medication errors can be reported to ISMP by telephone or through a secure website, https://www.ismp.org/orderforms/reporterrortoISMP.asp. ISMP staff prefers that reporters use their on-line form for submission as this helps ISMP to communicate back with them and ask follow-up questions as needed. This forum should be used to communicate information about interesting medication errors and preventable adverse drug events as they occur at the local practice site with an emphasis on events that have a high educational value or require action by manufacturers and/or the Food and Drug Administration (FDA).

Because of the educational focus, rather than representing the entire spectrum of medication errors, reports to the ISMP MERP tend to focus on unsafe conditions (such as look-alike names and drug packages) as well as serious or fatal errors (high-harm events). The impact of cumulative reports to this system includes early warning nationwide alerts about hazards, the dissemination of trends in error-prone situations as well as error reduction strategies, and, as a result, numerous changes in practice in individual organizations as well as drug/device packaging, labeling, and nomenclature changes.

Health care organizations may also participate in reporting to other PSOs in conjunction with their risk management reporting software, as part of a state-based consortium or other alliance, or develop their own health-system PSO. AHRQ maintains a list of PSOs on their website at http://www.pso.ahrq.gov.

Benchmarking Medication Safety—What About Error Rates?

It is challenging to use medication errors as a measure of health care safety or quality because of the limits of medication error reporting and detection. To use the iceberg analogy in a slightly different context, only a small proportion of medication errors are reported (detected) even in the best performing health care organizations. Numbers used for benchmarking are simply a measure of medication error *reporting* rates rather than a measure of medication errors. Trends in the number and types of medication errors may actually be more of a reflection of changes in your reporting, or other detection method(s), than an actual change in events. For example, after The Joint Commission highlighted the importance of collecting data on omitted respiratory treatments, albuterol became one of the most frequently reported medications associated with error as institutions began to focus on this particular type of event. Another inherent difficulty is the selection of a standard denominator. Should it be based on the number of doses of medications? If so, are doses counted when they are ordered, charged, dispensed, or administered? What about patient days, adjusted patient days, or some other measure as the denominator? Counting doses is particularly problematic because floor stock medications and drugs not dispensed by the pharmacy often are not captured, and multi-ingredient or multi-dose products (total parenteral nutrition, complex admixtures, and patient-controlled analgesia) generate different charges and may be considered as a single item or numerous doses depending on organizational preference.

The NCC MERP has also recognized significant variability among organizations in how the numerator and denominator are determined to calculate a medication error rate, and in 2002 issued a statement, "Use of Medication Error Rates to Compare Health Care Organizations Is of No Value," that was reaffirmed in June 2008 (Figure 9-10).[22] One of the key messages of that statement is that there is no acceptable incidence rate for medication errors. There is danger that if error rates are used to judge individual or institutional performance that the result will simply be to discourage reporting of medication errors, or even conceal evidence of errors. The NCC MERP contends that the true value of medication error reports and other data-gathering strategies is to provide the information that allows an organization to identify weaknesses in its medication-use system and to apply lessons learned to improve the system.

The rate of events resulting in serious patient harm (raw number of medication error index levels F through I) may be a more accurate barometer and consistent measure over time. Tracking the number and rate of events that did not result in

Use of Medication Error Rates to Compare Health Care Organizations Is of No Value

(Adopted June 11, 2002; reaffirmed June 24, 2008)

The use of medication error rates to compare health care organizations is not recommended for the following reasons:

1. Differences in *culture* among health care organizations can lead to significant differences in the reporting of medication errors. Organizations that encourage medication error reporting by providing incentives and resources to report within a non-punitive, continuous quality improvement arena will likely report more medication errors than organizations that wish to conceal errors and punish individuals who are involved in or report errors.
2. Differences in the *definition* of a medication error among health care organizations can lead to significant differences in the reporting and classification of medication errors. For example, some organizations may only consider actual errors that reach the patient as errors. Other organizations also will include potential errors and errors that do not reach the patient. The latter organizations will likely collect more medication errors, and information from reports of potential errors can sometimes be more useful in prevention efforts than reports of actual errors.
3. Differences in the *patient populations* served by various health care organizations can lead to significant differences in the number and severity of medication errors occurring among organizations. For example, tertiary care hospitals generally may serve more severely ill patients than rehabilitation hospitals. In addition, the intensity of drug therapies, the types of drugs used, and the methods of drug distribution may be substantially different in these environments, thereby leading to differences in number and types of errors.
4. Differences in the *type(s) of reporting and detection systems* for medication errors among health care organizations can lead to significant differences in the number of medication errors recorded. Passive reporting systems, relying upon voluntary reports from staff, are known to

Figure 9-10 (continued).

result in far fewer medication error reports than active surveillance systems are able to detect. Also, the number of error reports can be significantly different, depending on the type of active surveillance system (e.g., direct observation versus retrospective review of medical records versus computer-based data gathering from electronic medical records and order entry systems).

The National Coordinating Council for Medication Error Reporting and Prevention believes there is no acceptable incidence rate for medication errors. Use of medication error rates to compare health care organizations is of no value. The goal of every health care organization should be to continually improve systems to prevent harm to patients due to medication errors. Health care organizations should monitor actual and potential medication errors that occur within their organization, and investigate the root cause of errors with the goal of identifying ways to improve the medication use system to prevent future errors, and potential patient harm. The value of medication error reports and other data gathering strategies is to provide the information that allows an organization to identify weaknesses in its medication use system and to apply lessons learned to improve the system. The sheer number of error reports is less important than the quality of the information collected in the reports, the health care organization's analysis of the information, and its actions to improve the system to prevent harm to patients.

Figure 9-10. Statement from the National Coordinating Council for Medication Error Reporting and Prevention. Available at: http://www.nccmerp.org/council/council2002-06-11.html.
Source: Reprinted with permission.

patient harm and reports of unsafe conditions (index levels A through D) is a useful measure of the patient safety culture in the organization. Senior administration, hospital board members, and other key health care decision makers need to be educated that the only error numbers on a quality scorecard that should be considered negatively are events where the patient was harmed.

Using a consistent methodology to measure or sample medication errors over time in a *single organization* (or in a single practice site) is a more appropriate use of error rates as a medication safety measure. The observation method and IHI ADE tool kit are two examples of focused error detection methodologies used to create control or run-charts of institutional medication error rates. The approach of consistently measuring medication error rates over time has been used before and after the introduction of new technology, such as bar code verification or computerized provider order entry, as well as other health care process changes, and is a useful way to assess if a change had the desired impact.

Summary

Establishing consensus on what is considered a medication error is essential for any medication safety program. Monitoring medication errors that occur within an organization is one internal benchmark of medication safety; however, relying on incident reports is insufficient. Efforts are needed to encourage medication error reporting, including involving staff in determining root causes and opportunities for improvement. Detection, measurement, and analysis of medication errors require an active rather than passive approach. The MSO should not spend an excessive amount of time tracking and trending numbers and types of medication errors, but instead focus on what can be learned from medication errors, particularly through examination of the narrative associated with individual events. Root cause analysis of medication errors to understand the causes and contributing factors is an important first step to implement changes that can prevent future events. If the organization can develop a highly sensitive approach to detecting medication errors and near misses, it will be able to evaluate the success of efforts to improve medication safety.

PRACTICE TIPS

1. *Potential for harm—an important area of focus.* Don't focus just on harmful events when reviewing medication error reports. Events, whether near miss or actual, with a high potential for harm are often overlooked but can provide valuable focus for improvement efforts that proactively prevent harm. Close calls with chemotherapy, anticoagulants, or other medications where a single error reaches the patient can easily result in a Sentinel Event.
2. *Proactive medication error measurement and reporting.* In addition to retrospective error review, incorporate concurrent and prospective monitoring components to improve safety. Review bypassed computer alerts and infusion pump overrides in real time. Medication administration direct observations can detect errors that previously went unrecognized. A concurrent approach could identify a potential error or adverse drug event in a way that the error, or at least harmful effects of the error, might be averted.
3. *Practical considerations for a reporting program.* When designing or customizing a database for medication errors, maximize reporting by balancing the quantity with the quality and value of the data you will be collecting. Minimize the information the reporter must submit while encouraging a detailed narrative of what happened.
4. *Being effective.* Carefully consider the amount of time you spend collecting and documenting medication errors versus the resources you devote to process improvement activities. It is easy to get bogged down in large numbers of low value reports—keep the focus on medication-use improvement activities.

References

1. National Coordinating Council for Medication Error Reporting and Prevention. About medication errors: definition. Available at: http://www.nccmerp.org/aboutMedErrors.html. Accessed August 20, 2011.
2. Battles JB. Disaster prevention: lessons learned from the Titanic. *BUMC Proc.* 2001;14:150-153.
3. Kaplan HS, Battles JB, Van der Schaaf TW, et al. Identification and classification of the causes of events in transfusion medicine. *Transfusion.* 1998;38:1072-1082.
4. Battles JB, Lilford RJ. Organizing patient safety research to identify risks and hazards. *Qual Saf Health Car.* 2003;12:2-7.
5. Phillips MA. Voluntary reporting of medication errors. *Am J Health Syst Pharm.* 2002;59:2326-2328.
6. Gragg DN. Designing an internal reporting and learning system. In: Manasse HR, Thompson KK, eds. *Medication Safety: A Guide for Health Care Facilities.* Bethesda, MD: American Society of Health-System Pharmacists; 2005:171-193.

7. Sump LS. Re-engineering the medication error-reporting process: Removing the blame and improving the system. *Am J Health Syst Pharm*. 2000;57:S10-S17.
8. American Hospital Association and American Society of Health-System Pharmacists. Medication safety issue brief: A fully stocked toolkit. *Hosp Health Netw*. 2003;77(6): suppl 2 p. following 24.
9. Weissman JS, Schneider EC, Weingart SN, et al. Comparing patient-reported hospital adverse events with medical record review: Do patients know something that hospitals do not? *Ann Intern Med*. 2008:149:100-108.
10. Barker KN, McConnell WE. The problems of detecting medication errors in hospitals. *Am J Health Syst Pharm*. 1962;19:360-369.
11. Barker KN, Flynn EA, Pepper GA. Observation method of detecting medication errors. *Am J Health Syst Pharm*. 2002;59:2314-2316.
12. Dean B, Barber N. Validity and reliability of observational methods for studying medication administration errors. *Am J Health Syst Pharm*. 2001;58:54-59.
13. Department of Health and Human Services Centers for Medicare & Medicaid Administration. Medication Pass Worksheet. Available at: http://www.cms.hhs.gov/cmsforms/downloads/CMS677.pdf Accessed August 20, 2011.
14. Flynn EA, Barker KN, Pepper GA, et al. Comparison of methods for detecting medication errors in 36 hospitals and skilled nursing facilities. *Am J Health Syst Pharm*. 2002;59:436-446.
15. Kaushal R. Using chart review to screen for medication errors and adverse drug events. *Am J Health Syst Pharm*. 2002;59:2323-2325.
16. Bates DW. Using information technology to screen for adverse drug events. *Am J Health Syst Pharm*. 2002;59:2317-2319.
17. Lesar TS. Practitioner intervention-reporting systems for measuring the quality of drug use. *Am J Health Syst Pharm*. 2002;59:2320-2322.
18. National Coordinating Committee for Medication Error Reporting and Prevention. NCC MERP taxonomy of medication errors. Copyright 1998. Available at: http://www.nccmerp.org/pdf/taxo2001-07-31.pdf. Accessed August 20, 2011.
19. USP Center for the Advancement of Patient Safety (CAPS). CAPSLink™. Access to archives available at: http://www.usp.org/hqi/practitionerPrograms/newsletters/capsLink/ Accessed April 3, 2011.
20. Hartwig SC, Denger SD, Schneider PJ. Severity-indexed, incident report-based medication error-reporting program. *Am J Health Syst Pharm*.1991;48:2611-2616.
21. David U. Medication error reporting systems: Problems and solutions. *New Medicine*. 2001;1(2):41-65.
22. National Coordinating Council for Medication Error Reporting and Prevention. Statement on Medication Error Rates. Available at: http://www.nccmerp.org/council/council2002-06-11.html. Accessed August 20, 2011.

Event Management

Kathryn A. Crea

CHAPTER 10

Key Terms

Common Cause Analysis—A technique used to review information from multiple events to identify their common causes; also referred to as an aggregate root cause analysis.

Inattentional Blindness—The person performing the task fails to see what should have been plainly visible and, later, he or she cannot explain the lapse.[1]

National Coordinating Council for Medication Error Reporting and Prevention (NCC MERP)—This is an independent body of 27 national organizations (e.g., The Joint Commission, American Hospital Association) whose mission is to maximize the safe use of medications and to increase awareness of medication errors through open communication, increased reporting and promotion of medication error prevention strategies.

Root Cause—Any identified reason in the sequence of events that, if prevented, will stop a recurrence of the particular event. There must be a clear cause and effect such that if you eliminate the identified cause, future events will be prevented.

Root Cause Analysis (RCA)—A systematic process utilized to determine the primary cause of system failures. The goal is to define the root causes and develop an action plan to prevent recurrence or mitigate a future event.

Introduction

When an event occurs it's important to have a process in place to appropriately manage occurrences. The initial actions taken can set the tone for the health care system that events are taken seriously, and the culture of the organization is such that the immediate care of the patient and his or her family is foremost in our minds. It is equally important to provide support for the affected health care professionals. The steps involved with event review and analysis are discussed. Communication, action, and follow-up are all important processes for successfully managing events. To keep staff engaged in the reporting process, it is important that staff are not left wondering if or how the report was utilized to improve systems and processes. Regular review of events, further analysis on selected events, and feedback to hospital departments and individual reporters are essential in ensuring that hospital staff are aware of the follow-up that is completed and what further steps are taken to prevent recurrence.

Initial Actions Following Event Occurrence

The medication safety officer (MSO) must be able to guide appropriate actions for staff at the time of discovery of an adverse drug event (ADE) by following these steps:

- Confirm that the patient is cared for appropriately
- Assess the risk to other patients
- Communicate the event to unit leadership
- Report the event

Consider this case example: A patient develops significant hypotension following an incorrect infusion rate of nicardipine.

Confirm That the Patient Is Cared for Appropriately

The patient should be the focus of this first activity. Following discovery of an event, the patient must be assessed and treated if indicated. If emergent care is required, this may involve contacting a rapid response team (RRT) or calling a "code." Organizational protocols may be followed for antidote administration if indicated (for example, naloxone for narcotic overdose). The physician should be contacted to determine appropriate treatment. In this case, the nicardipine drip was placed on hold and the physician ordered a liter fluid bolus, followed by a repeat bolus in 1 hour. The patient was briefly placed on a pressor and transferred to the intensive care until (ICU) for further monitoring.

Assess the Risk to Other Patients

Determining the extent of condition involves determining the actual or potential applicability for the same condition to exist somewhere else in the organization for another patient. In this case, one consideration would be to review and double check any other medications infusing via pump that the nurse may have programmed, just to confirm this was an isolated programming error. Another consideration would be to check the pump library to ensure the values (e.g., maximum dose/infusion rate) are correct for nicardipine. Reviewing and determining who else may be at risk for this same problem enables the team to determine and take necessary actions to prevent a similar event from occurring until an analysis can take place. These are known as *remedial actions*. Remedial actions are interim actions intended to prevent recurrence of similar events in the near future, while a robust action plan to address the **root cause(s)** is being finalized and implemented. Remedial actions are not adequate to serve as a long-term corrective action and are generally considered temporary.

Communicate the Event to Unit Leadership

It should be noted that these three steps can occur concurrently, especially when more than one staff member is assisting with patient care and/or error follow-up. Unit leadership can include a charge nurse, team leader, or shift supervisor level. Organizational protocols are often specified for events with immediate significant outcome, such as advising the risk manager and/or higher leadership levels. Leaders can assist with provision of patient care and assessing risk to other patients, or they can redirect resources as needed to accomplish these steps.

Preservation of evidence is an important step in the process at the front line to ensure that equipment, medications, or other devices are sequestered from further use if there is any suspicion of malfunction or misuse. This step often requires reinforcement of all department supervisors, managers, and other leadership who will be available in the off hours when an event may occur. It is also important that devices and equipment not be directly turned over to the manufacturer for assessment of functionality. Many organizations involve risk management and an independent third party to determine any potential malfunctions associated with the equipment.

Report the Event

After the patient has been cared for and staff/leaders ensure other patients are not at risk, the event should be reported through the established organizational process. The person who discovered the event should be encouraged to report. Because most systems have a method for handling duplicate reports, there is no harm if more than one person reports the same event. The value of reporting has been discussed in Chapter 9, Medication Error Reporting and Analysis.

The MSO will want to ensure follow-up when reviewing a report received after the event occurred. In this case, the report received indicated the nurse misprogrammed the rate in the smart pump. The manager had not yet provided comments on the event report. The actions taken once the error was identified were not included on the event report. Therefore, a call to the manager was made. The manager had just been informed of the error and was in the process of obtaining additional information. There should be an expectation that the manager of the area responds to an event report with a defined time frame, perhaps through a policy. The manager, or designee such as a clinical manager, is responsible for reviewing the event report, investigating and discussing the event with staff that was involved to discern additional detail on what took place during the occurrence, and evaluating whether appropriate follow-up was completed. This information should be communicated within the event report when possible. In this case, the manager of the unit was not informed of the event over the weekend and did not have an opportunity to obtain further details. This delay in communication is an item of concern and should be addressed with the staff on the unit—to notify a supervisor or management team member at the time of the occurrence to assist in confirming that adequate follow-up and communication, either with the patient or family, is completed.

When evaluating an event report, the MSO must realize the report is reflective of the reporter's perspective. In other words, it presents only one side of the story. Assess whether additional information or data are available to evaluate the event. Depending on the event, reports can be generated for the automated dispensing cabinets (ADCs) (e.g., misfills, misdispenses, staff access) and smart pumps infusion details (e.g., rate/dose). In the scenario above, the reporter states the nurse misprogrammed the pump. The reality may be quite different—perhaps the nurse programmed the pump correctly but it malfunctioned, or the library was incorrect. Although the MSO is rarely the only person investigating events, he or she must be alert to the subjective nature of reporting and assess accordingly. If your role involves direct follow-up, request feedback from those involved in the event. Be aware of inattentional blindness—the person involved may not be able to explain a rationale for the error although he or she can plainly see it when asked. Listen objectively and refrain from jumping to conclusions or assuming you already know what occurred. You may be quite surprised at what you hear!

The MSO should consider each step in the medication-use process when assessing an event report. As improvement opportunities are noted, the MSO can facilitate communication with key leaders to discuss potential actions. Submission of a MedWatch[2] report may be appropriate. In this case, sequestration of the pump and a request to bioengineering to review the machine's functionality was completed. With many infusion pumps, it is possible to obtain a report of the keystrokes and overrides on a pump related to the case.[3] If the specific pump information is forwarded to the company with additional information about the case, they may be able to extract details that are important in understanding the error and potential action plan. This has proven to be quite useful in cases of significant concern.

Health Care Professional Support

As it is important to provide care and support for patients and their families when an error occurs, it is equally important to provide supportive care for the health professionals involved in the event. Frequently, staff will become upset upon recognition of their error. Recently a nurse, distraught after a mathematical calculation error led to an overdose of calcium chloride and subsequent death of an infant, committed suicide.[4] The MSO often collaborates with other key leaders in the organization such as a Nursing Director, physician leader, and human resources associates in ensuring that all the emotional needs of the health care professionals involved are met. One opportunity to do this in a confidential manner is during the interview process. As the information is being gathered, it is important to be cognizant of the mood and demeanor of the associate. After collection of the information, this is often a good time to discuss how the associate is handling the event and to provide information and encourage him or her to reach out, recognizing that it often is useful just to talk about it with someone. A brochure and/or business card to an Employee Assistance Program and/or chaplain with a phone number and contact name—ensuring confidentiality— is often more accepted and considered during these initial discussions. Emphasize that although they may feel they can handle the emotional aspect on their own, it can be very difficult for anyone. Reinforce that good people make errors and asking them to help identify the system issues is the goal of the analysis. Unfortunately, some professionals choose not to continue in their career due to the guilt and subsequent disconnect from colleagues after a serious error has occurred.

When to Take a Closer Look

A thorough analysis of safety events is key to learning from our mistakes in an effort to prevent recurrence. Because it is not possible to complete a thorough analysis on every report that is generated, it is recommended that criteria be developed to assist in determining the level of analysis that should occur for a reported event. The role of the MSO is often to review reported medication-related events and make a recommendation for further analysis. Examples of criteria include potential for significant patient harm, actual patient harm, severity level of patient harm, recurrent events, events associated with high-alert medications, and deviation from safe practices that may impact other processes. Be aware that restricting in-depth analysis to just events with very poor outcomes keeps us from learning from the lesser harm events. Generally, the causes of the sentinel and serious events are the same causes as the precursor events (those with minimal harm). Therefore, learning from precursor and near miss events (those that do not reach the patient) is a vital component of risk mitigation.[5] We may celebrate the "good catch" when an error does not reach the patient because our barriers were effective. On the other hand, we should also examine the factor that initiated the event, why it occurred, and how to prevent it from recurring because next time, perhaps, our barrier will not be effective.

The use of a system to rate the severity of event reports is recommended. Application of a rating system allows the most serious events to rise to everyone's attention in rapid fashion. Immediate action can be taken for critical events and the analysis process can be initiated. The use of the **National Coordinating Council on Medication Error Reporting and Prevention (NCC MERP)** Index for categorizing medication errors[6] is one method for prioritizing further review and action. The index and algorithm for its use are reproduced in Chapter 9. Review of event categorization should be completed and finalized by the MSO to ensure inter-rater reliability across the organization.

Many facilities routinely conduct an in-depth investigation on events resulting in patient harm; others will focus resources on investigations for events rated G or above (permanent patient harm). A **root cause analysis (RCA)**, as discussed in the next section, is required by The Joint Commission (TJC) for events that are classified as sentinel events. A *sentinel event* is defined by TJC as "an unexpected occurrence involving death or serious physical or psychological injury, or the risk thereof. Serious injury specifically includes loss of limb or function. The phrase *or the risk thereof* includes any process variation for which a recurrence would carry a significant chance of a serious adverse outcome.[1] The expectation is that the organization will conduct a timely, thorough, and credible RCA in response to a sentinel event, develop and implement an action plan to reduce the risk of recurrence, and monitor the effectiveness of the plan and its implementation.

An RCA can also be conducted on events other than sentinel events, such as when a trend of similar precursor or near miss events is identified. When several precursor events are identified that have not harmed a patient but have identified a recurring process gap, an aggregate RCA can be completed. An aggregate RCA collates data from several common events in an effort to identify the recurring variation(s).[7,8] This is a tool that has been used for falls, medication errors, and other similar events.

The level of risk to the involved patient and others should be defined through discussions held at the leadership level to determine the appropriate type of analysis. The MSO is an important resource in assisting in this discussion and determination. In the nicardipine example, the manager and MSO interviewed the nurse involved in the care of the patient to better understand the error. A concern with the infusion label and the method of programming the pump was identified. The nurse reviewed a similar infusion bag and showed how it was confusing and, in fact, was in the opposite formatting of what was required to be entered into the pump. Upon this discovery that there may have likely been a system contribution to the human error, this would be an appropriate case for a deeper analysis. Usually a small team makes a decision to conduct an RCA. Members of this small team may include:

- Medical Director for Quality and Safety
- Director for Quality and Safety
- Chief Nursing Officer
- Medication Safety Officer
- Vice President of Medical Affairs
- Risk Management
- Other similar roles

In this case, it was decided to do an RCA, due to the system implications with the medication label and pump programming requirements.

Steps in the Root Cause Analysis Process[9]

A structured approach to RCA is necessary to ensure all steps are accomplished in a thorough and timely manner. The goal of the RCA is to investigate the event in such detail that the true **root cause**(s) of the event are identified. This requires that the team takes the time to truly understand the processes as they exist and how they contribute to the event.

Determine Team Members

Once the decision is made to do an RCA, determining the composition and size of the RCA team is very important.

- *Team Sponsor/Champion*—A senior leader in the area of the event should serve as the champion or sponsor, ensuring that they are aware, involved, and have the ability to ensure timely and thorough implementation of the action plan. In this case, the Chief Nursing Officer and/or designated Nursing Director may serve as the team sponsor.
- *Facilitator*—A trained skilled facilitator generally investigates and guides the process. The facilitator should have formal training in RCA as well as experience in the performance of such analyses.
- *Unit Manager*—The unit manager is often included to provide information related to the culture and norms of the unit, as well as to provide feedback to the unit staff on what the RCA process involves. While the RCA process may be perceived as very intimidating and burdensome, it provides great value in educating managers and frontline staff on the benefits of in-depth analysis and action planning.
- *Content Experts*—As an RCA facilitator, it is not possible to be the content expert in every type of event that may occur. Including an expert in the field is very important. The MSO is considered the content expert for medication errors. The inclusion of a biomedical engineer in this instance would likely be appropriate as well as a hospital or system associate who works closely with the smart pumps, if the MSO is not the most knowledgeable person.
- *Risk Management*—Risk management often works closely with the safety and quality team in reviewing and investigating events. Although their focus also includes protecting the assets of the organization, close integration of the areas is beneficial in preventing future occurrences.
- *Physician Leader(s)*—Often a physician leader, such as Vice President of Quality and Safety, Vice-President of Medical Affairs, or comparable physician leader is involved or co-leads the analysis, providing the benefit of the physician perspective. Inclusion of residents is a great way to provide young physicians with early experience to safety and quality efforts within the facility.
- *Staff Member(s)*—The inclusion of a staff member from pertinent involved departments, such as a nurse from the floor, or a staff or clinical pharmacist, is vitally important for several reasons. Some managers have a more accurate perception of the functioning of their unit than others and involving staff can provide additional insight. Often, the manager of an area has a perception of how the unit functions, when in reality there may be some unexpected variation within the unit. A more subtle benefit to including

staff members is the culture change that may begin with exposure to process improvement in a multidisciplinary and rigorous process such as RCA[10] focused on identifying system problems. Including staff involved in the event in the RCA can be controversial. Initial experience including all of the involved staff in the RCA found that people tended to be defensive, were not appropriately engaged in the discussion, and were often more traumatized by recalling and discussing the events several times. For some staff, participation provides an outlet and a feeling of being involved in creating change for the organization. This is a case-specific decision and, for the most part, interviewing the affected staff separately and then keeping them informed of the team's progress and the final action plan tends to bring a feeling of resolution without being subjected to the entire process.

Preparation and Analysis

The investigation and analysis of the event begin with interviews of involved staff and physicians, medical record review, and identification of facts from various resources of information.

- *Confirm information as fact.* Much of the initial information that is relayed is not necessarily an accurate depiction of the events or includes the perceptions of only one group of practitioners. Key pieces of information must be validated in a thorough and objective review to be confident it is accurate.
- *Conduct interviews with all involved associates as soon as possible, to preserve the immediate memories*. The longer after an event the interviews occur, the increased chance that the story changes in some way (unintentionally through talking with others or assuming other stories are accurate). Interviews should be prefaced with the understanding that the goal of the RCA is to identify process gaps that contribute to error, not to blame or assess individual performance issues.[11] In this case, the following people were interviewed as soon as the manager was notified of the error: the nurse who programmed the pump, other nurses on the unit for the shift, the pharmacist, and the physician who was called to treat the patient.
  - *Open-ended questions should be used*, allowing moments of silence while the associate recalls the events and conversations.
  - *It is very important that the interviewer not ask questions until later in the discussion*—just allow the associate to recall everything he or she can.
  - *Once the associate can no longer recall additional information, it is appropriate to ask a more pointed question* (developed after the chart review or other interviews). In this case, the nurse was able to state that she was referencing the bag when programming the pump. She entered the fluid volume first (200 mL), followed by the drug dosage (40 mg), as was stated on the bag. The site used a real pump and asked the nurse to demonstrate how she programmed the pump, at which point it was discovered that the pump asks for the drug dosage first, followed by the fluid. She did recall

getting a warning of some type, which was bypassed. She stated there are so many nonsense warnings on the pump that rarely is there a warning of significance.

Develop a Timeline or Sequence of Events

Structured methods should be used to determine the sequence of events. The use of Events and Causal Factors diagrams, Barrier Analysis, Change Analysis, or Stream Analysis are examples of structured approaches to error investigation.[12] In this case the timeline is relatively succinct as there was a limited time period of activity. The use of a software product such as Visio, PowerPoint, or commercially available RCA software may be used to develop a timeline.

Identify Where Actions Deviated from What Was Expected

There should be no determination of fault or culpability up to this point—merely identification of what steps did not happen as they should have. One way to determine deviation is to compare the normal process (guided by policy and/or identified through observation) with the sequence of events to determine where things did not go as one would expect. These may be referred to as unsafe acts, inappropriate acts, deviations, or variations from the standard process. It is important to also consider whether the current policy/procedure meets accepted standards of care, for example, as described in professional organization documents or accreditation standards. If your policy is substandard (e.g., outdated) in comparison to others, this may be considered a deviation.

Determine whether the deviation was an individual deviation or whether others with similar experience and knowledge have or could have made the same choice or action. One way to do this is to provide information to several peers to determine what their course of action would likely have been—preferably without knowledge of the event and its causes so as not to skew their responses. This is an important step because the action plan for an individual deviation should look much different than an action item for a more comprehensive deviation or issue. In this case, ask several other nurses how they program the pump and about any warnings they receive and subsequent actions. The answers you receive may provide insight into whether this is a more global problem than just one practitioner, which changes the action plan significantly.

Identify Why the Unsafe Acts May Have Occurred[13]

There are many methods to accomplish this. Many utilize the *5 Whys* method of investigation. This is a questioning technique used to help identify the underlying reason for a particular problem. Begin by asking why the event occurred (why did the patient become hypotensive?), and continue to ask "why" until the most elemental reason is reached. It is perfectly acceptable to ask "why" more than five times if needed; however, five "whys" are generally sufficient to identify a root cause. Be sure to consider management oversight, human and environmental factors, ineffective or poor implementation of policies or procedures, or inadequate training or supervision. In this case, the nurse was utilizing the bag to program the pump, yet the two were not designed to be matched up when programming and, in fact, provided the information in an opposite manner. In addition, there were so many nuisance alarms leading to alarm fatigue that many practitioners were bypassing the warnings without placing full attention on the concern identified.

Identify Root Causes

Root causes are acts that if eliminated would have prevented an event from occurring. There must be confirmation of a clear cause and effect to be determined as a root cause of an event. Certainty around these causes is necessary. If changing this cause *might* prevent it from happening again—rethink whether this is a true root cause. There are on average two root causes in most cases, with a range of one to three. In this case, there were two root causes identified:

1. The design of the pharmacy label was not considered during the build of the drug library. Staff used the pharmacy label to guide programming of the pump, resulting in confusion. There was not adequate testing when designing and programming the drug library elements (e.g., dose/rate units) before implementing the smart pump.
2. Practitioners did not respond to smart pump alarms. They perceived that there was a high volume of "nonsense" alarms conditioning them to ignore alerts and miss valid warnings.

Extrapolating the causes to one that would absolutely prevent human error in programming the pump may require consideration of this possible cause: lack of adequate interfaces between the infusion pumps, the pharmacy computer programs, and computerized provider order entry systems increases the risk that a practitioner may misprogram a pump.

Develop an Action Plan to Prevent Recurrence

The action plan should be developed with the intent of preventing the recurrence with certainty. Risk reduction strategies such as re-educating the department staff, asking staff to be more careful, and developing or editing a policy and procedure are rarely sufficient. It is now recognized that although these may be necessary activities, they are weak action plans that will not prevent recurrence without some change to the processes. The concepts of mistake-proofing, standardization, and forcing functions are important considerations in the development of risk reduction strategies. Make it easy to do the right thing and hard to make an error. There is often not one single fix to resolve an issue, and using multiple strategies and several barriers or layers of protection to prevent patient harm may be appropriate. Define a responsible person for each action item, the expected time frame for implementation (expected completion date), and develop a measure of success. Be sure to include a follow-up assessment several months after implementation to confirm the action plan is working effectively as designed.

Share the Knowledge Through Transparency

Report the findings to hospital/facility leadership for approval and provide summary findings to various committees and medical staff groups (patient safety or quality council, process improvement teams, patient safety coaches, operations teams, shared governance teams, Pharmacy and Therapeutics committees, medication safety committees, Medical Executive Committee, and others). Work to bring the lessons learned from these events to the frontline staff. This demonstrates commitment to safety and develops a culture of transparency.

Regularly Review Previous Action Plans

Regular review should be performed to confirm previous action plans have been implemented and are functioning as intended. The key causes of event recurrence are not identifying the true root cause(s), developing an action plan that does not address the root cause, or inadequate implementation of the plan.

The MSO can adapt this framework to conduct a "mini" RCA for events that may not meet organizational criteria for a full RCA team analysis. This is best attempted after the MSO has had experience in participating in or facilitating RCAs, or by teaming with an experienced RCA facilitator. A template for preparing and documenting a mini RCA is provided in Figure 10-1. A method for an effective "one-meeting RCA" has also been described.[14]

Lessons Learned

One of the key challenges in facilitating RCAs is coordinating time for key frontline staff and management team members (e.g., physicians, vice-presidents, and others) to attend. One strategy is to have predetermined times designated for a team meeting used if and when an RCA is indicated. This ensures that those with busy schedules have adequate time allotted for this most vital activity.

The MSO roles for RCA may include interviewing involved parties, supporting staff involved in an error, and investigating the facts of a case. Investigation may be achieved as a participant on the team, as a medication safety expert, or as a team facilitator if trained and mentored appropriately. The MSO may also be responsible for implementing and communicating the action plan with the pharmacy team and other key associates or multidisciplinary teams. The MSO at a system level may also be responsible for conducting assessments at other sites within the system for the potential risk of a similar event, sharing the lessons learned, and facilitating improvements to avoid a repeat event within a system. In some cases, particularly involving pharmacy errors, the MSO may be involved with family/caregiver meetings to discuss error investigation details and identified system improvements.

An important factor in preventing recurrence is monitoring the action plan to ensure that it is implemented in a timely fashion. Measures should be defined as part of the action plan and revisited to assess the implementation and effectiveness of the action plan. A poorly designed action plan will be discovered if follow-up is timely.

Mini Root Cause Analysis (RCA) Template

Steps:

1. Select the team.
2. Review RCA and goals with team.
3. Summarize the event facts as known to date.
4. Diagram, or list, steps of the process *as they occurred*.
5. Compare process steps with process *as designed.*
6. Identify risk points in the process, asking "why" to understand thoroughly.
7. Develop actions to address contributing factors.

Summary of Completed RCA

Participants: List all members

Summary of event, as reported: Date, short objective description of event, outcome

Additional information: For example, demonstration of equipment used during event

Steps in process, as they occurred: Diagram, flow chart, or list—ask *Is this what "normally" happens?*

Steps in process, *as designed*: What do policies/procedures specify?

Contributing Factors:

- People (e.g., knowledge, skill)
- Organization (e.g., training, policies/procedures)
- Environment (e.g., surroundings)
- Tasks/practices (e.g., workflow)
- Tools/technology (e.g., equipment)

Action Plan:

Topic	Action	Responsible	Complete By

Confidential—Performance Improvement

Figure 10-1. Mini root cause analysis (RCA) template.
Source: D. Saine, Winchester Medical Center.

Use of a computer program that can provide reminders related to the completion of action items is beneficial in preventing inadvertent oversight.

The RCA team members tend to come into the process with a preconceived notion of the cause and what actions should be taken. It is important to work from the facts backward to determine the real reason(s) the event occurred. The team facilitator and/or sponsor are responsible for ensuring that the team remains focused and does not jump to solutions as teams often do.

Scope-creep is another risk of reviewing safety events. Be sure to keep the scope appropriate to the problem, even when tempted to solve other variances identified during the RCA process that did not contribute to the event.

One particularly common challenge within the RCA process is hindsight bias.[15] *Hindsight bias* is defined as a tendency people have to view events as more predictable than they really are—generally after an event. When one is aware of a poor outcome, the tendency to judge the actions that led up to the event as inappropriate is quite common. It is easy to assume that when in the midst of decision making and emergent need for action that a professional should have known that the stated action would lead to a bad outcome; however, this is not usually the case. The interview process is especially important here in determining what else was going on at the time of the event and what thought processes were used in the decision-making process. It is important to remind the team of this phenomenon.

A thorough literature search should be completed related to the type of event and processes involved. Identification of best practices may assist the team in devising an action plan or in determining whether an action was outside the standard of care. Of equal importance is to go to the location of the event and observe practices and processes in the area. The team members (managers and staff) may be so used to a process that they may not identify it as deviant from what is expected. Similarly, bringing an example of the equipment or products involved to the meeting gives all team members a common understanding of the product and how it functions. In the example case, bringing a nicardipine bag and a pump to demonstrate the screens and information required for programming is useful in ensuring all participants have a common understanding of the process.

It is important to the continued development of a safety culture to be transparent within the organization, and between organizations that are a part of a system, about the lessons learned from events. Information about the event and the action plan should be shared within the facility through structured meetings and communications—all the way to the staff level. This enables the organization to translate the lessons learned to other applicable areas of the facility (e.g., an event in a catheterization laboratory may provide key learnings for other similar procedural areas such as endoscopy, radiology, etc.).

Common Cause Analysis

Learning from multiple events is very powerful; however, determining where to focus limited resources becomes a challenge. At times it is necessary to prioritize the approach to the vulnerabilities in our systems. Identifying the common causes of multiple events provides a deeper look at the true system vulnerabilities. The use of **common cause analysis** (CCA)[16] provides a way to recognize trends and establish common themes within events. This process also referred to as an *aggregate root cause analysis*,[8] pools information from multiple events and identifies their common causes.

Devising an action plan for common causes may have a larger impact on safety events than an action plan focused on one case. Factors such as technologies that have not been optimized for use, poorly designed processes, and normalized deviance that is undetected by the manager are important to consider. The findings of a CCA provide a new level of confidence that the issues identified are truly important vulnerabilities within our system as they are risks that were seen in multiple events.

One example where a MSO can play a key role in CCA is collating ADEs as a result of anticoagulation therapy (or another high-risk medication class) to identify common causes across multiple cases. One method to identify these is through use of the ADE Trigger Tool.[17] The ADE trigger tool identifies cues, often through computer-generated reports, that an adverse event may have occurred. Examples include the use of a reversal agent such as naloxone, or an abnormal laboratory value such as an elevated internal normalized ratio (INR). Once the trigger is identified, the patient chart is reviewed to determine potential harm to a patient and to assess if the event was preventable. Key data elements are aggregated to identify common themes or causes to these events, from which an action plan can be generated.[8,9]

Just Culture and Individual Culpability

A *culture of safety* is the common beliefs, attitudes, and behaviors of a team or group of people related to safe health care. An area with a good culture of safety has staff that is willing to raise a concern about the safety of an activity, and management and physician teams that support this behavior, thanking them for clarifying any uncertainty that may result in harm to a patient. The use of critical language meant to "stop the line" in times of great concern is very important. Conflict resolution and teamwork skills are intentionally taught in organizations who have demonstrated strong safety culture. Regular measurement and improvement of safety culture is now a requirement of TJC as well as a recommendation from the National Quality Forum as a Safe Practice. Other important aspects of a safe culture include a focus on learning from events and defects in the process—often identified through event reporting. Developing safety culture requires a commitment from leadership, management, and staff as a long-term value.

A Just Culture

Consider the headlines: "Child dies from medication error," "Journalist dies of chemotherapy error." The rest of the story usually involves details about what happened (on the surface) and who was fired or reprimanded. What disciplinary action should be taken in these cases—if any? It depends on the circumstances entirely. We must have a good understanding of exactly what happened and the "whys" behind the decisions and actions taken. The culture in the health care industry in the 1990s shifted away from a focus on blame and shame. The culture shifted, perhaps a bit too far, to a blame-free culture in an effort to promote reporting. *Blame-free culture* recognized that humans will err, that most unsafe acts are slips or lapses, and that weaknesses in our systems and environments contribute significantly to error in medicine.

A *Just Culture* exists somewhere between two extremes, with blaming individuals on one end, blame-free culture on the other end, and a Just Culture that balances human error and accountability for intentional unsafe actions in the middle of the spectrum. It is thought to be inappropriate to discipline for all errors regardless of their circumstances and is likely just as inappropriate to be non-punitive in the face of individuals who are intentionally ignoring safe operating principles. A Just Culture is one in which discipline is applied in a consistent manner based on the intentions of the individual and the situation in which they were working—not the outcome.[18]

It is critically important, and can at times be difficult, to distinguish between those who make a conscious decision to complete an unsafe action despite knowledge that it is unsafe and those who usually work in a safe manner and experienced a slip or lapse. The use of a *substitution test* has proven to be useful in these instances.[19] When dealing with a serious event and a person who is implicated in an unsafe act, describe the scenario to several other individuals (at least three) of the same qualifications and experience (optimally who are not aware of the actual incident) and ask them under the circumstances at the time what decision(s) they would have made. If they would have made the same decision(s) and completed the same actions, then blaming any one individual is not likely appropriate as in this scenario there seems to be a system or cultural component as a contributing cause to the event. Another way to determine potential intent of the person is to observe individuals in the same situations (if possible) to determine how others behave in similar instances. This helps one determine whether the problem may lie with an individual, an expanded group (perhaps a unit or department), or a more global problem across the facility. This also helps in the development of an action plan. There is no need to retrain an entire department on a process if there is only one individual that is in need of coaching.

The use of a series of questions helps determine the culpability and accountability of a person's actions and have been developed from the Culpability Decision Tree (see Chapter 5, Figure 5-2).[20] It is key in developing a culture of safety that any decisions related to discipline are not made only when there's an adverse outcome.

Appropriate disciplinary actions, when warranted, should be taken when unsafe behaviors are identified regardless of the outcome.[20] *Pertinent questions include:*

- *Were the actions as intended?* This question differentiates intentional acts of malice to cause harm. Individuals involved in activities of this sort are culpable and need to be held accountable. Fortunately, this type of deviant behavior is uncommon.
- *Is there evidence of illness or substance abuse?* This question may reveal an individual with substance abuse problems or perhaps someone under treatment for a medical condition.
- *Did they knowingly violate a safe operating procedure? If so, was the procedure available, workable, intelligible, and correct?* This gets at those procedures that staff feel make no sense (not intelligible) and hence do not recognize or understand the value in their workflow. Step(s) in a procedure may be difficult to accomplish (not workable) so could be skipped for that reason. In these types of situations there is a component of system-induced error.
- *Do they pass the substitution test?* Would someone else have done the same thing? If so, then they are less likely to be culpable. *If not, were there deficiencies in training or experience?* If so, then a system induced error placed the individual at risk by expecting them to perform their duties without proper training.
- *Does the individual have a history of unsafe acts?* If not, again they are less likely to be culpable. If they do have a history of previous unsafe acts and intentional decisions to subvert safe practices, the question falls back to the management team to evaluate performance and accountability.

The use of these questions and a decision algorithm assists in determining the level of culpability of an individual. The actions in the first few questions bear more culpability than those that occur in the last several questions. Therefore, disciplinary actions are more likely to be appropriate for those acts that are intended and/or undertaken while under the influence of unauthorized substances, although there is a gray area where there may be system-induced errors along with the practitioner's culpability for not following established safe practices.

In this case example, the nurse did not intend to make an error nor harm the patient, she was not under the influence of unauthorized substances, and she did not intentionally subvert a safe practice. She made an unintentional human error. In this instance, a system issue was identified as a contributor; therefore, disciplinary action is less appropriate and recognizing and fixing the system issue is the most appropriate action.

Summary

The MSO has a critical role in event management—from the time the event occurs through evaluation and action planning phases. Ensuring that information provided by staff through event reports or other mechanisms are acted on is a key step in this process. Involving staff in the review and analysis of events brings a fresh perspective on what is actually occurring in everyday practice. This avoids any bias by managers into how they feel the process should be occurring versus how it is actually occurring. In addition, engaging frontline staff in the development of action plans to prevent recurrence ensures they feel a part of the process and the solution—a true part of the team.

PRACTICE TIPS

1. Learning from precursor and near-miss events (those that do not reach the patient) is a vital component of risk mitigation as causes are often similar to those of events that cause harm.
2. During an RCA, do not lead the interviewee on. Let him or her talk about what happened from start to finish and ask follow-up questions after the interviewee finishes providing information.
3. Be as empathetic as possible when investigating an event. Never assume you know what happened. An accusatory tone could antagonize someone and he or she might not be as forthcoming about the details of an event.
4. Be sure to review any reports/data related to technology use (e.g., ADCs, carousels, etc.) to clarify and potentially support or refute an interviewee's statements.

References

1. Green M. Inattentional blindness and conspicuity. Visual Expert 2004. Available at: www.visualexpert.com/Resources/inattentionalblindness.html.
2. MedWatch: The FDA Safety Information and Adverse Event Reporting Program. Available at: http://www.fda.gov/Safety/MedWatch/default.htm. Accessed July 27, 2011.
3. Proceedings from the ISMP Summit on the Use of Smart Infusion Pumps: Guidelines for safe implementation and use. Available at: http://www.ismp.org/tools/guidelines/smartpumps/comments/. Accessed July 27, 2011.
4. ISMP Newsletter. Too many abandon the 'second victims' of medical errors. July 14, 2011. Available at: http://www.ismp.org/newsletters/acutecare/articles/20110714.asp. Accessed July 31, 2011.
5. Barach P, Small SD. Reporting and preventing medical mishaps: Lessons from non-medical near miss reporting systems. *Br Med J.* 2000March 18;320(7237):759-763.
6. NCCMERP Index for Categorizing Medication Errors. National Coordinating Council for Medication Error Reporting and Prevention (NCC-MERP). Available at: http://www.nccmerp.org. Accessed July 24, 2011.
7. Using Aggregate root cause analysis to reduce falls. *Jt Comm J Qual Patient Saf.* 2005Jan;31(1):21-31.
8. Neily J, Oqrinc G, Mills P, et al. Using aggregate root cause analysis to improve patient safety. *Jt Comm J Qual Patient Saf.* 2003Aug;29(8):434-9, 381.
9. Woloshynowych M, Rogers S, Taylor-Adams S, et al. The investigation and analysis of critical incidents and adverse events in healthcare. *Health Technol Assess.* 2005;9:37-63.

10. Carroll JS, Rudolph JW, Hatakenaka S. Lessons learned from non-medical industries: Root cause analysis as culture change at a chemical plant. *Qual Saf Health Care.* 2002;11:226-269.

11. Root Cause Analysis Investigation Tools. National Patient Safety Agency. Available at: www. NRLS-0769D-RCA-tools-inve~iew-guide-2008-09-v1.pdf. Accessed July 31, 2011.

12. Corbett C, Clapper C, Johnson K, et al. *Maximize Patient Safety with Advanced Root Cause Analysis.* Marblehead, MA: HCPro, Inc.; 2004.

13. Spath PL. *Error Reduction in Health Care: A Systems Approach to Improving Patient Safety.* San Francisco, CA: Jossey-Bass; 2011.

14. Montanya, KR. Conducting a one meeting root cause analysis, In: Saine D, ed. *Safety and Quality Pearls 2.* Bethesda, MD: American Society of Health-System Pharmacists; 2009.

15. Henrikson K, Kaplan H. Hindsight bias, outcome knowledge and adaptive learning. *Qual Saf Health Care.* 2003:12(Suppl II):ii46-ii50.

16. Clapper C, Crea K. Common cause analysis. *Patient Saf Qual Healthcare.* May/June 2010;7:30-35.

17. Rozich JD, Haraden CR, Resar RK. Adverse drug event trigger tool: A practical methodology for measuring medication related harm. *Qual Saf Health Care.* 2003;12:194-200.

18. ISMP Newsletter: Our long journey towards safety-minded Just Culture. Part I: Where we've been. September 7, 2006. Available at: www.ismp.org/newsletters/acutecare/articles/. Accessed December 30, 2008.

19. Reason J. *Managing the Risks of Organizational Accidents.* Burlington, VT: Ashgate; 1997.

20. GAIN Working group E, Flight Ops/ATC Ops Safety Information Sharing. A roadmap to a Just Culture: Enhancing the safety environment. Available at: www.flightsafety.org/gain/just_culture.pdf . Accessed December 30, 2008.

Error Prevention Strategies and Staff Education

Kathryn A. Crea and Deb Saine

CHAPTER 11

Key Terms

Forcing Function—A design feature that, when employed by the user, will automatically guide the proper use of a device or process to prevent error.

Handoff—The process of transferring responsibility for care; the interactive transfer of information, allowing for questioning between the giver and receiver(s).

High-Reliability Organization—A complex organization with high risk for catastrophic error, with a very successful track record of maintaining a high level of safety over a long period of time.

Human Factors—"The scientific discipline concerned with the understanding of interactions among humans and other elements of a system, and the profession that applies theory, principles, data, and methods to design in order to optimize human well-being and overall system performance."[1]

Simulation—Imitation of the operation of a system or process, using a model that represents key characteristics of the selected system or process.

Standardize—To remove variations and irregularities; to bring into conformity with another.

System—A set of interacting, interrelated, or interdependent elements that work together in a particular environment to perform the functions required to achieve the system's aim.[2]

Introduction

This chapter begins with a review of human error and **systems** error to frame the relationships of these concepts to error prevention methods and staff education. We then move on to discuss broad strategies that can be employed to reduce error and resultant patient harm. The medication safety officer (MSO) will draw on these ideas and techniques quite often in daily work, while designing processes, developing education, or assessing errors, near misses, and adverse events. Effective education on medication safety is critical to providing safe patient care and establishing a culture of safety. Developing and maintaining a medication safety orientation and training program for pharmacy and other staff members is an important function for the MSO.

Human Error

Humans will most likely commit errors at an unacceptable rate despite our best efforts to understand and remedy their occurrence. With this in mind, it is necessary to develop systems of medication management that acknowledge human error and have processes in place to reduce the possibility of error and patient harm. See Chapter 5 for a more comprehensive discussion on this topic.

There are three modes of human performance: skill-based (SB), rule-based (RB), and knowledge-based (KB). It is important for the staff to have education regarding these basic concepts to understand why, despite the best of intentions, bad things can happen. The staff can get a better understanding why different tools (e.g., checklists, forms, policies, etc.) are utilized to improve safety.

- **Skill-based:** When in *skill-based level of performance*, humans are doing very routine tasks that are very practiced and automatic. People are very good at these tasks, as they do them all the time. In skill-based mode, a decision has been made on what the intended action is and the individuals are now in the process of executing a task. Activities such as checking a batch of compounded antibiotics or separating medication labels before labeling the products fit into this category. Experienced pharmacists or technicians who regularly perform these activities on a daily basis become proficient, and it requires very little effort or attention on their part and yet they are still able to detect a variance and prevent an error. However, if the routine process is interrupted, problems can occur. Skill-based errors are generally termed *slips* or *lapses*. They are easily identified. Slips are usually associated with attentional or perceptual failures and lapses generally involve memory failures.
    - A *slip* occurs when, for example, you are checking a report generated for a total parenteral nutrition (TPN) bag from a compounder and you miss the fact that the sodium chloride injection was listed as an ingredient to be added manually. Due to a drug product shortage, the product was removed from the pump in order to conserve supply. You fail to recognize this, and the drug is not added into the TPN. Checking TPNs

is something you do all the time, but you weren't aware of the shortage and miss the information on the report.
  - A *lapse* occurs when, for example, you are in the process of checking a compounded product and you are interrupted by a phone call. When you return to your task, you think you had completed your review, when in reality you had not. Unfortunately, you may have missed that the label was switched between two different medications.
- **Rule-based:** Humans perform in *rule-based mode* when problem-solving or making decisions. Perhaps there has been a change in the situation such as a patient may begin having renal dysfunction. We begin to problem-solve, realizing that we have been in this situation before. We have been trained to deal with many situations and, perhaps, learned a policy or procedure. Our thought processes focus on which rule to apply to the situation we have encountered. This is called an *if-then scenario*—if this situation, then do this action. In this situation, the patient may require adjustments to their medication therapy based on their decreased renal function. *Rule-based problems include:*
  - A wrong rule may be chosen because one misperceives the situation and applies the wrong rule.
  - If one misapplies a rule, a rule-based error has occurred. It is possible to unconsciously pull the wrong pattern or rule from our memory. Memory may be biased for many reasons: overgeneralization, recent occurrences (causing one to choose the first answer that comes to mind despite available evidence that would lead us to another conclusion), or other factors.
  - There is also intentional rule-based noncompliance in which an individual chooses an action despite the knowledge that he or she should take a different action (a nurse administers a medication without checking the patient's armband because he is sleeping soundly or the bar-code reader is not conveniently located).
- **Knowledge-based:** The other decision-making mode is *knowledge-based*. Knowledge-based errors occur when the individual is in a situation to which he or she has never been exposed or has no pre-programmed rules to apply. The person has a lack of required knowledge to complete the task or has possibly misinterpreted the problem. "You don't know what you don't know" is a representative phrase in the situation where you move forward without the necessary information. When we are in knowledge-based mode, we are much more likely to make an error than when we are in skill-based or rule-based mode. The best scenario is that we recognize that we are lacking the information that is needed and take the time to consult with other sources (colleagues, texts, policies, or literature) to determine the next course of action.

System Error

Systems have common characteristics, which generally include technology, tools and machines, interfaces, processes, products, user interaction with the system, and people. The health care system has become, and continues to become, very complex. There are many components that define the health system including individuals and teams of people, policies and procedures (generally for each individual entity), regulations, devices and equipment, communications, leadership, and management. It would be optimal if all of the parts of the system were integrated with seamless communication and coordination, but that is not the case. In addition, each of the components is likely to have their own "culture"; that is, common goals, values, beliefs, and behaviors. It is rare that each component of the system has similar cultures, even when speaking of departments or units within an individual entity, such as the patient care areas of a hospital. Poor coordination and communication contribute to a significant number of adverse outcomes. Optimization of systems and processes is essential to health care safety.

There are a variety of intrapersonal, interpersonal, and environmental factors that may contribute to errors in the medication-use process. These factors influence the occurrence of slips or performance lapses and mistakes committed by individuals as described in Chapter 5. They do not address failure of a system or failure of a safety net as a whole process. The medication-use process involves multiple health care professionals, nonprofessional staff, patients, and multiple physical environments. The safety net should work with all professionals and in all environments and may consist of multiple checks by individuals of other people's work, computer systems that screen for errors, barcode scanning systems, quality assurance measures, extra-organizational measures (e.g., to minimize ordering medications from companies with similar packaging), and multiple other systems. To adequately address the causes of errors, failures in the system must also be addressed. Although it is important to address the problem of individuals committing errors through a Just Culture, adequately developed safety systems should be in place to minimize the number of errors reaching patients. When errors do occur, it is necessary to address the event in the context of failure of the system or safety net.

The best way to provide education related to system errors is to provide case scenarios of actual occurrences and other examples of lessons learned from outside sources. Be sure that while highlighting what happened you also include information on how to proactively report risky or unsafe conditions before an error occurs.

Swiss Cheese Model

The Swiss Cheese Model of error is a visual depiction of system errors and how human errors reach the patient to potentially cause harm. The sequence usually begins with an error made by a human that proceeds through multiple barriers designed to prevent such errors from reaching the patient. In health care, as well as many other high-risk industries, processes are purposefully designed with the use of multiple defensive layers or barriers. Examples of these barriers are alarms, **forcing functions**, physical barriers, automatic shutdowns, and policies/procedures. These barriers prevent an error from reaching the patient. Ideally, these barriers would have no faults; however, holes often develop in these barriers due to *active* and *latent errors*. Picture the slices of cheese as the barriers described above, with the holes representing gaps that develop over time. An *active error* is an error made by a human, such as slips, lapses, mistakes, or procedural violations. These active errors are usually the first step in a chain of errors that eventually reaches the patient. *Latent conditions* are often conditions that exist due to the decisions of designers, procedure writers, and management within an institution. These decisions are often made with good intention but without the full understanding of **human factors** and safety principles. These may be equipment issues, gaps between policies and actual practice, unworkable procedures, and/or introduction of new staff without adequate orientation (see Figure 11-1). The figure illustrates the failed barriers in a drug-drug interaction that contribute to an adverse drug reaction. The holes in the Swiss cheese are dynamic, continuously changing over time. They are unpredictable and at times unnoticed. Occasionally, the holes in the Swiss cheese line up perfectly, allowing an initial error to reach the patient and potentially cause harm. Looking at the gaps within the barriers is a necessary step when investigating adverse outcomes. Placing blame on the first unsafe act neglects all of the contributing factors that may have played a role in individual decisions made by staff and places the next person in that role

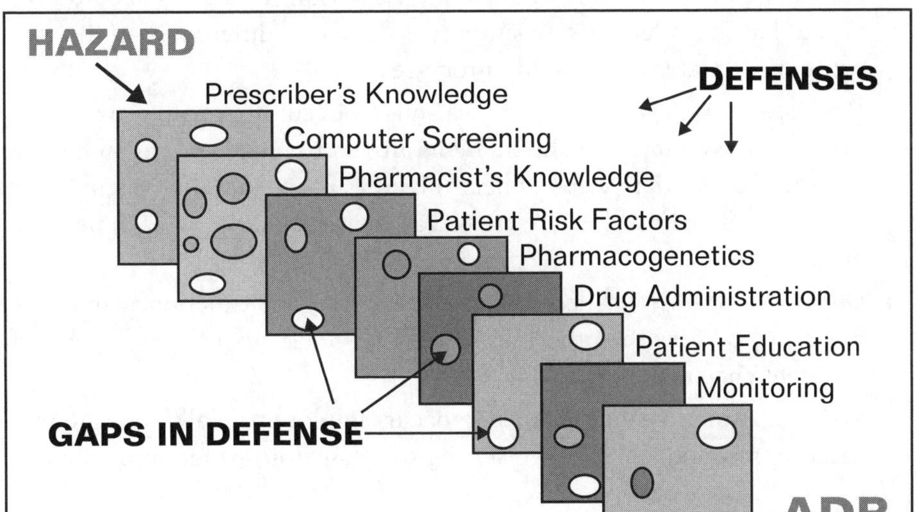

Figure 11-1. The Swiss Cheese Model of adverse drug outcomes.
ADR = adverse drug reaction
Source: Reprinted with permission of *Pharmacy Times*. John R. Horn and Philip D. Hansten, "Sources of error in drug interactions; The Swiss Cheese Model." *Pharmacy Times*. March 2004.

into the same risk of error. Examining the weaknesses in our systems (barriers) is a necessary step in ensuring that the error does not happen again.

High-Reliability Organizations

A **high-reliability organization** (HRO) may be thought of as a very complex organization at high risk for catastrophic accidents, yet has been very successful at maintaining a high level of safety (avoiding catastrophe) over a long period of time (i.e., reliable). Two of the most often quoted examples are nuclear power plants and the air traffic control system. HROs are continuously learning organizations reaching for high performance in everything they plan to do and effectively (often creatively) managing unexpected events to prevent harm. An increasing number of hospitals are using the same concepts applied by HROs to improve safety and quality. Leaders at all levels, including the MSO, can benefit from understanding and applying "high-reliability thinking." This section serves to briefly introduce the MSO to the HRO as we transition into error prevention strategies.

HROs share five key concepts, which the Agency for Healthcare Research and Quality (AHRQ) states are "essential for any improvement initiative to succeed."[3]

1. *Sensitivity to operations*. Leaders and staff are constantly aware of those systems and processes we use to provide patient care. This is essential to identifying risk and preventing harm.
2. *Reluctance to simplify*. Reliance on simplistic explanations for why things work or do not work is risky. One must understand the many factors that contributed to a failure to understand the reasons for risk. It should be noted that this reluctance to simplify is distinctly different than the error prevention strategy to simplify processes.
3. *Preoccupation with failure*. "When near-misses occur, these are viewed as evidence of systems that should be improved to reduce potential harm to patients. Rather than viewing near-misses as proof that the system has effective safeguards, they are viewed as symptomatic of areas in need of more attention."[3]
4. *Deference to expertise*. Leaders and managers value the experience and insight of staff who know the processes best. High-reliability culture depends on this deference to expertise.
5. *Resilience*. When system failures do occur, employees at all levels are prepared to respond and recover, setting the stage for further improvement.

Error Prevention Strategies

Health care has learned many lessons from other HROs, although at a slower rate than one would prefer. Many of the strategies described here are drawn from, or modified from, these other industries. Many key error prevention techniques involve the *incorporation of human factors principles into the design of processes*. Human factors research applies knowledge of human strengths and limitations to design things people use (systems, processes, equipment) in order to enhance performance and minimize errors. Put simply, it is "making it easy to do the right thing, and hard to do the wrong thing." Designing processes with human factors principles in mind is an effective way to improve the safety of the process and an important part of implementing an error reduction strategy. As James Reason notes, "we cannot change the human condition, but we can change the conditions under which humans work."[4]

In this section, we discuss a number of strategies that, when implemented, will form the structure for your organization's error reduction program.

Core principles of human factors design include:

- Simplify
- Reduce reliance on memory
- Standardize
- Error-proof
- Improve information access
- Make errors visibile
- Reduce **handoffs**
- Automate wisely
- Mitigate unwanted side-effects of change
- Improve communication
- Provide adequate training

Simplify

"Success in a coordinated activity requires that people simplify in order to stay focused on a handful of key issues and key indicators."[5] When simplifying processes or tasks, seek to reduce opportunity for error occurrence, as well as facilitating error detection and recovery, should an error occur.[1] Limiting the choice of medications available for use within the organization, otherwise known as a *formulary*, is one example of this strategy. Reducing the number of options to select from will reduce the potential for errors.

Complexity contributes to errors. Processes with a greater number of steps are more complex; the error rate for a process will increase as the number of steps increase. Consider a single-step process with an error rate of 1%. Assuming this same base error rate of each step, a 100-step process will have an error rate of 63%![6] In reality, it is unlikely that the error rates at each step will be identical; however, this does give you a picture of the relationship between complexity and error. Thus, reducing the number of steps in a process, the number of choices, or the time it takes to perform a task will help reduce the potential for error.

Of note, each of these strategies cannot be applied in isolation. For example, it may be less complex (simple) to purchase and implement an emergency department order management system without worrying about interfaces to other systems in the hospital. However, few would argue that such a stand-alone system used in isolation from all other hospital areas such as pharmacy, laboratory, imaging, etc., would provide safe processes for patient care. The challenge is to consider the application of strategies within the context of the system or work process.

Reduce Reliance on Memory

The human mind can hold only a limited amount in short-term memory; about four to seven items depending on which source you read.[7,8] In the absence of reminders, the probability of a human error of omission is 1%. However, if the necessary steps are embedded within a process, the probability for forgetting something drops by 70%.[6]

A number of strategies may be used individually, or combined, to reduce reliance on memory. These include checklists, protocols, pre-packaging, and automated reminders. Figure 11-2 illustrates an example which combines the first three concepts for "pre-packaged alteplase." In this instance, the process was created for a low-volume, time-dependent, and high-risk activity: preparing alteplase for a stroke patient. To reduce reliance on memory, all the necessary supplies (pre-packaging) are gathered together in one resealable, labeled plastic bag, as listed in the figure. A protocol for preparation is listed in stepwise fashion and may be used as a checklist for preparation. The dosing protocol is also included, again to reduce reliance on memory as well as to reduce research time that may be needed to confirm correct dosing.

Standardize

This principle is often closely linked with *simplify*. Standardization may be used to limit choices in products or performance of tasks or procedures, ultimately resulting in decreased complexity or reliance on memory. Communication between health care professionals and/or patients can be improved (e.g., accuracy, clarity, completeness, timeliness) by using **standardized** scripts or outlines. A pharmacy technician's use of a script for interviewing patients to obtain medication histories is one example. Use of a standardized format for documenting progress notes in a patient's medical record can assist pharmacists in providing clear, concise, and complete information to other care providers. Other examples of standardization to decrease error, such as establishing standardized concentrations and purchasing commercially available products (e.g., dopamine 400 mg/250 mL bags) for parenteral infusions and using standardized physician order sets, are discussed in other chapters.

Error-Proofing

Error-proofing, also called *mistake-proofing*, is the use of process or design features that prevent errors or automate the inspection of process outcomes to determine if error is present.[9] Mistake-proofing is also known as *poka-yoke* (pronounced pokayokay), Japanese slang for "avoiding inadvertent errors."[10] One example is the file cabinet: have you ever opened one file drawer, and then a second drawer, just to find the entire cabinet falling over on top of you? If more than one file drawer is opened at a time, the center of gravity moves, causing the file cabinet to fall. Modern file cabinets are designed to avoid this type of injury, as opening one drawer locks the rest. The design forces correct behavior and only allows for proper use. Two of the most reliable forms of error-proofing are *constraints* and *forcing functions*.

Alteplase (t-PA) for Stroke

Kit Supplies:

1 – box 100-mg vial Alteplase with Sterile Water for Injection vial and transfer device
1 – 10 mL syringe
1 – dispensing spike
1 – pack syringe caps
2 – needles
2 – 60-mL syringes
1 – 100-mL empty IV bag
1 – foil security seal
2 – alcohol prep pads

Preparation:

1. Use aseptic technique throughout. Prepare in laminar flow hood.
2. Disinfect vials. Insert transfer device into vial of sterile water.
3. Holding vial of alteplase upside down, spike vial with other end of transfer device.
4. Invert the two vials so that the alteplase vial is now on the bottom (upright) and the sterile water vial is upside down.
5. Allow sterile water to flow down through transfer device. Fluid should be transferred in approximately 2 minutes. Approximately 0.5 mL of sterile water will remain in vial. Alteplase concentration = 1 mg/mL
6. Remove empty sterile water vial and transfer device.
7. Gently swirl to dissolve drug. **DO NOT SHAKE!**
8. Insert a dispensing pin into vial of alteplase into same hole created by the transfer device.
9. In a 10-mL syringe, withdraw a bolus dose of alteplase. Cap syringe and label with bolus label.
10. Look at infusion label. Determine volume of infusion and draw up in syringes. Inject into an empty bag. Label IV bag with infusion label and apply foil seal to injection port.
11. Complete pharmacist check. Syringe and bag to be hand-delivered to ER as soon as possible.

Usual IV dosage:

- Total dose 0.9 mg/kg; MAXIMUM 90 mg
  - 10% of this dose administered as IV bolus over 1 minute
  - Remaining 90% of dose administered IV over 60 minutes

Label Samples:

Bolus in Syringe

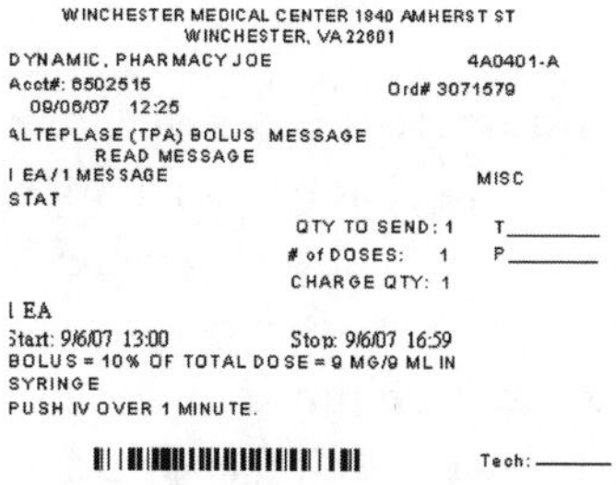
WINCHESTER MEDICAL CENTER 1840 AMHERST ST
WINCHESTER, VA 22601
DYNAMIC, PHARMACY JOE 4A0401-A
Acct#: 6502515 Ord# 3071579
09/06/07 12:25
ALTEPLASE (TPA) BOLUS MESSAGE
READ MESSAGE
1 EA/1 MESSAGE MISC
STAT
QTY TO SEND: 1 T______
# of DOSES: 1 P______
CHARGE QTY: 1
1 EA
Start: 9/6/07 13:00 Stop: 9/6/07 16:59
BOLUS = 10% OF TOTAL DOSE = 9 MG/9 ML IN SYRINGE
PUSH IV OVER 1 MINUTE.
Tech: ______

Infusion in Bag

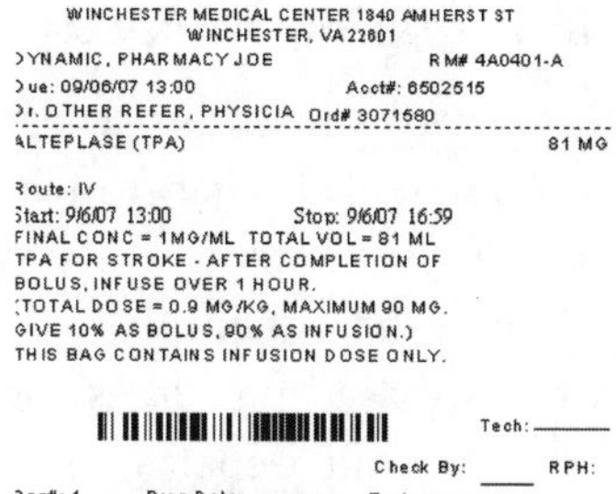
WINCHESTER MEDICAL CENTER 1840 AMHERST ST
WINCHESTER, VA 22601
DYNAMIC, PHARMACY JOE RM# 4A0401-A
Due: 09/06/07 13:00 Acct#: 6502515
Dr. OTHER REFER, PHYSICIA Ord# 3071580
ALTEPLASE (TPA) 81 MG
Route: IV
Start: 9/6/07 13:00 Stop: 9/6/07 16:59
FINAL CONC = 1MG/ML TOTAL VOL = 81 ML
TPA FOR STROKE - AFTER COMPLETION OF BOLUS, INFUSE OVER 1 HOUR.
(TOTAL DOSE = 0.9 MG/KG, MAXIMUM 90 MG. GIVE 10% AS BOLUS, 90% AS INFUSION.)
THIS BAG CONTAINS INFUSION DOSE ONLY.
Tech: ______
Check By: ____ RPH:
Bag#: 1 Prep Date: ______ Expires: ______

Figure 11-2. Combination of the first three concepts for "pre-packaged alteplase." *Source:* Courtesy D. Saine, Winchester Medical Center.

1. *Constraints*—A constraint restricts certain actions, so that certain errors cannot occur even if the worker is distracted. Constraints may be physical, procedural, or cultural.[9] The file cabinet scenario above is an example of a physical constraint. The free-flow protection feature on IV pumps is a physical constraint we are used to in health care. Procedural constraints may be used widely throughout the organization to prevent error and are often relatively simple and inexpensive to implement. You may recognize the removal of concentrated potassium chloride from patient care units as a procedural constraint. Use of order forms or electronic order sets with limited sets of medications is another example of a procedural constraint, as is computerized ordering software that doesn't allow a medication to be ordered for a route that is not appropriate for that medication. For example, vincristine should not have an intrathecal route available as a choice during the ordering process. Industrial safety programs have successfully used cultural constraints by "defining unsafe acts and rigidly censuring those who perform them."[9] In health care, scheduling pharmacists or nurses to work consecutive shifts would be considered unacceptable; thus, a cultural constraint for patient safety.
2. *Forcing function*—A forcing function is very similar to a constraint, but it requires the person to use the process or device correctly in order to derive the benefit. For example, oral syringes have specially designed hubs that will not securely or easily connect to IV lines. This safety feature is designed to prevent inadvertent intravenous administration of oral liquids. When oral syringes are used, this is an effective forcing function. However, if the oral syringe is not used, the safety feature (the forcing function) is not present.

Error-proofing may also involve automating the inspection of process outcomes to determine if error is present. For example, including a temperature-sensitive color indicator in a medication package or delivery tote will immediately identify incorrect storage (the "error") of the medication. Another common example is use of a special tape wrap that will display black stripes to indicate adequate sterilization. Absence of these stripes makes it obvious that an error has occurred.

Improve Information Access

Providing up-to-date and easily accessible information resources can help prevent errors. This will also reduce reliance on memory (see above). Drug information resources should be readily available to everyone involved in the medication-management process. This may be accomplished by providing organization-wide access to electronic or web-based resources, or by locating printed reference materials on all patient care areas and departments. Responsibility for maintaining and updating printed material must be assigned. Web-based or electronic resources generally have the advantage of automated, rapid information updates, avoiding the time-consuming tasks associated with manual reference upkeep. Integrating information into point-of-care technologies, such as computerized provider order entry (CPOE) systems or automated dispensing cabinets (ADCs) are very effective methods for information access. Whichever method is selected, staff must be made aware of these resources and how to use them.

Make Errors Visible

A safe system employs redundancies and safeguards to detect errors, so they can be corrected before causing patient harm. Examples may include use of bar-coding, automated reminders, and independent verification (double-checking). In the case of bar-coded medication administration or verification (BCMA/BCMV), imagine that the incorrect medication has been dispensed for the patient. When scanning the patient and medication bar codes, the nurse will receive an alert that there is a mismatch—effectively making the dispensing error that occurred *visible* to the nurse. Once it is visible, actions can be taken to correct the error before administration to the patient.

Independent double-check systems. Performing independent double-checks can reduce the risk of error by having one person independently check another's work. When this procedure is properly carried out, the likelihood that two individuals would make the same error with the same medication for the same patient is quite low. Thus, double-checks can be a barrier to preventing human errors from reaching the patient. The intended meaning of a double-check must be well-defined and carefully taught to staff. Common pharmacy processes that employ double-checks include preparation of TPN, chemotherapy orders, and pediatric and neonatal medications. See Chapter 7 for more specifics.

Reduce Handoffs

A *handoff* is an interactive transfer of information, allowing for questioning between the giver and receiver(s). Handoffs contribute to error through communication failures and by increasing the number of process steps. Suggestions for reducing communication errors are discussed later in this chapter. As noted in the *Simplify* section above, reducing the number of steps in a process will reduce the probability of error. By reducing handoffs, you reduce the number of people involved and reduce the number of steps, e.g., reducing the need to communicate the information multiple times. Work schedules may be created to avoid handoffs at critical times. Cross-training is another strategy to avoid handoffs from one specialist to another.[11]

Automate Wisely

Technology may be used to support tasks (e.g., CPOE), perform tasks (e.g., robotic dispensing), and to collect or present information (e.g., pharmacy information system drug interaction alerts). To avoid unintended consequences and errors associated with the use of technologies, keep in mind the three principles for the wise application of technology:[6]

- Keep the aim focused on system improvement rather than automating what is technologically feasible
- Use technology to support rather than supplant the human worker
- During the design and implementation phase, recognize and reduce new cognitive demands required by the technology, especially those demands that occur at busy or critical times

The MSO, with his or her expertise in knowledge/application of safety strategies and change management, can be tremendously helpful in "automating wisely." For example, while duplicate medication checking may be *technologically* feasible for a CPOE system, the MSO needs to assess the effectiveness of this feature. If it provides such a high number of alerts that no one will pay attention to any of them, essentially creating an unsafe system, the MSO will help weigh the risks and benefits of implementing this feature, keeping the aim focused on system improvement. Chapter 8 presents additional information on technology and safety.

Mitigate the Unwanted Side Effects of Change

Change often involves learning something new and altering familiar routines, and during this learning curve the chance for error is increased. The MSO may employ three strategies to mitigate error and harm:[6]

- Use a formal process to predict opportunities for error and harm before making the change and eliminate them, if possible, or develop contingency plans
- Test changes on a small scale with minimum risk and devote resources to redesign the procedure as problems are identified
- Monitor the clinical outcomes, errors, and adverse events over time during testing and implementation

Improve Communication

There is no doubt that communication plays a role in the majority of safety events. Statistics from The Joint Commission related to sentinel events support this notion. While this is widely recognized, it also appears to be one of the most difficult tasks to improve upon as communication crosses so many professions, shifts, and types of handoffs. Stress to the staff that effective communication is complete, clear, brief, and timely. (The MSO should use all of these attributes of communication as well!) *There are several methods of structured communication techniques:*

- *SBAR* is a communication framework adapted from the U.S. Navy by Michael Leonard, MD, and colleagues for use in the Kaiser Permanente health system. The SBAR (**S**ituation-**B**ackground-**A**ssessment-**R**ecommendation) technique provides a framework for communication between members of the health care team about a patient's condition. SBAR is an easy-to-remember structured method for framing any conversation. It is especially useful in critical situations, which require a clinician's immediate attention and action. It allows for an easy and focused way to set expectations for what and how it will be communicated between members of the team. It is an essential component of teamwork and a culture of patient safety. Additional information and downloads are available at: http://www.ihi.org/knowledge/Pages/Tools/SBARToolkit.aspx.

- *Three-Way Communication* is the standard communication protocol used by the military, air traffic controllers, and nuclear operators. It is required by The Joint Commission for verbal orders and critical test result communications. The read-back requires the sender to communicate the information, the receiver to write down (or enter electronically) the information and repeat it back to the sender, and thirdly the sender confirms that the information is accurate. The repeat-back is the same except that the information is not required to be written down before it is repeated back. This method provides confirmation that what we are hearing is accurate. Role-play is helpful to demonstrate the correct technique for this requirement.
- *I PASS the BATON* is a structured communication for handoffs that is recommended by TeamSTEPPS™, a teamwork system designed for health care professionals by the Department of Defense Patient Safety Program and the Agency for Healthcare Research and Quality (AHRQ).[12] Simulated research in surgical patients determined that all data were lost in a verbal handoff of 12 patients, 31% of data were lost when notes were taken during verbal handoff, and the use of a form for handoff resulted in minimal loss of information.[13] The elements include:
    - **I**ntroduction—Introduce yourself and your role
    - **P**atient—Identifiers, age, sex, and location
    - **A**ssessment—Present chief complaint, vital signs, symptoms, and diagnosis
    - **S**ituation—Current status, level of uncertainty, recent changes, code status, and response to treatment
    - **S**afety—Critical lab values/results, allergies, alerts (falls, isolation)
    - **The B**ackground—Co-morbidities, previous episodes, current medications, family history
    - **A**ctions—What actions were taken or are required, with brief rationale
    - **T**iming—Level of urgency, timing, and prioritization of actions
    - **O**wnership—Who is responsible (doctor, pharmacist, nurse)? Include patient and family responsibilities
    - **N**ext—What will happen next? Anticipated changes? What is the plan? Are there contingency plans?

- *The 5 Ps* method was developed by Sentara Health Care in Virginia in 2004 to clarify communications during the transfer of responsibility from one caregiver to another.[14] It is a more simple mnemonic that condenses the communication elements into fewer categories, and it can be adapted for pharmacist's communications in the following way:
  - **P**atient: Name, identifier(s), location
  - **P**lan: Drug therapy plan, next steps
  - **P**urpose: Rationale for the care plan
  - **P**roblems: What problems might you anticipate, or watch for?
  - **P**recautions: What precautions are necessary (for example, drug levels)?

Provide Adequate Training

Adequate orientation and training is essential in ensuring that all staff members (new and current employees) have the requisite knowledge to perform their duties in a safe and efficient manner. Integrating safety education into new employee orientation and continuing through staff meetings and other venues help all levels of staff to comprehend the risks in health care. Staff members need to be able to recognize risks, understand methods to reduce the risk of error, and intervene appropriately when others are at risk.

Staff Education

Ideally, medication safety education will begin with a new employee's orientation, and will continue throughout his or her employment with the organization. While the MSO will typically oversee the medication safety portion for orientation and training, it is also essential to facilitate its inclusion for process changes and as a routine part of quality improvement. The latter concepts have been discussed in earlier chapters, so we will concentrate on the education that should be provided at the entry level.

Orientation refers to the relative position or direction of something: it introduces the new staff member to the organization's mission, vision, and values, among other basics. Safety has become a top priority in today's health care world and is sure to be a part of the mission/vision/values triad. The MSO can capitalize on this strength to emphasize the importance of medication safety concepts.

Training goes beyond the introductory elements of orientation and will focus on performance of the job safely, effectively, and efficiently. It is important to include these elements of training for all members of the pharmacy department, including pharmacists, technicians, interns, support staff, and students.

Basic Outline of Topics

A basic outline of topics for medication safety during the orientation and training process follows and is illustrated in Figures 11-3 and 11-4. The information you provide should be tailored to your organization as much as possible, and meaningful for the new employee's work environment. Information on content for the training program may be found in this chapter and throughout the book.

1. **Why errors occur**
   a. Human error
   b. Systems error
2. **Medication errors, adverse drug reactions (ADRs), and adverse drug events (ADEs)**
   a. Definitions
   b. Severity ranking
   c. Reporting
   d. Follow-up and feedback
   e. Just Culture
3. **Analysis of errors**
   a. Root Cause Analysis (RCA)
   b. Failure Modes and Effects Analysis (FMEA)
   c. Organization-specific trends
4. **Event management**
   a. Disclosure of adverse outcomes
   b. Emotional support around errors and events
5. **The medication-management process**
   a. Pharmacy staff roles
   b. Teams and committees
   c. Integrating medication safety into daily practice
6. **Regulations, standards, and accreditation**
   a. Medication management chapter
      i. Organization—specific policies and procedures
      ii. Organization—specific risks and avoidance strategies
   b. National Patient Safety Goals
      i. Patient identification
      ii. Labeling medications
      iii. Anticoagulation
      iv. Medication reconciliation
      v. Health care–associated infections
7. **Technology and medication safety**
   a. Unintended consequences of technology use
8. **Error prevention techniques**

New Pharmacist Orientation: Understanding, Recognizing, and Preventing Errors

Learning Objectives

- Define *medication error* and *adverse drug event.*
- Identify characteristics of people that impact on their ability to perform (human factors).
- Define *latent* and *active* failures.
- Define *confirmation bias.*
- Identify types of medication errors that can occur during the ordering process.
- Identify types of medication errors that can occur during the preparation and dispensing processes.
- Describe problems with detecting sterile admixture errors.
- Identify medication error root causes.
- Describe the role patient education plays in preventing errors.
- Describe ways that pharmacists can prevent errors.
- Identify Just Culture responsibilities.
- Describe medication error reduction reactive and proactive approaches.
- Describe relationship of safety management to human resources.

Program

- View "Beyond Blame" videotape.
- View MSO medication safety inservice on DVD covering the learning objectives.
- Meet with MSO to go over questions related to the recordings and learning objectives.
- In meeting with MSO, review resources available to staff to provide assistance with job performance (e.g., clinical care guidelines and policies and procedures related to medication safety) and problem-solving (e.g., chain of command).

Figure 11-3. New pharmacist orientation: understanding, recognizing, and preventing errors.
Source: Courtesy C. Larson, University of Illinois Hospital & Health Sciences System.

Topic	Methods	Date Completed	Completed By (initial)
Safety Basics ■ Define safety ■ Human error, system error ■ Just Culture	■ Video: "Beyond Blame," "Chasing Zero," "Josie King Story" ■ Discussion ■ Case study: "Swiss Cheese"		
Event reporting (risk reports) ■ Medication error ■ ADR ■ Near miss ■ Analysis of errors ■ Current trends, issues ■ Just Culture	■ Discussion ■ Tutorial: reporting system ■ Demonstration: event report ■ Review summary report ■ Review posters, resources regarding current issues (e.g., HYDROmorphone dosing)		
Medication Management System ■ Review ■ Opportunities for error ■ Order clarification process ■ Standard administration times ■ Medications that "never leave pharmacy" ■ Integrating safety into your daily practice ■ P&T Committee role	■ Readings: ASHP Guidelines (Preventing Medication Errors in Hospitals, Preventing Medication Errors with Antineoplastic Agents) ■ Discussion ■ Case scenarios		
Accreditation ■ Agencies, purpose ■ NPSG ■ Medication reconciliation ■ Hospital policies related to accreditation standards • Sound-alike • High-alert • U-500 insulin • Patient's own meds • Standard administration times	■ Read TJC Pharmacy Guide ■ Discuss TJC Pharmacy Guide ■ Complete TJC Competency ■ Review related documents ■ Case scenarios		
Technology ■ Dispensing technologies ■ ADCs, overrides ■ CPOE, eMAR, pumps ■ Alerts, warnings, messages ■ Unintended consequences	■ Discussion ■ Demonstration		
Med Safety Resources ■ Role of MSO ■ Safety teams ■ ISMP newsletters, MedWatch ■ Bulletin boards	■ Discussion ■ SafeMed charter, annual summary ■ Review samples		
Questions/Suggestions	■ Discussion		

Figure 11-4. Medication safety orientation topics, pharmacy staff.
Source: Courtesy Deb Saine, Winchester Medical Center.

The mechanism(s) by which this material is presented is important in ensuring that the learner successfully achieves your objectives for medication safety orientation and training. Learning styles encompass visual (seeing), auditory (hearing), and kinaesthetic (doing). Try to match your teaching style to the learner's preferred learning style. Reflect on this proverb as you create your training program:

I hear, I know.
I see, I remember.
I do, I understand.

—*Confucius*

By using a variety of active teaching and learning approaches you will increase the opportunities to learn in the preferred method. Suggestions include:

- Use of videos to engage emotional response
- Storytelling—discussion of errors that have occurred within and external to the organization
- Presentations with discussion
- Personal reflection and recall activities
- Demonstrated use of the event reporting system, or other process/technology
- Role-play and practice scenarios—most importantly for error prevention techniques and problem solving
- Simulation—The use of **simulation** in health care has become relatively widespread. Simulation does not require a high-fidelity simulation lab with realistic human simulators. It can, in fact, be very low-tech and classroom-based. There are debates related to which method is better, and this is somewhat dependent on the objective(s) of the simulation. A mock code can be conducted in a simulation lab or can be simulated in an emergency room bay with a specific focus on one element of the code, perhaps having pharmacists calculating and preparing medications. Other examples of low-tech simulation include mock patient cases intended to assess the accuracy of computer order entry, conflict resolution scenarios, and medication reconciliation simulations for students and practitioners.[15]

The MSO should endeavor to include the topic of medication safety into orientation and training programs for *all* professionals who engage in the medication-management process. This would include not only pharmacy staff, but also prescribers, nurses, and respiratory therapists. This is most commonly done as part of new employee orientation. As an alternative, these components can be broken into individual modules and covered in department meetings or other venues. Strategies to overcome limited resources for providing this education include creative use of video resources, involving pharmacy residents in presentations, or including written resources that may be reviewed by other pharmacy colleagues. Consider inviting new personnel to tour the pharmacy department and deliver aspects of medication safety education at that time. Schedule a one-to-one meeting with new prescribers to orient them to pharmacy services, while integrating safety topics. Be creative. Use eye-catching posters or slogans. You may also utilize web-based technologies, organizational electronic learning programs, point-of-care messaging, and existing tutorials to enhance medication safety training.

Summary

Understanding concepts of human and systems error is a precursor to understanding safe system design. Incorporating human factors principles into the design of medication management processes will help prevent error and reduce patient harm. These error prevention strategies include standardizing, reducing reliance on memory, error-proofing, improving information access and communication, and providing adequate training. Designing appropriate educational sessions that emphasize the practical application of core processes is important. Include real-life scenarios of errors and focus on system issues identified and the actions taken to minimize/prevent further risk and patient harm. Practicing the desired error prevention technique is the key to habit formation. Communication is one of the key contributing factors to many safety events and can always be improved, either through teamwork implementation and/or through development of structured communication processes. These skills, along with integration of best practices, work to enhance the culture of patient safety in all health care institutions.

PRACTICE TIPS

1. Incorporate error prevention strategies into work processes with the input and feedback of the staff performing the job.
2. Role-play and practice scenarios can be very effective training mechanisms to provide education on a complex process that may not happen very frequently.
3. Meet with all new staff so they get to know you and they learn how you can help them do their job to the best of their abilities.
4. Utilize organization-specific error examples during training/education sessions.
5. Check with other organizations to see what tools they use that may be helpful to your organization.

References

1. Carayon P. *Handbook of Human Factors and Ergonomics in Health Care and Patient Safety*. Mahwah, NJ: Lawrence Erlbaum Associates Publishers; 2007.
2. Bertalanffy LV. General system theory: Foundations, development, applications. New York: George Braziller, Inc; 1968.
3. U.S. Department of Health and Human Services. Agency for Healthcare Research and Quality. Becoming a high reliability organization, executive summary. Available at: http://www.ahrq.gov/qual/hroadvice/hroadviceexecsum.htm. Accessed September 4, 2012.
4. Reason J. Human error: models and management. *Br Med J*. 2000;320:768-770.
5. Weick KE, Sutcliffe KM. *Managing the Unexpected: Assuring High Performance in an Age of Complexity*. University of Michigan Business School Management Series. Jossey-Bass; 2001.
6. Nolan TW. System changes to improve patient safety. *Br Med J*. 2000;320:771-773.
7. Cowan N. The magical number 4 in short-term memory: A reconsideration of mental storage capacity. *Behav Brain Sci*. 2001;24:87-114.
8. Miller GA. The magical number seven, plus or minus two: Some limits on our capacity for processing information. *Psychol Rev*. 1956;63:81-97.
9. Graban M. *Lean Hospitals: Improving Quality, Patient Safety and Employee Engagement*. 2nd ed. Boca Raton, FL; CRC Press; 2012.
10. Grout J. Mistake-proofing the design of health care processes. Rockville, MD, AHRQ Publication No. 07-0020, 2007. Available at: http://www.ahrq.gov/qual/mistakeproof/. Accessed August 29, 2012.
11. Porto GG. Safety by design: ten lessons from human factors research. *J Healthc Risk Manag*. 2001;21(4):43-50.
12. Pocket Guide: TeamSTEPPS. Strategies & tools to enhance performance and patient safety. AHRQ Publication No. 06-0020-2, November 2008. Agency for Healthcare Research and Quality. Rockville, MD. Available at: http://www.ahrq.gov/teamsteppstools/instructor/essentials/pocketguide.htm#communication. Accessed August 30, 2012.
13. Pothier B, Montiero P, Mooktiar M, et al. Pilot study to show the loss of important data in nursing handover. *Br J Nurs*. 2005;14:1090-1093.
14. Virginia Business Coalition on Health. Sentara Virginia Beach General Hospital: Creating a culture of safety: behavior based expectations for human error prevention. Available at: http://vbch.stratum.net/documents/TROIANONQFSafePracticesLeapURBANVBCH2006DEC7.pdf Accessed March 17, 2013.
15. Lindquist LA, Gleason KM, McDaniel MR, et al. Teaching medication reconciliation through simulation: a patient safety initiative for second year medical students. *J Gen Intern Med*. 2008;23:998-1001.

Essential Websites and Other Resources

Joanne G. Kowiatek

CHAPTER 12

Introduction

It is important for every medication safety officer (MSO) to have a list of resources at hand. The information provided in this chapter includes a brief description of the role of organizations and/or how information they present on the website or publication might best be utilized. The following journals, articles, books, websites, apps, and newsletters provide a wealth of information for the MSO on essential background information to the field of medication safety, research activities, best practices, and useful information for everyday practice. Because of the nature of the subject and the continued availability of changed or new information, this list is not intended to be exhaustive. Table 12-1 provides a brief summary of some helpful tools available on the Web.

PRACTICE TIPS

1. Share medication safety–related apps, websites, resources, and tools with other clinicians in your organization (pharmacists, nurses, physicians, risk managers, patient safety officers, etc.). Don't keep safety to yourself; engage others to understand and promote patient safety.
2. Bookmark or make a "shortcut" for your favorite medication and patient safety websites you use most often.
3. Network with other MSOs using listservs or other professional online connections or communities.
4. Build your MSO library with key reference books, resources, and tools identified in this chapter.

Table 12-1. Key Websites with Tools

Organization	Key Website	Toolkit, Tools, Forms (etc.)
Association of periOperative Registered Nurses (AORN)	http://www.aorn.org/Clinical_Practice/Toolkits/Tool_Kits.aspx	Safe Medication Administration Toolkit and many other toolkits (some available only with membership)
AHRQ	http://teamstepps.ahrq.gov/abouttoolsmaterials.htm_	TeamSTEPPS™ Tools
ASHP Foundation	http://www.ashpfoundation.org/MainMenuCategories/Education/SpecialPrograms/BarCodeGuide.aspx_	Implementing a Bar-Coded Medication Safety Program: A Pharmacist's Toolkit
IHI	http://www.ihi.org/IHI/Programs/AudioAndWebPrograms/WebandACTIONUsingtheIHIGlobalTriggerToolApril2009.htm?player=wmp	IHI Global Trigger Tool for Measuring Patient Safety
ISMP	■ http://www.ismp.org/tools/abbreviations/default.asp ■ http://www.ismp.org/Consult/ruralhospital/default.asp ■ http://www.ismp.org/Tools/communitySafetyProgram.asp ■ http://www.ismp.org/Tools/FMEA.asp ■ http://www.ismp.org/Tools/anticoagulantTherapy.asp	■ Abbreviations Toolkit ■ ISMP Rural Hospital Medication Safety Connection™ Resource Kit ■ Community Pharmacy Medication Safety Tools and Resources ■ Failure Mode and Effects Analysis Tool and Guide ■ Improving Medication Safety with Anticoagulation Therapy Tools
Massachusetts Coalition for the Prevention of Medical Errors	http://www.macoalition.org/	Reconciling Medications Toolkit
Purdue University	http://excellence.acforum.org/sites/default/files/Purdue%20Univ%20Anticoag%20Toolkit.pdf	Anticoagulation Toolkit
VA National Center for Patient Safety (NCPS)	■ http://www.va.gov/NCPS/SafetyTopics.html#HFMEA ■ http://www.va.gov/ncps/CogAids/RCA/index.html#page=page-1	■ Healthcare Failure Mode and Effects Analysis (HFMEA) ■ NCPS Root Cause Analysis Tools

Websites

Professional Organizations

- **American Academy of Pediatrics** (AAP) (www.aap.org) is an organization of pediatricians committed to the attainment of optimal physical, mental, and social health and well-being for all infants, children, adolescents, and young adults.
  - This site provides helpful educational offerings for medication safety such as: Simple Solutions to the Complicated Problem of Home Medication Use, Medication Safety in Ambulatory Care and Automatic Surveillance and Pediatric Trigger Tools. (http://www.aap.org/saferhealthcare).
- **American Hospital Association** (AHA) (www.aha.org) is the national organization that represents and serves all types of hospitals, health care networks, and their patients and communities. Close to 5000 hospitals, health care systems, networks, other providers of care, and 40,000 individual members come together to form the AHA.
  - This site has a Resources page under Quality and Patient Safety (http://www.hpoe.org/resources?topic=40) that provides toolkits (e.g., Strategies for Leadership: A Toolkit for Improving Patient Safety) and reports (e.g., Legislating Medication Safety: The California Experience and Addressing Medication Errors in Hospitals: A Framework for Developing a Plan). The site also provides case studies in Improving Medication Safety and Leading the Quest for Quality: 2010 Profiles in Quality and Patient Safety (http://www.hpoe.org/case-studies/8988057069); (http://www.hpoe.org/case-studies/resources/hanys-new-island-hospital-2.pdf). Membership may provide additional benefits and resources.
- **American Medical Association** (AMA) (www.ama-assn.org) is an organization which promotes the art and science of medicine and the betterment of public health, with a concerted effort to help doctors help patients by uniting physicians nationwide to work on the most important professional and public health issues.
  - On this site under Resources/Clinical Practice Improvement/Patient Safety/ are sections titled Medication Safety: The Physician's Role in Medication Reconciliation; Medication Safety: Pharmacogenomics; and Making Strides in Safety: Communication Tools for Safer Healthcare. Membership may provide additional benefits and resources.

- **American Organization of Nurse Executives** (AONE) (http://www.aone.org/aone/edandcareer/home.html) is the voice of nursing leadership in health care, seeking to advance nursing practice and patient care, promote nursing leadership excellence, and shape public policy for health care.
  - This site provides medication and patient safety presentations on medication administration, medication infusion safety, and other topics as well as news updates on safety. Membership may provide additional benefits and resources.
- **American Society of Health-System Pharmacists** (ASHP) (www.ashp.org) is a 40,000-member national professional association representing pharmacists who practice in hospitals, ambulatory care settings, health maintenance organizations, long-term care facilities, home care, and other components of health care systems. It is the only national organization of hospital and health-system pharmacists and has a long history of improving medication use and enhancing patient safety.
  - This website has several free resource centers related to patient safety and quality. The purpose of the ASHP Resource Center on Patient Safety (http://www.ashp.org/patientsafety) is to foster fail-safe medication use in health systems through the leadership of pharmacists. The Center fulfills its mission through advocacy, education, and research. This resource site provides many patient and medication safety resources (e.g., tools, recommended readings including books and patient safety articles), guidelines, policies, best practices, training, and education for MSOs, alerts, news, hospital accreditation, announcements, patient and consumer education, and access to ASHP Connect. ASHP Connect is the Society's online community exclusively for members to connect with each other and share ideas.
  - The ASHP Quality Improvement (QI) Resource Center (http://www.ashp.org/qii) provides resources to support pharmacist leadership and engagement in health care quality initiatives that improve patient outcomes and reward performance excellence. The site includes a primer on quality improvement and has sections for advanced practitioners, managers (featuring a toolkit), and clinicians.
- **American Society of Health-System Pharmacists** (ASHP) **Research and Education Foundation** (http://www.ashpfoundation.org/) is the philanthropic arm of ASHP, the national professional organization representing health-system pharmacists. The foundation offers more than 25 research grant, educational, and awards programs that assist and recognize pharmacists providing care to patients in our nation's health systems, leading to optimal medication outcomes.
  - A section on Useful Resources includes Implementing a Bar-Coded Medication Safety Program—A Pharmacist's Toolkit, and My Medicine List™. Also on this site is information on the application process for the Award for Excellence in Medication-Use Safety, and videos and stories

of past winners. http://www.ashpfoundation.org/MainMenuCategories/Awards/AwardforExcellenceinMedicationUseSafety.aspx.

- **American Society for Healthcare Risk Management** (ASHRM) (http://www.ashrm.org/) is a personal membership group of the American Hospital Association with members representing health care, insurance, law, and other related professions. ASHRM promotes effective and innovative risk management strategies and professional leadership through education, recognition, advocacy, publications, networking, and interactions with leading health care organizations and government agencies.
  - A free document available for download is Risk Management Pearls for Medication Safety. (http://www.ashrm.org/ashrm/online_store/files/PearlsMedSafety_sample.pdf). Also on this site is a page for Patient Safety Resources with organizations and links.
- **American Society of Medication Safety Officers** (ASMSO) (http://www.asmso.org/) is a society devoted to medication safety officers and leaders in medication management. The mission of ASMSO is to advance and encourage excellence in safe medication use by providing communication, leadership, direction, and education among its members. This site provides a free listserv (registration required).
  - This site has an online newsletter with free access and provides links to patient safety–related web resources, Institute of Medicine reports, journal articles, state safety initiatives, conference presentations, consumer and patient information, and other resources. The site provides information on medication safety residency and fellowships.
- **Anesthesia Patient Safety Foundation** (APSF) (http://www.apsf.org/) was the first independent multi-disciplinary organization (practitioners, equipment, drug manufacturers, and many related professionals) created expressly to help avoid preventable adverse clinical outcomes, especially those related to human error. APSF has been the leader in the proactive, successful efforts to dramatically improve the safety of anesthesia administration and reduce adverse events.
  - This site provides clinical patient safety tools for anesthesia.
- **Association of periOperative Registered Nurses** (AORN) (http://www.aorn.org/) is the national association committed to improving patient safety in the surgical setting. AORN promotes safe patient care and is recognized as an authority for safe operating room practices and a definitive source for information and guiding principles that support day-to-day perioperative nursing practice.
  - This site provides toolkits such as Safe Medication Administration, Just Culture, and Human Factors in Healthcare. Membership is required for access to some toolkits.

Government Agencies

- **Agency for Healthcare Research and Quality** (AHRQ) (http://www.ahrq.gov/) is the lead U.S. federal agency charged with improving the quality, safety, efficiency, and effectiveness of health care for all Americans. As one of 12 agencies within the Department of Health and Human Services, AHRQ supports health services research that will improve the quality of health care and promote evidence-based decision-making.
    - This site has a Quality & Patient Safety page (http://www.ahrq.gov/qual/) with many resources and tools, including surveys to measure patient safety culture and a re-engineered discharge toolkit. You can sign up for various e-mail updates or newsletters (e.g., Medical Errors & Patient Safety, Patient Safety and Health Information Technology E-Newsletter, Surveys on Patient Safety Culture). The AHRQ Patient Safety Network (http://www.psnet.ahrq.gov/) provides book reports, journal articles, newspaper/magazine articles, and meetings and conferences. Related to pediatrics, this site provides the tool Twenty Tips to Help Prevent Medical Errors in Children (http://www.aap.org/saferhealth care/files/5907_20tipkid.pdf).
- **Aviation Safety Reporting System** (http://asrs.arc.nasa.gov/) is a program aimed at maintaining and improving aviation safety via voluntarily submitted aviation safety incident/situation reports.
    - While this site does not discuss medication safety, it has articles and newsletters related to human factors. "Cockpit Interruptions and Distractions," which includes case examples (http://asrs.arc.nasa.gov/publications/directline/dl10_distract.htm) may be a very useful tool if applied in many areas of hospital medication-use processes.
- **Centers for Disease Control and Prevention** (CDC) (http://www.cdc.gov/; http://www.cdc.gov/medicationsafety/) is one of the major operating components of the U.S. Department of Health and Human Services. It is dedicated to protecting health and promoting quality of life through the prevention and control of disease, injury, and disability.
    - This site has a Medication Safety Program webpage (http://www.cdc.gov/medicationsafety/) that provides many helpful resources on topics such as Medication Safety Basics, Program Focus and Activities (adverse drug event monitoring, adverse drug events from select medication classes such as antibiotics and opioids, and adverse drug events in children as well as older adults), campaigns and initiatives, a resource library (publications by year and topic), the Protect Initiative (strategies to keep children safe from unintentional medication overdoses), and related links. Resources for safe injection practices may be found at http://www.cdc.gov/injectionsafety/

- **Centers for Medicare & Medicaid Services** (CMS) (http://www.cms.hhs.gov/) plays a key role in the overall direction of the U.S. health care system. Its mission is to ensure effective, up-to-date health care coverage and to promote quality care for beneficiaries.
  - Regulations and Condition of Participation (COP) may be accessed in the State Operations Manual Appendix A at http://www.cms.gov/Regulations-and-Guidance/Guidance/Manuals/downloads/som107ap_a_hospitals.pdf Accessed March 27, 2013. Relevant COPs include: 482.22 Medical Staff, 482.23 Nursing Services and 482.25 Pharmaceutical Services. Proposed changes and final updates for Rules and Regulations are released via the *Federal Register*.
- **Food and Drug Administration** (FDA) (http://www.fda.gov/default.htm) is one of the oldest and most respected consumer protection agencies in the United States. It is responsible for protecting public health by ensuring the safety, efficacy, and security of human and veterinary drugs, biological products, medical devices, the national food supply, cosmetics, and products that emit radiation.
  - The FDA site provides helpful patient safety news videos/audio broadcasts with a variety of topics (http://www.accessdata.fda.gov/psn/), safety alerts (MedWatch) (http://www.fda.gov/Safety/MedWatch/SafetyInformation/default.htm), and the FDA Drug Safety Newsletter (free push mail) that provides post marketing information to health care professionals to enhance communication of new drug safety information, raise awareness of reported adverse events, and stimulate additional adverse event reporting (http://www.fda.gov/Drugs/DrugSafety/DrugSafetyNewsletter/default.htm). The FDA website also provides information on drug recalls and shortages. http://www.fda.gov/Safety/Recalls/default.htm
- **National Institute for Occupational Safety and Health** (NIOSH) (http://www.cdc.gov/niosh/) is part of the CDC and provides national and world leadership to prevent workplace illnesses and injuries. An area of focus on this site for pharmacists and MSOs is the NIOSH list for hazardous drugs that require safe labeling and handling. http://www.cdc.gov/niosh/docs/2012-150/pdfs/2012-150.pdf
- **VA National Center for Patient Safety** (NCPS) (http://www.patientsafety.gov/); (http://www.va.gov/NCPS/) was established in 1999 to develop and nurture a culture of safety throughout the Veterans Health Administration. Their goal is the nationwide reduction and prevention of inadvertent harm to patients as a result of their care.
  - This site provides useful tools such as Healthcare Failure Mode and Effects Analysis (HFMEA) (http://www.va.gov/NCPS/SafetyTopics.html#HFMEA) and Root Cause Analysis (http://www.va.gov/ncps/CogAids/RCA/index.html#page=page-1), which are all free. Also available on this website is *VA Topics in Patient Safety (TIPS)* bimonthly newsletter with helpful articles and free toolkits (http://www.patientsafety.gov/pubs.html#tips).

State Safety Initiatives

- **Betsy Lehman Center for Patient Safety and Medical Error Reduction** (Massachusetts) (http://www.mass.gov/dph/betsylehman) serves as a clearinghouse for the development, evaluation, and dissemination of best practices for patient safety and medical error reduction. This includes but is not limited to the sponsorship of training and education programs.
    - This site has a page on medication error prevention (best practice recommendations, flash facts, medication error study, patient medication list, a description of a state board of pharmacy program to reduce prescription errors and promote optimum pharmaceutical care, and a Report on Analysis of Quality Related Events (medication errors).
- **California Hospital Patient Safety Organization** (CHPSO) (http://www.chpso.org/) is one of the largest PSOs in the nation, and through its alliances with other PSOs has access to the experience of over 700 hospitals. It is dedicated to eliminating preventable harm and improving the quality of health care delivery in California hospitals.
    - This is an excellent website. Free medication safety resources on this site include addressing drug recalls, infusion pumps, safe naming labeling and packaging, specific error reduction initiatives (e.g., IV medication concentrations standardization, ICU sedation guidelines, patient-controlled analgesia, and preventing microbial contamination), specific implementation examples (e.g., improving medication reconciliation, high-alert medication program), and health services advisory group resources.
- **Colorado Patient Safety Coalition** (http://coloradopatientsafety.org/reading.html) is a non-profit corporation dedicated to promoting patient safety through education, communication, collaboration, and encouraging best practices.
    - This site provides free safety resources such as readings, tools (e.g., 30 Safe Practices for Better Healthcare), and links.
- **Massachusetts Coalition for the Prevention of Medical Errors** (http://www.macoalition.org/) is a public-private partnership whose mission is to improve patient safety and eliminate medical errors in Massachusetts. The Coalition's membership includes consumer organizations, state agencies, hospitals, professional associations, health plans, employers, policymakers, and researchers. It promotes a systems-oriented approach to improving patient safety, identifying the causes of medical errors, and developing and supporting implementation of strategies for prevention.
    - Downloads of safety initiatives, presentations, protocols, tools (e.g., medication reconciliation), sample forms, and general resources are available free of charge.

- **Maryland Patient Safety Center** (MPSC) (http://www.marylandpatientsafety.org/) is recognized as a national leader in patient safety. MPSC engages patients and providers in improving care and communication, voluntary reporting of patient safety events and near misses that do not result in harm, and provides education and training on patient safety issues.
  - Resources available on this site include TeamSTEPPS™, patient safety links, and safety publications, tools, reports, and presentations.
- **Minnesota Alliance for Patient Safety** (MAPS) (http://www.mnpatientsafety.org/) is a partnership among the Minnesota Hospital Association, Minnesota Medical Association, Minnesota Department of Health and more than 50 other public-private health care organizations working together to improve patient safety.
  - Interesting finds on this site are video consumer stories, safety toolkits, links and resources.
- **Missouri Center for Patient Safety** (MOCPS) http://www.mocps.org/ is a private, not-for-profit corporation dedicated to fostering change throughout Missouri's health care delivery systems and across the continuum of care. It was established by The Missouri Hospital Association, the Missouri State Medical Association, and Primaris (a nonprofit health care business solution organization) in response to recommendations from the Governor's Commission for Patient Safety. The Center's vision is "a health care environment safe for all patients, in all processes, all the time."
  - General resources include websites and provider resources, free toolkits, recent safety headlines, and studies and research. The website also provides safety alerts and safety alert websites.
- **New York State Department of Health Patient Safety Center** (http://www.health.state.ny.us/nysdoh/healthinfo/patientsafety.htm).
  - This site provides patient safety tips, reports, presentations, initiatives, and a free *Quality & Safety Newsletter.* Also on this website is information on the Pharmacy Safety Forum 2010.
- **Ohio Patient Safety Institute** (OPSI) (http://www.ohiopatientsafety.org/) is an organization dedicated to improving patient safety in Ohio. The Institute is a subsidiary of the Ohio Health Council, which was founded by the Ohio Hospital Association, the Ohio State Medical Association, and the Ohio Osteopathic Association. Through this collaboration and common effort, OPSI has the ability to work with over 180 hospitals and 9000 physicians in Ohio to improve patient safety. OPSI was designated by the Agency for Healthcare Research and Quality as a patient safety organization (PSO) in February 2009.
  - This site has a medication safety section with free medication safety brochures, medication safety cards, brownbag toolkit, medication safety resources, and a section on health literacy.

- **Pennsylvania Patient Safety Authority** (http://www.patientsafetyauthority.org) is an independent state agency charged with decreasing medical errors by identifying problems and recommending solutions that promote patient safety in health care facilities. The Authority's role is non-regulatory and non-punitive.
  - This is an excellent free site with numerous patient safety articles, patient safety tools (e.g., insulin measures worksheet), and focus areas (e.g., culture of safety, operating room safety, high-alert medications, human factors engineering). It contains discipline-specific topics, patient safety advisories produced by ECRI and ISMP, patient and consumer tips, and medication error specific advisories. The subscription to the educational patient safety advisories is also free.

Websites Focused on Safety

- **Black Box RX** (http://blackboxrx.com/)
  - This website provides information on black box drug warnings by drug name and therapeutic class. Additional resources include safety labeling information from the FDA. This is a subscription service.
- **Emergency Care Research Institute** (ECRI) (www.ecri.org) is a nonprofit organization dedicated to bringing the discipline of applied scientific research to discover which medical procedures, devices, drugs, and processes are the best in enabling clinicians to improve patient care.
  - The Patient Safety Center (https://www.ecri.org/PatientSafety/Pages/default.aspx) provides public access to a few of their patient safety resources and services. Some of the free patient safety resources are derived from their membership services, including the Healthcare Risk Control (HRC) System and Health Devices Alerts. Free e-mail newsletters are available once you have registered. ECRI became a patient safety organization (PSO) in 2008 and has a website (https://www.ecri.org/pso) with information on PSO membership and support.
- **Institute for Safe Medication Practices** (ISMP) (www.ismp.org) is the nation's only nonprofit organization devoted entirely to medication error prevention and safe medication use. ISMP represents over 30 years of experience in helping health care practitioners keep patients safe, and it continues to lead efforts to improve the medication-use process. The organization is known and respected worldwide as the premier resource for impartial, timely, and accurate medication safety information.
  - It is one of the most comprehensive sites for medication safety issues and alerts, safety tools ("Do Not Crush" list, Error-Prone Abbreviations list, ISMP Assess-ERR™, to name just a few), resources, and self-assessments of safety practices. There are 4 ISMP MEDICATION SAFETY ALERT!® newsletters available for health care professionals and consumers. The ISMP *Nurse Advise-ERR* is a free newsletter available on the website. Other

ISMP newsletters, including *Acute Care Edition*, *Community/Ambulatory Care Edition*, and *Safe Medicine* (a consumer medication safety newsletter) require a paid subscription. http://www.ismp.org/Newsletters/default.asp

- **Institute of Medicine** (IOM) (http://www.iom.edu/) is an independent, non-profit organization that works outside of government to provide unbiased and authoritative advice to decision makers and the public. Their aim is to help those in government and the private sector make informed health decisions by providing evidence upon which they can rely. Many of the studies that the IOM undertakes begin as specific mandates from Congress, and others are requested by federal agencies and independent organizations.
    - There is a page on Quality and Patient Safety with Clinical Practice Guidelines, Standards for Systematic Reviews, and Innovations in Health Literacy. On this site you download them for free to read online (e.g., Standardizing Medication Labels: Confusing Patients Less; Workshop Summary; Preventing Medication Errors: Quality Chasm Series; and many more).
- **The Joint Commission** (TJC) (http://www.jointcommission.org/) is an independent, not-for-profit organization which accredits and certifies more than 18,000 U.S. health care organizations and programs. TJC accreditation and certification is recognized nationwide as a symbol of quality that reflects an organization's commitment to meeting certain performance standards.
    - This site provides accreditation and standards information, the National Patient Safety Goals; Look-alike, Sound-alike Drug List; and topics such as Sentinel Event Alerts, patient safety, dangerous abbreviations, and a Failure Mode Effect and Criticality Analysis worksheet. Some information is accessible only to accredited sites. Sign up on this site for free news and alerts.
- **The Just Culture Community** (http://www.justculture.org) was formed with the help of partners in health care and aviation to combine resources to allow for the development of increasing better methods and tools for operational safety and performance.
    - The Just Culture Algorithm, which must be purchased as part of a training product, is a structured process to guide managers through the evaluation of an event, near miss, or the analysis of a risky behavior. It is a process for conducting an investigation of the event, for identifying system contributions, and for assessing accountability (whether remedial or punitive) for those involved in the event. To use this site, you must register.
- **National Coordinating Council for Medication Error Reporting and Prevention** (NCC MERP) (www.nccmerp.org) is an independent body comprised of 27 national organizations. In 1995, the United States Pharmacopeial Convention (USP) spearheaded the formation of the NCC MERP. Leading national health care organizations collaboratively address the interdisciplinary causes of errors and to promote the safe use of medications.

- This is a valuable site for MSOs because it includes information about medication errors: definition, taxonomy, category index, and dangerous abbreviations. Numerous Council recommendations from 1996 to the present, information on how to report a medication error, and a page on consumer information for safe medication use may also be accessed.

- **National Patient Safety Agency** (NPSA) (http://www.npsa.nhs.uk/) leads and contributes to improved, safe patient care by informing, supporting, and influencing the health sector in the United Kingdom. The NPSA has a National Reporting and Learning Service.
  - Some of the helpful pages on this site include alerts and tools (includes patient safety resources), patient safety data, and the Good Practice Toolkit.
- **National Patient Safety Foundation** (NPSF) (http://www.npsf.org/). As a central voice for patient safety in the United States, NPSF is committed to a collaborative, inclusive, multi-stakeholder approach to improve the safety of care provided to patients. Free membership is needed to access many programs.
  - Its website has an extensive list of patient safety links, patient information, annual patient safety congress announcements, research funding, and a listserv archive. It has a collection of patient safety topics that is easily searchable. Also available is the *FOCUS on Patient Safety Newsletter*, NPSF's online quarterly publication covering critical issues in patient safety.
  - Patientsafety-L is a moderated listserv (online discussion forum using e-mail) devoted to thoughtful conversation toward the development of a safer health care system. Members of the NPSF patient safety listserv represent diverse backgrounds and an impressive array of knowledge and experience. A variety of individuals, including patients and families, researchers, providers, administrators, and those in the boardroom make up the listserv community.
- **Partnership for Patient Safety** (p4ps®) (www.p4ps.org) is a patient-centered initiative to advance the reliability of health care systems worldwide. p4ps® initiates focused partnerships and joint ventures with organizations and individuals that share our core values and objectives of achieving a health care system that is authentically patient-centered and systems-based.
  - The site includes information about the Partnership symposia, links, the latest health care news, products (such as patient safety books and *First, Do No Harm* film series) and projects. Resources on the site point you to the Agency for Healthcare Research and Quality's Patient Safety Network (PSNet) and Consumers Advancing Patient Safety online resource collection.
- **Pathways for Medication Safety** (http://www.medpathways.info/). This site provides a coordinated, extensive set of tools designed to reduce medication errors with a process-driven, system-based approach. The tools were developed

by the American Hospital Association, the Health Research and Educational Trust, and the Institute for Safe Medication Practices with support from The Commonwealth Fund. Tools on the site include Leading a Strategic Planning Effort, Looking Collectively at Risk, and Assessing Bedside Bar-Coding Readiness.

- **World Health Organization** (WHO) Patient Safety Center (http://www.who.int/patientsafety/en/) WHO is the directing and coordinating authority for health within the United Nations system. It is responsible for providing leadership on global health matters, shaping the health research agenda, setting norms and standards, articulating evidence-based policy options, providing technical support to countries, and monitoring and assessing health trends.
  - Their patient safety web page is found under Programmes and Projects. There are features such as a Patient Safety Solutions Survey, a free booklet, and the video "Learning from Error and Case Studies in Patient Safety Research" (measuring harm, understanding causes, identifying solutions, evaluating impact, and translating evidence into safer care).

Health Care Quality

- **Institute for Healthcare Improvement** (IHI) (http://www.ihi.org/ihi) works with health care providers and leaders throughout the world to fulfill the promise that everyone deserves safe and effective health care. It is an independent not-for-profit organization that focuses on building the will for change, identifying and testing new models of care, and ensuring the broadest possible adoption of best practices and effective innovations.
  - This site has a wealth of safety and quality programs, resources and tools, including an Adverse Drug Event Trigger Tool, Culture of Safety, Root Cause Analysis, Failure Modes and Effects Analysis, and sections on high-hazard medications, medication reconciliation, medication core processes, and more.
- **The Leapfrog Group** (http://www.leapfroggroup.org/) is a voluntary program aimed at mobilizing employer purchasing power to alert the U.S. health industry that big leaps in health care safety, quality, and customer value will be recognized and rewarded. Among other initiatives, Leapfrog rewards hospitals that have a proven record of high-quality care.
  - This site provides hospital resources (e.g., Ten Case Studies of Improving Patient Safety, Mistake-Proofing the Design of the Healthcare Process) and consumer resources (Leapfrog hospital ratings).

- **National Quality Forum** (NQF) (http://www.qualityforum.org/) operates under a three-part mission to improve the quality of U.S. health care by building consensus on national priorities and goals for performance improvement and working in partnership to achieve them, endorsing national consensus standards for measuring and publicly reporting on performance, and promoting the attainment of national goals through education and outreach programs.
  - It has a patient safety page with projects (e.g., Serious Reportable Events in Healthcare, Patient Safety Measures and Safe Practices), standards (Patient Safety Measures) and resources (Safe Practices in Better Healthcare).
- **National Center for Human Factors Engineering in Healthcare** (NCHFEH) (http://chfeh.org/); (http://medicalhumanfactors.net/)
  - These sites are related, and they define human factors engineering (HFE) and its application to health care. They provide numerous publications, presentations, and HFE-related links. Courses and conferences are also highlighted. This site also provides a link (http://chfeh.org/epharm/index.html) called the "Emergency Pharmacist Research Center," aimed at increasing the use of clinical pharmacists in emergency medicine.
- **Texas Medical Institute of Technology** (TMIT) (http://www.safetyleaders.org/) is a medical research organization dedicated to accelerating performance solutions that save lives, save money, and build value in communities. TMIT applies the Institute of Medicine's (IOM) design principles of patient centeredness, evidence-based medicine, and systems performance improvement.
  - Use of the site requires free registration. This site links to emotionally powerful patient safety documentaries such as "Chasing Zero" (with Dennis Quaid), "Out of the Danger Zone," "Greatness by Accident," and "Staying Alive." (http://www.safetyleaders.org/pages/chasingZeroDocumentary.jsp). Other helpful resources include the Global Trigger Tool, free safety workshops and webinars, and safety podcasts with free subscriptions to electronic concepts and a tools and resources feed.
- **University HealthSystem Consortium** (UHC) (http://www.uhc.edu/) is an alliance of academic medical centers and their affiliated hospitals representing approximately 90% of the nation's non-profit academic medical centers. Its vision of the future is to help members attain national leadership in health care by achieving excellence in quality, safety, and cost effectiveness. Membership provides additional benefits to resources.

- **U.S. Pharmacopeial Convention** (USP) (http://www.usp.org/) is a non-governmental authority that sets official public standards for prescription and over-the-counter medicines and other health care products manufactured or sold in the United States. USP's standards are recognized and used in more than 130 countries around the globe.
  - On this site is a page with patient safety tools and resources (http://www.usp.org/hqi/patientSafety/resources/) including USP's Drug Error Finder (a free tool for accessing look-alike/sound-alike drug names), posters and presentations (e.g., Medication Errors in the Operating Room, Emergency Department, Patient's Home, Day Surgery Settings, and Post Anesthesia Care Unit), congressional testimonies, published articles, USP patient safety newsletters, alerts, recommendations, and resources.

Websites Focused on Consumers

- **BeMedWise** (http://www.bemedwise.org/) is a public education initiative by the National Council on Patient Information and Education (NCPIE) (see below). BeMedWise seeks to promote a better understanding that over-the-counter drug products are serious medicines and must be taken with care.
  - This site provides pages such as Know Your Medicine, Drug Facts Label, Be MedWise, tips, a quiz, FAQs, a brochure, a toolkit, and public service announcements. It also has a helpful resource center for the consumer (e.g., FDA Consumer Education: Over-the-Counter Medicine) with many helpful resources.
- **Consumers Advancing Patient Safety** (CAPS) (http://www.patientsafety.org/) is a consumer-led nonprofit organization formed as a collective voice for individuals, families, and healers who wish to prevent harm in health care encounters through partnership and collaboration.
  - The website shares patient stories of medical errors, provides a CAPS Toolkit called "Taking Charge of your Healthcare: Your Path to Being an Empowered Patient," and patient safety, general medical information, and communication and education resources.
- **Consumer Med Safety** (http://www.consumermedsafety.org/)
  - This site is made available to consumers by the Institute for Safe Medication Practices (ISMP). It provides drug alerts to consumers, tools, and resources (commonly confused drug names, drug information, medication identification), and consumer safe-medicine articles. This is a great medication safety site for consumers.

- **Medication Use Safety Training** (MUST) for Seniors™ (http://www.mustforseniors.org/)
    - From the NCPIE (see below) this program is designed as an interactive, national initiative to promote safe and appropriate medicine use by older adults. It has web pages such as Facts: Older Adults and Medicine Use, program materials, and other resources.
- **My Medicine List™** (http://www.ashpfoundation.org/MainMenuCategories/PracticeTools/MyMedicineList/MyMedicineListREFLogo.aspx)
    - This is a tool that patients can use to keep track of the medications they are taking, including the medication's name and dose. The list is a result of the ASHP Foundation's Continuity of Care in Medication Use Summit and was developed by a health literacy expert from Emory University.
- **National Council on Patient Information and Education** (NCPIE) (http://www.talkaboutrx.org/) is a coalition of over 125 diverse organizations whose mission is to stimulate and improve communication of information on appropriate medicine use to consumers and health care professionals. It is the nation's leading authority for informing the general public and health care professionals about safe medicine use through better communication.
    - This site has pages with tools for consumers, educational resources for purchase or free download, and medication use statistics, publications, and patient medication information.
- **Persons United Limiting Substandards and Errors in Healthcare** (PULSE) (www.pulseamerica.org) is a nonprofit support group and organization dedicated to raising awareness about patient safety and reducing medical errors through advocacy, education, and support. They work to empower the public to make informed decisions, increase effective communication and respect between health care providers and the public, and create community partnerships leading to safer health care environments.
    - On the website you can find: advocacy (Patient/Survivor Advocacy), education (Medical Error Research and Patient Safety Tips), news and events, true stories regarding patients who have been harmed, and a True Stories Pictorial (faces of medical errors).
- **Safe Medication** (http://www.safemedication.com/) is a consumer site made available by the American Society of Health-System Pharmacists (ASHP).
    - It features complete, easy-to-read information on more than 12,000 drug products. This information is based on the ASHP's drug information resources that are developed independently by pharmacists and other medication experts. The site provides Medication Tips and Tools, Pharmacist's Journal, How to Administer, and My Medicine List™.

- **Safe Patient Project** (http://www.safepatientproject.org/2009/11/voice4patients.html/) is a Consumers Union campaign focused on eliminating medical harm, improving FDA oversight of prescription drugs, and promoting disclosure laws that give information to consumers about health care safety and quality. The campaign also works to improve drug safety by ensuring that consumers have full information about prescription drugs (such as in direct-to-consumer ads and access to clinical trial results), by strengthening oversight of the FDA, and by ending practices that create conflicts of interest (such as drug company gifts to doctors).
  - The site shares patient stories of medical errors and numerous drug safety topics.

Journals

- *American Journal of Health-System Pharmacy* (AJHP) http://www.ajhp.org/
- *Association of periOperative Registered Nurses (AORN) Journal* http://www.aorn.org/AORNJournal/
- *BMJ Quality & Safety* http://qualitysafety.bmj.com/
- *Hospital Pharmacy* http://www.thomasland.com/hospitalpharmacy.html
- *International Journal for Quality in Health Care* http://intqhc.oxfordjournals.org/ (search on "medication safety")
- *Joint Commission Journal on Quality and Patient Safety* http://store.jcrinc.com/the-joint-commission-journal-on-quality-and-patient-safety/
- *Journal of the American Medical Association* (JAMA) http://jama.ama-assn.org/
- *Journal of Clinical Outcomes Management* http://www.turner-white.com/jc/contentjc.php (search on "medication safety")
- *Journal of Patient Safety* http://journals.lww.com/journalpatientsafety/pages/default.aspx
- *Patient Safety & Quality Healthcare* http://www.psqh.com/

Applications (Apps)

- **Doctor's Digest** (free)—delivering real-time medical and safety alerts from ISMP and Practice Management tips from Doctor's Digest. www.doctorsdigest.net/
- **MedWatcher; Drug Safety Reporting** (free)—stay up to date with the latest news and government safety alerts for prescription medicines. Submit side effects experienced to the U.S. Food and Drug Administration (FDA) to make drugs safer for all. http://itunes.apple.com/us/app/medwatcher-drug-safety-reporting/id391767048?mt=8

- **Product Recalls** (from the FDA, free) http://apps.usa.gov/product-recalls-2/
- **Rx Shortages** (free/$)—searchable information on drug shortages, with capability to report new shortages; links to the ASHP website on drug shortages. http://mickschroeder.com/rxshortages/

Journal Articles

Adverse Drug Events (ADEs) and Adverse Drug Reactions (ADRs)

Bates DW, Boyle DL, Vander Vliet MB, et al. Relationship between medication errors and adverse drug events. *J Gen Intern Med.* 1995;10:199-205.

Bates DW, Cullen DJ, Laird N, et al. Incidence of adverse drug events and potential adverse drug events. Implications for prevention. ADE prevention study group. *JAMA.* 1995;274:29-34.

Bates DW. Drugs and adverse reactions: how worried should we be? *JAMA.* 1998;279(15):1216-1217.

Brennan TA, Leape LL, Laird NM et al. Incidence of adverse events and negligence in hospitalized patients. Results of the Harvard Medical Practice Study I. *N Engl J Med.* 1991;324(6):370-376.

Cavuto NJ, Woosley RL, Sale M. Pharmacies and the prevention of fatal drug interactions. *JAMA.* 1996;275(14):1086-1087.

Classen DC, Pestonik SL, Evans RS, et al. Adverse drug events in hospitalized patients. *JAMA.* 1997;277:301-306.

Cullen DJ, Sweitzer BJ, Bates, DW, et al. Preventable adverse drug events in hospitalized patients: A comparative study of intensive care and general units. *Critical Care Med.* 1997;25:1289-1297.

Gholami K, Shalviri G. Factors associated with preventability, predictability and severity of adverse drug reactions. *Ann Pharmocother.* 1999;33:236-240.

Golz G, Fitchett L. Nurses' perspectives on a serious adverse drug event. *Am J Health Syst Pharm.* 1999;56:904-907.

Gurwitz JH, Field TS, Harrold LR, et al. Incidence and preventability of adverse drug events among older adults in the ambulatory setting. *JAMA.* 2003;289:1107-1116.

Kaushal R, Bates DW, Landrigan C, et al. Medication errors and adverse drug events in pediatric inpatients. *JAMA.* 2001; 285:2114-2120.

Lazarou J, Pomeranz BH, Corey PN. Incidence of adverse drug reaction in hospitalized patients. *JAMA* 1998; 279:1200-1205.

Leape LL, Cullen DJ, Demspey-Clapp M et al. Pharmacist participation on physician rounds and adverse drug events in the intensive care unit. *JAMA.* 1999;282(3):267-270.

Leape LL. Preventing adverse drug events. *Am J Health Syst Pharm.* 1995;52(4): 379-382.

Leape LL, Bates DW, Cullen DJ et al for the ADE prevention group. Systems analysis of adverse drug events. *JAMA.* 1995;274(1):35-43.

Leape LL. Reporting of adverse events. *N Engl J Med.* 2002;347(20):1633-1638.

Nebeker JR, Barach P, Samore MH. Clarifying adverse drug events: A clinician's guide to terminology, documentation, and reporting. *Ann Intern Med.* 2004;140(10):795-801.

Raschke RA, Gollihare B, Wunderlich TA, et al. A computer alert system to prevent injury from adverse drug events. *JAMA.* 1998;280(15):1317-1320.

Rozich JD, Haraden CR, Resar RK. Adverse drug event trigger tool: a practical methodology for measuring medication related harm. *Qual Saf Health Care.* 2003;12:194-200.

Seeger JD, Kong SX, Schumock GT. Characteristics associated with ability to prevent adverse drug reactions in hospitalized patients. *Pharmacotherapy.* 1998;18(6):1284-1289.

Thomas EJ, Brennan TA. Incidence and types of preventable adverse events in elderly patients: population based review of medical records. *BMJ.* 2000;320:741-744.

Thomas EJ, Studdert DM, Burstin HR, et al. Incidence and types of adverse events and negligent care in Utah and Colorado. *Med Care.* 2000;38:261-271.

Weideman RA, Bernstein IH, McKinney WP. Pharmacist recognition of potential drug interactions. *Am J Health Syst Pharm.* 1999 Aug 1;56(15):1524-1529.

Costs of Error and Economic Impact

Bates DW, Spell N, Cullen DJ, et al. The costs of adverse drug events in hospitalized patients. *JAMA.* 1997;277:307-311.

Bootman JL, Harrison DL, Cox E. The health care cost of drug-related morbidity and mortality in nursing facilities. *Arch Intern Med.* 1997;157(18):2089-2096.

Classen DC, Pestotnik SL, Evans et al.. Adverse drug events in hospitalized patients. Excess length of stay, extra costs, and attributable mortality. *JAMA.* 1997;277(4):301-306.

Johnson JA, Bootman JL. Drug-related morbidity and mortality: A cost-of-illness model. *Arch Intern Med.* 1995;155(18):1949-1956.

Johnson JA, Bootman JL. Drug-related morbidity and mortality and the economic impact of pharmaceutical care. *Am J Health Syst Pharm.* 1997;54(5):554-558.

Rothschild JM, Federico FA, Gandhi TK. Analysis of medication-related malpractice claims: Causes, preventability, and costs. *Arch Intern Med.* 2002;162:2414-2420.

Schneider PJ, Gift MG, Lee YP, et al. Cost of medication-related problems at a university hospital. *Am J Health Syst Pharm.* 1995;52(21):2415-2418.

Thomas EJ, Studdert DM, Newhouse JP, et al. Costs of medical injuries in Utah and Colorado. *Inquiry.* 1999;36:255-264.

Error Management/Quality/Prevention and Culture

Berwick DM, Leape LL. Reducing errors in medicine: It is time to take this more seriously. *BMJ.* 1999;319(7203):136-137.

Cohen MR. Cooperative approaches to medication error management. *Top Hosp Pharm Manage.* 1991;11(Apr):53-65.

Cohen MR, Anderson RW, Attilio RM et al. Preventing medication errors in cancer chemotherapy. *Am J Health-Syst Pharm.* 1996;53:737-746.

Cohen, MR. Medication naming, labeling, and packaging. *Am J Health Syst Pharm.* 2002;59(9): 876-877; author reply 879.

Dang D, Feroli RE, Gill C, et al. Quest for the Ideal: A Redesign of the Medication Use System. *J Nurs Care Qual.* 2007;22(1):11-19.

Frankel A, Graydon-Baker E, Neppl C, et al. Patient safety leadership walkrounds. *Jt Com Qual Saf.* 2003;29:16-26.

Goldspiel BR, DeChristoforo R, Daniels CE. Continuous-improvement approach for reducing the number of chemotherapy-related medication errors. *Am J Health Syst Pharm.* 2000;57:S4-S9.

Henry TR, Azuma L, Shaban HM. Learning and process improvement after a sentinel event. *Hosp Pharm.* 1999;34 839-844.

Hsia DC. Medicare quality improvement: bad apples or bad systems? *JAMA.* 2003;289:354-356.

Hutchinson D. Getting to the bottom of a sentinel event. *Am J Health Syst Pharm.* 1999;56(30):2031-2032.

Knudsen P, Herborg H, et al. Preventing medication errors in community pharmacy: frequency and seriousness of medication errors. *Qual Saf Health Care.* 2007;16:291-296.

Kelly W, Rucker D. Compelling features of a safe medication-use system. *Am J Health Syst Pharm.* 2006;63:1461-8.

Manasse HR. Pharmacists and the quality-of-care imperative. *Am J Health Syst Pharm.* 2000;57(12):1170-1172.

Meyer-Massetti C, Cheng CM, Schwappach DLB et al. Systematic review of medication safety assessment methods. *Am J Health Syst Pharm.* 2011;68:227-240.

Myers CE. Medication misadventures: A policy of openness and learning. *Am J Health Syst Pharm.*56(9):863.

Nolan TW. System changes to improve patient safety. *BMJ.* 2000;320(7237):771-773.

Ovretveit J, Bate P, Cleary P, et al. Quality collaboratives: lessons from research. *Qual Safety Health Care.* 2002;11:345-351.

Ryan KD. Driving fear out of the medication-use process so that improvement can occur. *Am J Health Syst Pharm.* 1999;56(17):1765-1769.

Schneider PJ. Creating an environment for improving the medication-use process. *Am J Health Syst Pharm.* 1999;56(17):1769-1972.

Sirio CA, Segel KT, Keyser DJ, et al. Pittsburgh Regional Healthcare Initiative: A systems approach to achieving perfect patient care. *Health Aff (Millwood)* 2003;22(5):157-165.

Tucker LL, Cohen MR, Davis NM. Orientation teaching tool to prevent medication error. *Hosp Pharm.* 1994;29(11):984,986-988,991.

Error, ADE, and ADR Detection and Reporting

Betz RP, Levy HB. An interdisciplinary method of classifying and monitoring medication errors. *Am J Hosp Pharm.* 1985;42(8):1724-1732.

Cohen MR. Why error reporting systems should be voluntary. *BMJ.* 2000;320(7237):728-729.

Colodny L, Spillane J. Toward increased reporting of adverse drug reactions. *Hosp Pharm.* 1999;34:1179-1185.

Dean BS, Barber ND. A validated, reliable method of scoring the severity of medication errors. *Am J Health Syst Pharm.* 1999;56(1):57-62.

Dunn EB, Wolfe JJ. Medication error classification and avoidance. *Hosp Pharm.* 1997;32:860-865.

Edgar TA, Lee DS, Cousins DD. Experience with a national medication error reporting program. *Am J Hosp Pharm* 1994;51(10):1335-1338.

Flynn EA, Barker KN, Pepper GA, et al. Comparison of methods for detecting medication errors in 36 hospitals and skilled-nursing facilities. *Am J Health Syst Pharm.* 2002;59(5):436-446.

Handler S, Perera S, Olshansky EF, et al. Identifying modifiable barriers to medication error reporting in the nursing home setting. *J Am Med Dir Assoc.* 2007;8:568-574.

Handler SM, Nace DA, Studenski SA, et al. Medication error reporting in long-term care. *Am J Geriatr Pharmacother.* 2004;2(3):190-196.

Rozich JD, Haraden CR, Resar RK. Adverse drug event trigger tool: a practical methodology for measuring medication related harm. *Qual Saf Health Care.* 2003;12:194-200.

Santell JP, Hicks RW, McMeekin J, et al. Medication errors: experience of the United States Pharmacopeia (USP) MEDMARX reporting system. *J Clin Pharmacol.* 2003;43(7):760-767.

Savage SW, Schneider PJ, Pedersen CA. Utility of an online medication error reporting system. *Am J Health Syst Pharm.* 2005;62(21):2265–2270.

Schneider PJ, Hartwig SC. Use of severity-indexed medication error reports to improve quality. *Hosp Pharm.* 1994;29(3):205-206,208-211.

Human Factors

Gawron VJ, Drury CG, Fairbanks, RJ et al. Medical error and human factors engineering: Where are we now? *Am J Med Qual.* 2006;21(1):57-67.

Ginsburg G. Human factors engineering: A tool for medical device evaluation in hospital procurement decision-making. *J Biomed Inform.* 2005;38(3):213-219.

Gosbee JW. Human factors engineering and patient safety. *Qual Saf Health Care.* 2002;11:352-354.

Gosbee JW, Anderson T. Human factors engineering design demonstrations can enlighten your RCA team. *Qual Saf Health Care.* 2003;12:119-121.

Gosbee JW. Introduction to the human factors engineering series. *Jt Comm J Qual Saf.* 2004;30(4):215-219.

Hellier E, Edwirthy J, Derbyshire N, et al. Considering the impact of medicine label design characteristics on patient safety. *Ergonomics.* 2006;49(5-6):617-630.

Karsh BT, Holden RJ, Alper SJ, et al. Safety by design. A human factors engineering paradigm for patient safety: designing to support the performance of the health care professional. *Qual Saf Health Care.* 2006;15:59-65.

Leape LL. "Smart" pumps: A cautionary tale of human factors engineering. *Crit Care Med.* 2005;33(3):679-680.

Lin L, Vicente KJ, Doyle DJ. Patient safety, potential adverse drug events, and medical device design: A human factors engineering approach. *J Biomed Inform.* 2001;34(4):274-284.

IV Medication Safety

Adachi W, Lodolce AE. Use of failure mode and effects analysis in improving the safety of IV drug administration. *Am J Health Syst Pharm.* 2005;62(9):917-920.

ASHP Reports. Proceedings of a summit on preventing patient harm and death from IV medication errors. July 14–15, 2008. *Am J Health Syst Pharm.* 2008;65:2367-2379.

Eskew JA, Jacobi J, Buss WF, et al. Using innovative technologies to set new safety standards for the infusion of intravenous medications. *Hosp Pharm.* 2002;37:1179-1189.

Nicholas, PK. Toward Safer IV Medication Administration. *Am J Neurosci.* 2005;Supplement:25-30.

Sanborn MD, Moody ML, Harder KA, et al. Second consensus development conference on the safety of intravenous drug delivery systems-2008. *Am J Health Syst Pharm.* 2009;66:185-192.

Schneider PJ. A review of the safety of intravenous drug delivery systems. *Hosp Pharm.* 1999;34:1044-1056.

Just Culture

Connor M, Duncombe D, Barclay E, et al. Creating a fair and just culture: One institution's path toward organizational change. *Jt Comm J Qual Patient Saf.* 2007;33(10):617-624.

Frankel AS, Leonard MW, Denham CR. Fair and just culture, team behavior, and leadership engagement: The tools to achieve high reliability. *Health Serv Res.* 2006;41:1690-1709.

Khatri N, Brown GD, Kicks LL. From a blame culture to a just culture in health care. *Health Care Manage Rev.* 2009;34(4):312-322.

Smetzer JL, Cohen MR. Lessons from the Denver medication error/criminal negligence case: look beyond blaming individuals. *Hosp Pharm.* 1998;33:640-657.

Medication Errors (Prescribing, Dispensing, Administering)

Allan EL, Barker KN. Fundamentals of medication error research. *Am J Hosp Pharm.* 1990;47:555-571.

Ashley ES, Kirk K, Fowler VG. Patient detection of a drug dispensing error by use of physician provided drug samples. *Pharmacotherapy.* 2002;22:1642-1643.

Barker KN, Flynn EA, Pepper GA, et al. Medication errors observed in 36 health care facilities. *Arch Intern Med.* 2002;162:1897-1903.

Bond CA, Raehl CL. Pharmacist assessment of dispensing errors: risk factors, practice sites, professional functions, and satisfaction. *Pharmacotherapy.* 2001;21:614-626.

Bryony D, Schachter M, Vincent C, et al. Causes of prescribing errors in hospital inpatients: a prospective study. *Lancet.* 2002;359:1373-1378.

Cohen MR, Proulx SM, Crawford SY. Survey of hospital systems and common serious medication errors. *J Healthcare Risk Manage.* 1998;18(1):16-27.

Flynn EA, Barker KN, Carnahan BJ. National observational study of prescription dispensing accuracy and safety in 50 pharmacies. *J Am Pharm Assoc.* 2003;43:191-200.

Hasegawa GR. Responsibility for medication errors. *Am J Health Syst Pharm.* 1999;56(3):215.

Kistner UA, Keith MR, Sergeant KA, et al. Accuracy of dispensing in a high-volume, hospital-based outpatient pharmacy. *Am J Hosp Pharm.* 1994;51(22):2793-2797.

Kuiper SA, McCreadie SR, et al. Medication error in inpatient pharmacy operations and technologies for improvement. *Am J Health Syst Pharm.* 2007;64(9):955-959.

Leape LL, Berwick DM. Five years after to err is human: What have we learned? *JAMA.* 2005;293(19):2384-2390.

Lesar TS, Briceland L, Stein DS. Factors related to errors in medication prescribing. *JAMA.* 1997;277(4):312-317.

Lesar TS, Lomaestro BM, Pohl H. Medication-prescribing errors in a teaching hospital. A 9-year experience. *Arch Intern Med.* 1997;157(14):1569-1576.

Lesar TS. Tenfold medication dose prescribing errors. *Ann Pharmacother.* 2002; 36:1833-1839.

Manasse HR. Medication use in an imperfect world: drug misadventuring as an issue of public policy. Part 1. *Am J Hosp Pharm.* 1989;46:929-944.

Manasse HR. Medication use in an imperfect world: drug misadventuring as an issue of public policy. Part 2. *Am J Hosp Pharm.* 1989;46:1141-1152.

Means BJ, Derewicz HJ, Lamy PP. Medication errors in a multidose and a computer-based unit dose drug distribution system. *Am J Hosp Pharm.* 1975;32(2):186-191.

Phillips J, Beam S, Brinker A, et al. Retrospective analysis of mortalities associated with medication errors. *Am J Health Syst Pharm.* 2001;58:1835-1841.

Prot S, Fontan JE, Alberto C, et al. Drug administration errors and their determinants in pediatric in-patients. *Int J Qual Health Care.* 2005;17:381-389.

Santell JP, Kowiatek JG, Weber RJ, Hicks RW, Sirio CA: Medication errors resulting from computer entry by non-prescribers. *Am J Health Syst Pharm.* 2009;66:843-853.

Sellers JA. Too many medication errors, not enough pharmacists. *Am J Health Syst Pharm.* 2000;15:57:337.

Leadership, Medication Safety Officers, and Programs

Burgess LH, Cohen MR, Denham CR. A new leadership role for pharmacists: a prescription for change. *Patient Saf* 2010;6:31-37.

Kowiatek JG, Weber RJ, Skledar S, Sirio C. Medication safety manager in an academic medical center. *Am J Health Syst Pharm.* 2004;61:58-64.

Mark S, Weber RJ. Developing a medication patient safety program: Infrastructure and strategy. *Hosp Pharm.* 2007;42(2):149-154.

Mark S, Weber RJ. Developing a medication patient safety program, part 2: process and implementation. *Hosp Pharm.* 2007;42(3):249-254.

McCarthy ID, Cohen MR, Kateiva J, McAllister JC, Ploetz PA. What should a pharmacy manager do when a serious medication error occurs? A panel discussion. *Am J Hosp Pharm.* 1992;49(16):1405-1412.

Phillips MA. Institutionwide medication safety program. *Am J Health Syst Pharm.* 2003. 60(21):2198-200.

Rozich JD, Resar RK. Medication safety: one organization's approach to the challenge. *JCOM.* 2001;8(10):27-34.

Sanks RJ. A pharmacy manager's perspective on a serious adverse drug event. *Am J Health Syst Pharm.* 1999;56:907-909.

Schneider PJ. Five worthy aims for pharmacy's clinical leadership to pursue in improving medication use. *Am J Health-Syst Pharm.* 1999;56:2549-2552.

Weeks WB, Bagian JP. Making the business case for patient safety. *Jt Comm J Qual Saf.* 2003;29:51-54.

Technology and Automation (CPOE, e-MAR, Automated Dispensing Machines)

Bates DW. Using information technology to reduce rates of medication errors in hospitals. *BMJ.* 2000;320(7237):788-791.

Bates DW, Teich JM, Lee J, et al. The impact of computerized physician order entry on medication error prevention. *J Am Med Inf Assoc.* 1999;6:313-321.

Bates DW, Gawande AA. Improving safety with information technology. *N Engl J Med.* 2003;348(25):2526-2534.

Bates DW, Leape LL, Cullen, et al. Effect of computerized physician order entry and a team intervention on prevention of serious medication errors. *JAMA.* 1998;280(15):1311-1316.

Eskew JA, Jacobi J, Buss WF, et al. Using innovative technologies to set new safety standards for the infusion of intravenous medications. *Hosp Pharm.* 2002;37:1179-1189.

Hammond J, Bermann M, Chen B, et al. Incorporation of a computerized human patient simulator in critical care training: a preliminary report. *J Trauma.* 2002; 53:1064-1067.

Kaushal R, Bates DW. Information technology and medication safety: What is the benefit? *Qual & Saf in Health Care.* 2002;11:261-265.

Schiff GD, Rucker TD. Computerized prescribing: building the electronic infrastructure for better medication usage. *JAMA.* 1998;279(13):1024-1029.

Schneider P J. Using technology to enhance measurement of drug-use safety. *Am J Health Syst Pharm.* 2002;59:2330-2332.

Books

Aspden P, Wolcott JA, Bootman JL, et al., eds. *Preventing Medication Errors*. Washington, DC: National Academy Press; 2007.

Cohen MR, ed. *Medication Errors*. 2nd ed. Washington, DC: American Pharmaceutical Association; 2007.

Committee on Quality of Health Care in America, Institute of Medicine. *Crossing the Quality Chasm: A New Health System for the 21st Century*. Washington, DC: National Academy Press; 2001.

Cousins DD, ed. *Advancing Patient Safety in U.S. Hospitals: Basic Strategies for Success*. Rockville, MD: US Pharmacopeia; 2004.

Dekker S. *The Field Guide to Understanding Human Error.* Burlington, VT: Ashgate; 2006.

Joint Commission Resources. *The Pharmacist's Role in Patient Safety*. Oakbrook Terrace, IL: Joint Commission Resources; 2007.

Kohn LT, Corrigan JM, Donaldson MS. eds. *To Err Is Human, Building a Safer Health System*. Washington, DC: National Academy Press; 2000.

Kirschling TE, ed. *The Handbook on Storing and Securing Medications*. 2nd ed. Chicago, Illinois: Joint Commission Resources; 2009.

Manasse Jr HR, Thompson KK, ed. *Medication Safety: A Guide for Health Care Facilities*. Bethesda, MD: American Society of Health-System Pharmacists; 2005.

McNeil MJ, ed. *ASHP's Safety and Quality Pearls*. Bethesda, MD: American Society of Health-System Pharmacists; 2008.

Phelps, PK, ed. *Smart Infusion Pumps*. Bethesda, MD: American Society of Health-System Pharmacists; 2011.

Reason J, ed. *Human Error*. Cambridge: Cambridge University Press; 1990.

Saine DR, ed. *ASHP's Safety and Quality Pearls 2*. Bethesda, MD: American Society of Health-System Pharmacists; 2009.

Wachter, RM, Shojania KG. *Internal Bleeding*. New York: Rugged Land; 2004.

Zipperer L, Cushman S, eds. *Lessons in Patient Safety*. Chicago: National Patient Safety Foundation; 2001.

Medication Safety Blogs

Blogs typically include features such as comments and links to increase user interactivity. They are as good as the opinion and knowledge base of the blogger(s). Some are individuals and some blogs are part of organizational websites. A few examples related to medication safety are below:

- Jerry Fahrni, Pharmacy Informatics and Technology: http://jerryfahrni.com/category/medication-safety/
- ASHP Connect: http://connect.ashp.org/ASHP/ASHP/Blogs/Default.aspx
- Florence dot com: http://florencedotcom.blogspot.com/
- American Society of Medication Safety Officers blog: http://asmso.org/blog

Glossary of Terms

Accreditation—Voluntary process wherein a health care organization meets established standards or criteria as determined through initial and periodic reviews.

Adverse Drug Event—Harm resulting from use of a medication.

Adverse Drug Reaction—An idiosyncratic reaction or other adverse effect of a medication that is not preventable (i.e., not a medication error).

Adverse Event—An undesirable occurrence associated with the use of a medical product in a patient, directly associated with care or services provided within the jurisdiction of a medical facility.

Alert Fatigue—Tendency to disregard or not thoroughly review pop-up alerts/warnings in an information system due to high-volume, low-significance, or nuisance alerts.

Balanced Scorecard—A tool to display and link the organization's mission and vision to the strategic goals and objectives.

Blame and Train Culture—A culture in which the person is assumed to be able to perform without error, if properly educated and motivated. Latent failures are not considered. Errors are attributed to laziness, negligence, or incompetence, resulting in blaming and/or retraining the person that made the error.

Change—To transform or guide into a different direction.

Common Cause Analysis—A technique used to review information from multiple events to identify their common causes; also referred to as an *aggregate root cause analysis*.

Computerized Provider Order Entry (CPOE)—Direct entry of medical orders into a health care system's electronic health records by licensed independent practitioners or other staff with specific ordering privileges and not by clinical or administrative support staff; may or may not include direct integration with other information systems such as pharmacy, laboratory, or radiology.

Continuous Quality Improvement—A systematic, organized approach for continually improving processes to deliver quality services and products.

Dashboard—An "at-a-glance" visual display of selected metrics or key performance indicators often used to track the individual initiatives, goals, and objectives at a more local level.

Data Mining—The process of extracting meaningful (useful and potentially actionable) information from large databases such as administrative and clinical health records (sifting through volumes of data to find hidden material of value).

Detection Sensitivity Level—The rate at which errors that occur are actually reported and recognized by the organization. A high detection sensitivity level is demonstrated through a high error reporting rate.

End-User—Primary user of a technology product, often frontline staff involved in direct patient care.

Error Trap—Component of failure mode and effects analysis that seeks to prevent error through mechanisms aimed at detecting the error; elimination of alternatives or choices that may lead to error or potential mix-up/confusion; preventing actions that would result in or contribute to the error; and/or minimizing error consequence should it occur.

Failure Mode and Effects Analysis—Problem-solving tool used to analyze a process or system to identify possible modes of failure, and potential consequences of those failures.

Focused Standards Assessment (FSA)—The Joint Commission online tool for subscribers; annual process of performing a gap analysis between practice in your organization and regulatory requirements and correcting deficiencies by developing and completing actions plans with measures of success when indicated.

FOCUS-PDCA Cycle—A nine-step process (Find-Organize-Clarify-Understand-Select-Plan-Do-Check-Act) that emphasizes work teams, data-driven analysis, careful planning, organized implementation, and measurement of results.

Food and Drug Administration MedWatch—The Food and Drug Administration safety information and adverse event reporting program.

Forcing Function—A design feature that, when employed by the user, will automatically guide the proper use of a device or process to prevent error.

Gap Analysis—A process tool to evaluate and compare differences between two items; often used to compare actual performance with desired performance and to identify action steps needed to achieve the desired state.

Global Trigger Tool—A tool developed by the Institute for Healthcare Improvement that assists with identification of adverse events. This tool's methodology allows for the identification of various "triggers" when reviewing charts in order to determine the presence of adverse events. Examples of triggers include an abnormal lab result, a stop order, or administration of an antidote.

Handoff—The process of transferring responsibility for care; the interactive transfer of information, allowing for questioning between the giver and receiver(s).

High Reliability Organization—A complex organization with high risk for catastrophic error, with a very successful track record of maintaining a high level of safety over a long period of time.

High-Alert or High-Risk Medications—High-alert or high-risk medications have a greater capacity to cause significant patient harm if used incorrectly.

Hindsight Bias—The tendency for those evaluating an error to overestimate what they would have known, and what others should have known at the time of the error.

Human Error—The failure of planned actions to achieve their desired ends, without the intervention of some unforeseeable event. Human errors can be further divided into slips, lapses, and mistakes.

Human Factors—"The scientific discipline concerned with the understanding of interactions among humans and other elements of a system, and the profession that applies theory, principles, data, and methods to design in order to optimize human well-being and overall system performance."

Inattentional Blindness—The person performing a task fails to see what should have been plainly visible and, later, he or she cannot explain the lapse.

Just Culture—A culture that recognizes the contribution of systems in error along with a focus on behavioral choices and accountability. Just Culture distinguishes between acceptable and unacceptable behavior, between unsafe acts and the blatant disregard of safety procedures with which most peers would comply. Just Culture is one component of an overarching safety culture.

Look-Alike/Sound-Alike Medications—Similar medication names, either written or spoken, which may lead to potentially harmful medication errors when they are confused with each other.

Meaningful Use—Term used to describe a component of the 2009 American Recovery and Reinvestment Act that provides governmental monetary incentives for health care organizations that implement specific levels and elements of an electronic health record and various health care technologies.

Medication—According to The Joint Commission, any prescription medications, sample medications, herbal remedies, vitamins, nutraceuticals, vaccines, or over-the-counter drugs; diagnostic and contrast agents used on or administered to persons to diagnose, treat, or prevent disease or other abnormal conditions; radioactive medications, respiratory therapy treatments, parenteral nutrition, blood derivatives, and intravenous solutions (plain, with electrolytes and/or drugs); and any product designated by the Food and Drug Administration (FDA) as a drug. This definition of medication does not include enteral nutrition solutions (which are considered food products), oxygen, and other medical gases.

Medication Error—An error occurring in any step of the medication-use process; any preventable event that may result in incorrect medication use or patient harm.

Mistake/Error-Proofing—Implementation of fail-safe mechanisms to prevent errors from occurring with a process; for example, an ATM that gives the debit card back before the cash so that the card is not forgotten.

National Coordinating Council for Medication Error Reporting and Prevention (NCC MERP)—This is an independent body of 27 national organizations (e.g., The Joint Commission, American Hospital Association) whose mission is to maximize the safe use of medications and to increase awareness of medication errors through open communication, increased reporting, and promotion of medication error prevention strategies.

Near Miss—An error process that is stopped or interrupted either by chance or through a check-and-balance in the medication-use process, such as recognition of the problem and intervention by an experienced practitioner. Other similar terms include *close call* and *good catch*.

Non-Punitive—An approach that uses positive feedback to individuals who report errors (including self-reports) rather than punishment when an error is detected and contributes to a culture where open communication about errors is encouraged.

Override—A function related to patient-profiled automated dispensing cabinets (ADC) that allows the user (e.g., nurse) to have access to a medication prior to verification by a pharmacist.

Patient Safety Organizations—Entities registered with and listed with the Agency for Healthcare Research and Quality under the Patient Safety Act and Patient Safety Rule, which provide confidentiality and privilege protections for patient safety work product.

PDCA Cycle—A quality improvement methodology involving Plan-Do-Check-Act steps for planning, implementing, evaluating, and changing a process or system.

Regulation—A government-imposed requirement for which compliance is mandatory.

Requirement for Improvement (RFI)—Citation for a standard found that is out of compliance during an accreditation survey. Also referred to as a *finding*.

Risk Mitigation Strategies—Tactics utilized to avoid system failures and prevent errors. Risk mitigation strategies may be implemented in response to a recent event or utilized as a proactive strategy. Multiple risk mitigation strategies are often needed to fully address potential failure points. Examples include forcing functions, automation, double checks, and provider education.

Root Cause—Any identified reason in the sequence of events that, if prevented, will stop a recurrence of the particular event. There must be a clear cause and effect such that if you eliminate the identified cause, future events will be prevented.

Root Cause Analysis (RCA)—A systematic process utilized to determine the primary cause of system failures. The goal is to define the root causes and develop an action plan to prevent recurrence or mitigate a future event.

Safe Culture—Shared values and beliefs of an organization that result in a common goal among frontline staff and leadership to consistently improve and maintain a safe environment for both its workforce and patients. In a safe culture, the organization is committed to continuous improvement and encourages reporting of potential or actual hazards in this effort.

Safety—The degree to which the risk of an intervention (for example, use of a drug, or a procedure) and risk in the care environment are reduced for a patient and other persons, including health care practitioners. Safety risks may arise from the performance of tasks, from the structure of the physical environment, or from situations beyond the organization's control (such as weather).

Sentinel Event—"An unexpected occurrence involving death or serious physical or psychological injury, or the risk thereof," as defined by The Joint Commission.

Simulation—Imitation of the operation of a system or process, using a model that represents key characteristics of the selected system or process.

Slips and Lapses—A human error whereby the action deviates from the intention. A *slip* is when an action is carried forth, but deviated from the intention. A *lapse* is when there was an intention of an action, but the action was forgotten.

Stakeholder—A person, group, or organization that will be affected by or can themselves affect a process.

Standardize—To remove variations and irregularities; to bring into conformity with another.

Standards—A set of rules or principles established by consensus and approved by a recognized body that describes services, systems, or practices to meet a certain level of quality; in health care, to provide safe patient care in a secure environment.

Statistical Process Control Chart—A statistical graph that helps to detect process variation over time and is a tool for monitoring the ongoing stability of a process, distinguishing variation due to causes common to the process versus special (potentially actionable) causes.

Super-User—An individual, often an end-user, who has received additional training in use of a particular technology and functions as a resource for purposes of training or problem-solving/trouble-shooting.

Symmetry Bias—The tendency to assign blame for an error in a manner that is proportional to the severity of the outcome (also called *Severity Bias*).

System—A set of interacting, interrelated, or interdependent elements that work together in a particular environment to perform the functions required to achieve the system's aim.

Systems Thinking—Evaluating the whole process rather than a particular single part, since all parts are inter-related. This approach includes consideration of everyone who could potentially influence the process.

Taxonomy—The practice and science of classification. The National Coordinating Council for Medication Error Reporting and Prevention taxonomy is a classification system to describe and analyze the details around individual medication error events.

Team Charter—A written document defining a team's mission, scope, structure, and objectives; serves to communicate the team's focus and direction for team members, organizational leaders, and other work groups.

Tracer—An evaluation method that uses the medical record as a guide to follow a patient through transitions in the course of an episode of care to assess compliance with standards. This methodology may also be used to assess the medication management process and other organizational systems to provide or evaluate patient care.

Unit Dose—Medication to be given to a particular patient at a specific time packaged in the exact dosage required for that time.

Violation—The action of bypassing a rule, standard, or safe operating procedure. Violations can be further divided into optimizing violations, necessary violations, and routine violations.

Walk Round—A tool that assists with discussion between leadership and frontline staff in order to raise awareness of needed system changes, promote accountability for creating a safe environment, and support decisions for future system improvements and resource allocation.

Workaround—A method for achieving a task by not following proper procedures; a shortcut; often a creative solution to circumvent a problem without eliminating the problem.

Glossary of Acronyms

ACPE—Accreditation Council for Pharmacy Education

ADC—automatic dispensing cabinet

ADE—adverse drug event

ADR—adverse drug reaction

ADT—admission, discharge, transfer

AHA—American Hospital Association

AHRQ—Agency for Healthcare Research and Quality

APPE—advanced pharmacy practice experience

aPTT—partial thromboplastin time

ASHP—American Society of Health-System Pharmacists

ASMSO—American Society of Medication Safety Officers

BCMA—bar code medication administration

BCMSS—Board Certified Medication Safety Specialist

BCMV—bar code medication verification

CBPPS—Certification Board for Professionals in Patient Safety

CCA—common cause analysis

CCG—clinical care guideline

CDC—Centers for Disease Control and Prevention

CDS—clinical decision support

CE—continuing education

CEO—chief executive officer

CI—criticality index

CMS—Centers for Medicare & Medicaid Services

CNO—chief nursing officer

CONT—contingent (accreditation)

CoP—conditions of participation

CPHQ—Certified Professional in Healthcare Quality

CPO—chief pharmacy officer

CPOE—computerized provider order entry

CPPS—Certified Professional in Patient Safety

CQI—continuous quality improvement

CSG—clinical/service group

DNVHC—Det Norske Veritas

DSL—detection sensitivity level

EBOS—evidence-based order set

EC—environment of care (TJC standards)

ED—emergency department

EHR—electronic health record

EM—emergency management (TJC standards)

eMAR—electronic medication administration record

EMR—electronic medical record

EP—element of performance

EPA—Environmental Protection Agency

ESC—Evidence of Standards Compliance

FAQs—frequently asked questions

FDA—Food and Drug Administration

FMEA—failure mode and effects analysis

FOCUS—Find-Organize-Clarify-Understand-Select

FSA—Focused Standards Assessment

HAC—hospital acquired conditions

HEN—hospital engagement network

HFAP—Healthcare Facilities Accreditation Program

HR—human resources (TJC standards)

HRO—high-reliability organization

IC—infection control (TJC standards)

ICD—International Classification of Diseases

ICM—intracycle monitoring

IHI—Institute for Healthcare Improvement

IID—intelligent infusion device

IM—information management (TJC standards)

IOM—Institute of Medicine

ISMP—Institute for Safe Medication Practices

IT—information technology

IV—intravenous

KSA—knowledge, skill, ability

L & D—labor and delivery

LASA—look-alike/sound-alike

LD—leadership (TJC standards)

LMWH—low molecular weight heparin

MAR—medication administration record

ME—medication error

MERP—medication error reduction plan; medication error reporting program

MM—medication management

MOS—measure of success

MS—medical staff (TJC standards)

MSC—Medication Safety Committee

MSDS—material safety data sheet

MSO—medication safety officer

MUE—medication-use evaluation

NAHQ—National Association for Healthcare Quality

NCC MERP—National Coordinating Council for Medication Error Reporting and Prevention

NF—nonformulary

NHS—National Health Service (U.K.)

NIAHO—National Integrated Accreditation for Healthcare Organizations

NICU—neonatal intensive care unit

NIOSH—National Institute for Occupational Safety and Health

NNP—neonatal nurse practitioner

NPSA—National Patient Safety Agency (U.K.)

NPSF—National Patient Safety Foundation

NPSG—National Patient Safety Goals

NQF—National Quality Forum

OR—operating room

OSHA—Occupational Safety and Health Administration

P&T—Pharmacy and Therapeutics

PC—provision of care, treatment and services (TJC standards)

PDA—preliminary denial of accreditation

PDCA—Plan-Do-Check-Act

PFA—priority focus area

PGY1—postgraduate year one (residency)

PGY2—postgraduate year two (residency)

PI—performance improvement

PIS—pharmacy information system

POA—plan of action

POCT—point-of-care testing

PPMI—Pharmacy Practice Model Initiative

PP—policy and procedure

PSO—patient safety organization; patient safety officer

PT—prothrombin time

QI—quality improvement

RC—record of care, treatment, and services (TJC standards)

RCA—root cause analysis

RCRA—Resource Conservation and Recovery Act

REMS—risk evaluation and mitigation strategy

RFI—Requirement for Improvement

RI—rights and responsibilities of the individual (TJC standards)

RRT—rapid response team

RT—respiratory therapy

SAQ—Safety Attitudes Questionnaire

SBAR—situation, background, assessment, recommendation

SCIP—Surgical Care Improvement Project

SEA—sentinel event alert

SIG—Standards Interpretation Group

SOD—severity-outcome-detection

TJC—The Joint Commission

TPN—total parenteral nutrition

UFH—unfractionated heparin

UHC—University Health-System Consortium

USP—United States Pharmacopeia

VANCPS—Veterans Affairs National Center for Patient Safety

VBP—value-based purchasing

WT—waived testing (TJC standards)

Index

P

Q

R

S